Handbook of Integrative Pediatrics

Handbook of Integrative Pediatrics

Editor: Magan Gilbert

AMERICAN
MEDICAL PUBLISHERS
www.americanmedicalpublishers.com

AMERICAN
MEDICAL PUBLISHERS
www.americanmedicalpublishers.com

Cataloging-in-Publication Data

Handbook of integrative pediatrics / edited by Magan Gilbert.
p. cm.
Includes bibliographical references and index.
ISBN 979-8-88740-147-8
1. Children--Diseases. 2. Integrative medicine. 3. Pediatrics. I. Gilbert, Magan.
RJ27 .H36 2023
618.92--dc23

American Medical Publishers,
41 Flatbush Avenue,
1st Floor, New York,
NY 11217, USA

ISBN 979-8-88740-147-8 (Hardback)

Contents

Preface

Pediatrics refers to a branch of medicine concerned with the care, growth and illnesses of children, newborns and adolescents. The rising occurrence of diseases like metabolic syndrome, mental illness, attention deficit disorder, cancer, asthma, obesity, autism, diabetes, chronic pain and other inflammatory-mediated illnesses has drastically changed the landscape of pediatrics. These changes also have a negative impact on younger age groups and children today confront major health issues which have increased the need for pediatricians having new abilities and a stronger emphasis on preventative health. This has led to the emergence of pediatric integrative medicine, which is the result of changing pediatric illness patterns and patient demands. Integrative pediatrics uses a combination of traditional and alternative therapies to develop a tailored plan that meet the requirements of each child, family and circumstance based on the best available research. The objective of this book is to present the latest researches on integrative pediatrics. Those in search of information to further their knowledge will be greatly assisted by it.

The researches compiled throughout the book are authentic and of high quality, combining several disciplines and from very diverse regions from around the world. Drawing on the contributions of many researchers from diverse countries, the book's objective is to provide the readers with the latest achievements in the area of research. This book will surely be a source of knowledge to all interested and researching the field.

In the end, I would like to express my deep sense of gratitude to all the authors for meeting the set deadlines in completing and submitting their research chapters. I would also like to thank the publisher for the support offered to us throughout the course of the book. Finally, I extend my sincere thanks to my family for being a constant source of inspiration and encouragement.

Editor

1

Acupuncture and Lifestyle Myopia in Primary School Children—Results from a Transcontinental Pilot Study Performed in Comparison to Moxibustion

Xiaojuan Shang [1], Luquan Chen [1,*], Gerhard Litscher [1,2,3,4,*], Yanxia Sun [3], Chuxiong Pan [3], Cun-Zhi Liu [4], Daniela Litscher [2] and Lu Wang [1,2,3]

1 Department of Traditional Chinese Medicine, Beijing Tongren Hospital, Capital Medical University, Beijing 100730, China; joy_shang@hotmail.com (X.S.); lu.wang@medunigraz.at (L.W.)
2 TCM Research Center Graz, Research Unit of Biomedical Engineering in Anesthesia and Intensive Care Medicine, and Research Unit for Complementary and Integrative Laser Medicine, Medical University of Graz, 8036 Graz, Austria; daniela.litscher@medunigraz.at
3 Department of Anesthesiology, Beijing Tongren Hospital, Capital Medical University, Beijing 100730, China; sun00017@gmail.com (Y.S.); pandedao@126.com (C.P.)
4 Department of Acupuncture and Moxibustion, Dongfang Hospital Affiliated to Beijing University of Chinese Medicine, Beijing 100078, China; lcz623780@126.com
* Correspondence: chenluquan@hotmail.com (L.C.); gerhard.litscher@medunigraz.at (G.L.);

Abstract: Background: Lifestyle risks for myopia are well known and the disease has become a major global public health issue worldwide. There is a relation between reading, writing, and computer work and the development of myopia. **Methods:** Within this prospective pilot study in 44 patients aged between 6 and 12 years with myopia we compared possible treatment effects of acupuncture or moxibustion. The diopters of the right and left eye were evaluated before and after the two treatment methods. **Results:** Myopia was improved in 14 eyes of 13 patients (15.9%) within both complementary methods. Using acupuncture an improvement was observed in seven eyes from six patients out of 22 patients and a similar result (improvement in seven eyes from seven patients out of 22 patients) was noticed in the moxibustion group. The extent of improvement was better in the acupuncture group ($p = 0.008$ s., comparison before and after treatment); however, group analysis between acupuncture and moxibustion revealed no significant difference. **Conclusions:** Possible therapeutic aspects with the help of evidence-based complementary methods like acupuncture or moxibustion have not yet been investigated adequately in myopic patients. Our study showed that both acupuncture and moxibustion can improve myopia of young patients. Acupuncture seems to be more effective than moxibustion in treating myopia, however group analysis did not prove this trend. Therefore, further Big data studies are necessary to confirm or refute the preliminary results.

Keywords: acupuncture; moxibustion; evidence-based complementary medicine; myopia; primary school children; lifestyle; computer; eye diseases

---

1. Introduction

Myopia has become a major global public health issue worldwide. Lifestyle risk factors are well known and summarized in recent publications [1–3]. It has been shown that there is a relation between reading and writing from a short distance and the development of myopia. Computer work is also responsible for this relationship [4–7].

The constantly increasing number of eye diseases, as a result of too intensive personal computer work, increases the need for adequate treatment methods. In this context evidence-based complementary methods like acupuncture and/or moxibustion could be potential starting points for early intervention of myopia, which is defined as more than equal to −0.50 diopter (D) [3].

The purpose of this study was to investigate complementary medical methods (acupuncture and moxibustion) in school children with mild or moderate myopia because conventional medical therapies do not show sufficient improvements [1–3]. Acupuncture and moxibustion are among the most important methods used clinically in myopia in school age in China. Since this is an invasive method (needle acupuncture) on the one hand and a non-invasive procedure (moxibustion) on the other hand, it is obvious to compare both methods in one study. The aim is also to find out whether the methods differ significantly in terms of a possible improvement of myopia or not.

Within this transcontinental (Asia-Europe) prospective study in 44 children with low (<−3.0 D) and medium (between −3.0 D and −6.0 D) myopia [3] we compared possible treatment effects of acupuncture or moxibustion for the first time. The measurements were performed at the Tongren Eye Hospital affiliated to Capital Medical University in Beijing, China and the analysis was performed at the Traditional Chinese Medicine (TCM) Research Center at the Medical University of Graz, Austria.

2. Materials and Methods

2.1. Patients

A total of 44 patients aged between 6 and 12 years, with a mean age ± SD of 9.3 ± 1.4 years (27 female, 17 male) were treated either with acupuncture (group A) or with moxibustion (group B). The children suffer from mild-to-moderate myopia (−0.5 D to −4.25 D), and their lens-corrected vision was 100%. The average stature of the 44 subjects was 137.7 ± 9.4 cm (115–157 cm), and the average body weight was 33.2 ± 7.9 kg (21–53 kg). No person was under the influence of drugs. The treatments (needle acupuncture or moxibustion) were approved by the local ethics committee of the Tongren Hospital for treatment and research (EPU 5/2017) and performed in accordance with the recommendations of the Helsinki Declaration of the World Medical Association. Informed consent has been obtained from at least one of their parents.

Acupuncture treatment was used in group A, moxibustion in group B. Each group consisted of 22 patients. Age, sex, and basic demographic data are shown in Table 1.

Table 1. Demographic data of the 44 patients.

Parameter	Group A	Group B
	Acupuncture (N = 22)	**Moxibustion (N = 22)**
Age (years)	9.4 ± 0.9	9.3 ± 1.7
Sex (female, male)	14 f, 8 m	13 f, 9 m
Height (cm)	140.2 ± 6.8	137.2 ± 11.4
Weight (kg)	34.6 ± 8.0	31.8 ± 7.8
Treatment sessions	6.9 ± 1.7	9.1 ± 1.2

Randomization to one of the groups A or B has been done by an independent employee (medical doctor) from the Tongren Hospital using an envelope (group A, group B). The duration of one treatment (acupuncture or moxibustion) was 20 min. Altogether completion of 10 sessions was planned (~2 sessions per week) however not all participants could finish the examinations (compare treatment sessions in Table 1).

The following exclusion criteria were applied: (i) Less than −0.5 diopters; (ii) other eye diseases/disorders affecting visual acuity; (iii) secondary eye diseases (e.g., following diabetes); (iv) cardiologic, neurologic, nephrologic, hepatologic, hematologic, or psychiatric disorders; (v) chronic diseases requiring medication that must not be interrupted.

2.2. Treatment Methods

2.2.1. Acupuncture

All 22 patients in group A received needle acupuncture at traditional point locations (see Figures 1 and 2).

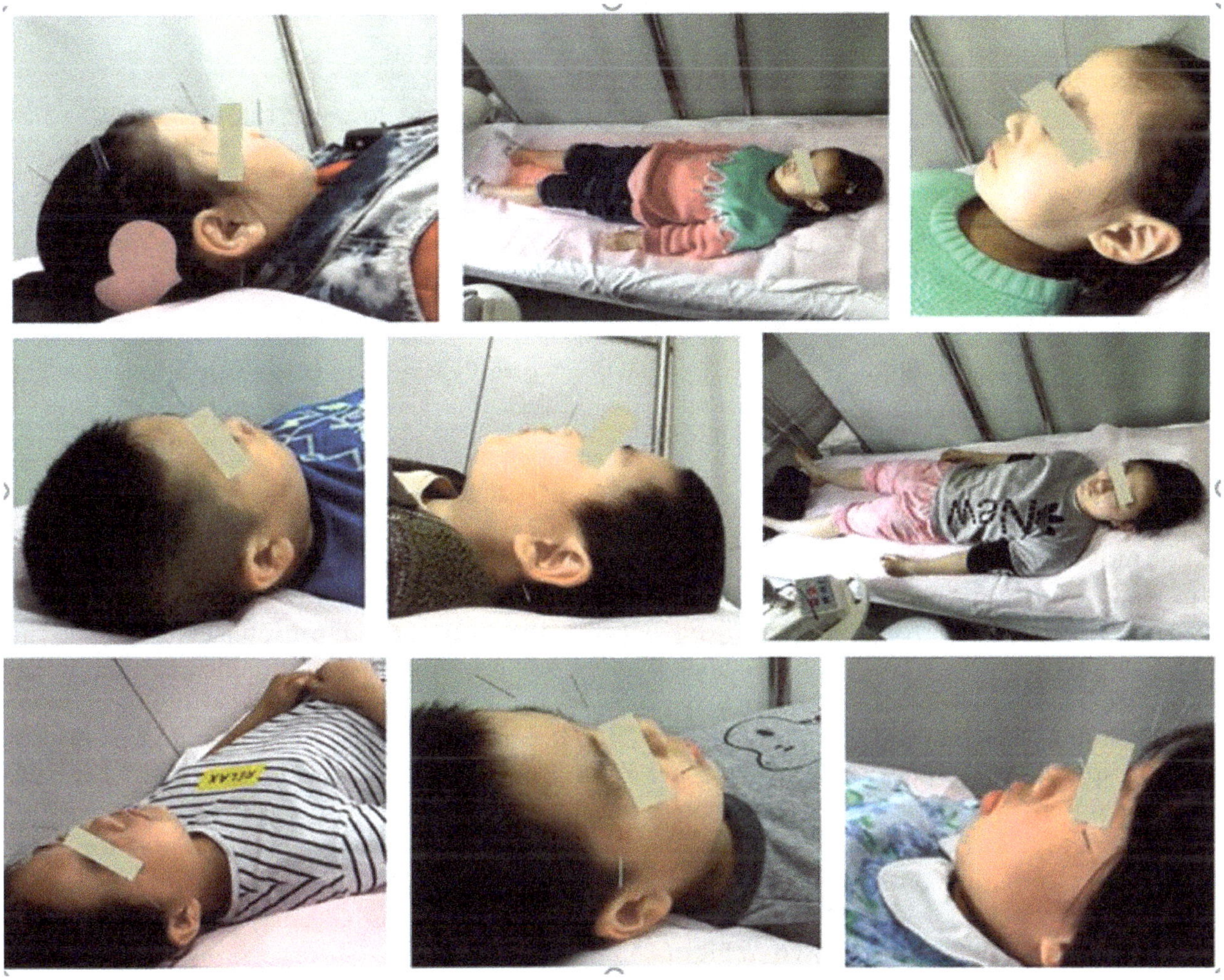

Figure 1. Acupuncture treatment in 22 young patients with myopia (group A).

After the patients lay down on a bed in a relaxed manner, the skin at the acupoint locations was disinfected with cotton which contains 75% alcohol. Disposable acupuncture needles (0.25 mm × 25 mm) were used. The needling method used is called mild reinforcing and attenuating, and was performed by inserting the needle at the appropriate depth. The angle of insertion was straight for the points on hands, body, and ankles, and oblique for the points on head, face, and neck. The depth of perpendicular needling was 25 mm, which of oblique is 15 mm. The needles were not stimulated and stayed in the body. After 20 min the needles were removed with dry cotton. An expert panel of acupuncturists from the Tongren Hospital in Beijing, China have reviewed and participated in the selection of the points. Acupuncture was always performed by the same highly experienced acupuncturist.

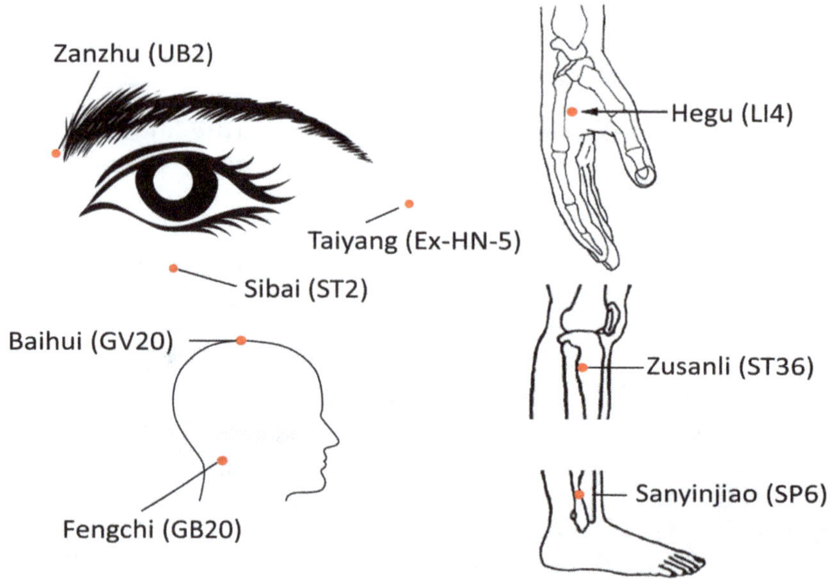

Figure 2. Acupuncture points for group A (acupuncture treatment). UB2 = Urinary Bladder 2; ST2 = Stomach 2; Ex-HN-5 = Extra Point Head/Neck 5; GV20 = Governing Vessel 20; GB20 = Gallbladder 20; LI4 = Large Intestine 4; ST36 = Stomach 36; SP6 = Spleen 6.

2.2.2. Moxibustion

For moxibustion treatment the patients sat down and closed their eyes. Then moxibustion on the forehead was performed for two minutes moving the stick in a horizontal direction (see Figure 3). Moxibustion was also performed around the eyes for duration of three minutes (moving the moxa in a horizontal direction for one minute, clockwise for one minute, vertical direction for one minute). Then sparrow-pecking Moxa on acupuncture points near the eyes (Ex-HN5, ST2 and UB2) was done for two minutes. This method is characterized by the ignited moxa stick being moved up and down over the point like a bird pecking or moving left and right, or circularly simultaneously. Acupressure was made on the same points simultaneously. In addition, moxibustion around the ears was made for two minutes moving the stick in vertical directions. Sparrow-pecking moxa on LI4 and simultaneous acupressure at the same point for one minute completed the Zhao's thunder-fire moxa (manufacturer: Chongqing Zhao's Thunder-fire Moxa Institute of Traditional Medicine, Chongqing, China) procedure. The points for moxibustion are shown in Figure 4.

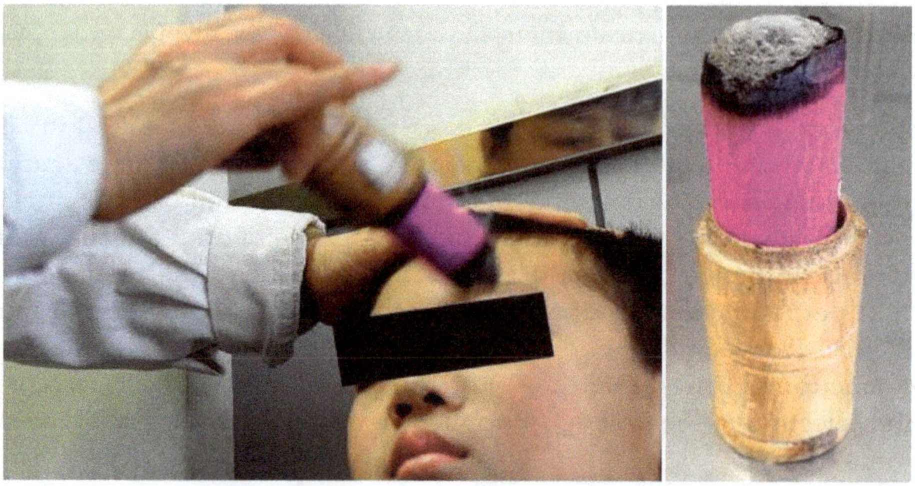

Figure 3. A part of the moxibustion treatment in 22 young patients with myopia (group B).

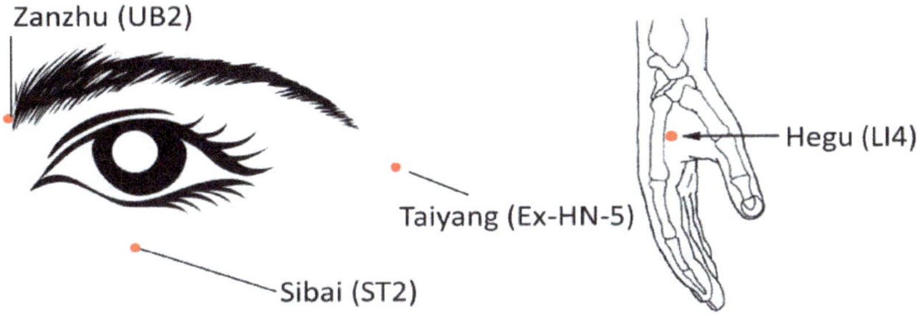

Figure 4. Points for group B (moxibustion treatment). UB2 = Urinary Bladder 2; Ex-HN-5 = Extra Point Head/Neck 5; ST2 = Stomach 2; LI4 = Large Intestine 4.

2.3. Evaluation Parameters

Axial lengths were observed before and after treatment with acupuncture or moxibustion. The diopters of the right (OD) and left (OS) eye were evaluated before and after the two treatment methods by a blinded assessor (medical doctor from Tongren Hospital). Compound tropicamide eye drops (0.5% tropicamide, 0.5% phenylephrine hydrochloride) were used before and after the last treatment session.

2.4. Statistical Analysis

The statistical analysis was carried out with the computer program SigmaPlot 14.0 (Systat Software, Chicago, IL, USA). Kruskal-Wallis One Way Analysis of Variance (ANOVA) on Ranks for group analysis and box plot analysis was used. In addition, paired t-tests before and after the treatments were carried out. The level of significance was set at $p < 0.05$. The original data can be found at the Department of Traditional Chinese Medicine & Acupuncture, Tongren Hospital affiliated to Capital Medical University, 100730 Beijing, China and at the TCM Research Center Graz, Medical University of Graz, 8036 Graz, Austria.

3. Results

All 44 patients finished at least five treatment session (mean sessions: 8.0 ± 1.8 (range: 5–10 treatments)). Due to time reasons, treatment in the children in Beijing was only possible during holiday time. Group analysis of the demographic data showed no statistical difference in age, sex, height, and weight. Acupuncture and moxibustion were accepted well and there were no side effects monitored by the medical doctors of the Tongren Hospital in any of the children. Table 2 demonstrates the mean ± SD of OD and OS from all patients and each from both groups (A and B) respectively.

Table 2. Diopters of the right (OD) and left (OS) eye before and after the two treatment methods (N = number of eyes).

N: Number of Eyes	Both Complementary Treatment Methods	Group A	Group B
		Acupuncture	Moxibustion
OD + OS before	-1.68 ± 1.03 (N = 88)	-1.57 ± 0.84 (N = 44)	-1.79 ± 1.18 (N = 44)
OD + OS after	$-1.67 \pm 1.08^{\#}$ (N = 88)	$-1.52 \pm 0.87^{**}$ (N = 44)	-1.81 ± 1.25 (N = 44)
OD before	-1.66 ± 1.03 (N = 44)	-1.53 ± 0.86 (N = 22)	-1.80 ± 1.20 (N = 22)
OD after	-1.72 ± 1.08 (N = 4)	-1.50 ± 0.88 (N = 22)	-1.80 ± 1.20 (N = 22)
OS before	-1.69 ± 1.03 (N = 44)	-1.60 ± 0.83 (N = 22)	-1.81 ± 1.20 (N = 22)
OS after	$-1.61 \pm 1.08^{*}$ (N = 44)	$-1.53 \pm 0.87^{+}$ (N = 22)	-1.71 ± 1.31 (N = 22)

$^{\#}$ $p = 0.011$; * $p = 0.002$; ** $p = 0.008$; $^{+}$ $p = 0.030$.

Altogether myopia was improved (diopters) in 14 eyes of 13 patients (15.9%) with both complementary methods. Using acupuncture, an improvement was observed in seven eyes from six patients out of 22 patients and a similar result (improvement in seven eyes from seven patients out of

22 patients) was noticed in the moxibustion group (group B). However the extent of the improvement was significantly different between the acupuncture (group A: $p = 0.008$) and the moxibustion (group B: No significance).

The results are graphically presented in Figure 5. The basic values before the treatment of both acupuncture and moxibustion are similar (see median values). Only needle acupuncture treatment changes the diopters in the sense of an improvement of myopic children significantly.

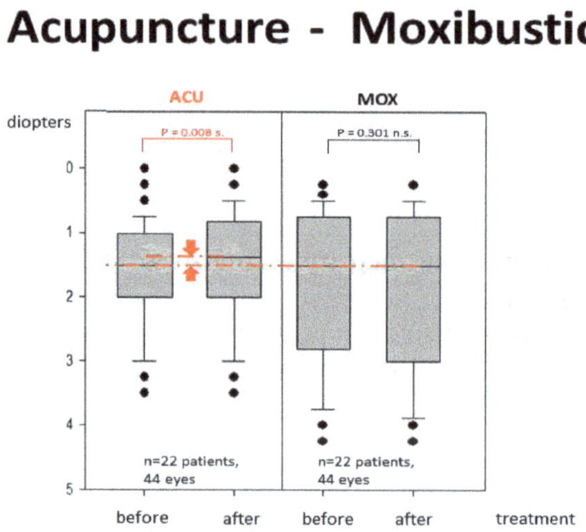

Figure 5. Box-plot of change in diopter values of all 44 subjects before and after treatment. The line in the box indicates the position of the median; the ends of the boxes define the 25th and 75th percentiles. The error bars show the 10th and 90th percentiles, and the dots represent "outliers". Note the significance ($p = 0.008$ s.) of the decrease in diopters after acupuncture treatment (left part).

In addition, a group analysis has been performed. The differences in the median values among the two treatment groups (acupuncture and moxibustion) was not great enough to exclude the possibility that the difference is due to random sampling variability; there was not a statistically significant difference ($p = 0.973$ n.s.) between the acupuncture and moxibustion group.

4. Discussion

A current literature analysis in the two databases PubMed and Cochrane Library regarding this important topic yielded the following results: up to now (1 June 2018) there are 28,106 published articles in PubMed under the search term "acupuncture" (11,464 at Cochrane Library). The term "myopia" provided 21,252 results in PubMed, and in Cochrane Library 1435 articles. The search term "personal computer" yielded 24,940 results in PubMed, and Cochrane Library 1905 published articles. The search with combined keywords yielded fewer results. The combined search terms "personal computer myopia", "personal computer acupuncture", and "acupuncture myopia personal computer" led to no results in Cochrane Library (in PubMed at least double-digit results, excluding "acupuncture myopia personal computer"). The only combined keyword which yielded more results in both databases was "acupuncture myopia". PubMed listed 46 articles, and in Cochrane Library 22 articles were found.

The result of the database analysis shows that until now there is very little research related to therapeutic aspects of eye diseases and screen handling. Therefore, new research like the present study is absolutely necessary. As already mentioned in the introduction, acupuncture or moxibustion could be possible starting points. The database analysis also clearly shows that acupuncture has already been used in myopia, but currently plays a very minor role in relation to PC-work induced disorders.

A study from Beijing which has been published in 2015 in PLoS One [2], deals with myopia in high school students. The title of the article is "*Prevalence and associated factors of myopia in high-school students in Beijing*". The authors came to the worrying result that students aged between 16 and 18 years have an 80% prevalence of myopia. They even speak of a 10% prevalence of severe myopia. When this generation which has grown up with PCs gets older, it will cause enormous costs for the health care system. Experts warn that myopia will win importance as a cause of visual impairment and blindness [2].

"*Acupuncture for teenagers with mild to moderate myopia: study protocol for a randomized controlled trial*" is the title of another important work. Especially the safety of acupuncture application in this field and its effectiveness should be investigated for a period of six months. Here is a brief excerpt from the study protocol: This randomized, parallel, blinded clinical trial will be conducted controlled. A total of 100 young people aged between seven and twelve years with mild to moderate myopia are recruited. The patients are randomized into two groups (control group and acupuncture group). Each group consists of 50 young people. In the acupuncture group, the five acupoints Zanzhu bilaterally, Tongziliao, Sibai, Muchuang and Hegu are stimulated daily for nine consecutive days. Then there is a one-day treatment break. Six of these treatment cycles are carried out continuously over a total of 60 days. After six months, a follow-up examination takes place. The primary endpoint is the determination of the diopter [8]. This is in context with our present study and also some acupoint are the same. The study could provide very interesting results. Another work that should be mentioned in the context of this discussion was written by Ming Yeung. According to this work, 3–4% of children are affected by tired eyes. Attention is drawn to a treatment with acupuncture. This method of treatment is according to the authors well tolerated by children and shows promising results [9].

In the following some important experiences from our own research should be mentioned briefly.

Myopia in children and adolescents up to the age of 21 is also well treatable with complementary medical methods. In adults, however, only little success has been recorded [10].

Our study has been performed as a transcontinental research pilot study. This means that two main research teams were involved; one team from Asia (Beijing, China) and one from Europe (Graz, Austria). Although it was a pilot study, the preliminary results are promising. The examinations showed that a total of 14 eyes of 13 patients out of 44 patients showed a significant improvement in myopia. The improvements were better with acupuncture than with moxibustion (comparison before and after treatment). The invasiveness of acupuncture seems to play a role over the non-invasiveness of moxibustion or acupressure.

However, the investigation has also limitations. Firstly, the sample size was very small and in the future sample size will be calculated according to rigorous methodology and considered in the improvement rate of this pilot study. Secondly, the average number of treatment sessions was lower in the moxibustion group than in the acupuncture group. Thirdly, because of ethical principles and actual clinical conditions in China, neither a control group of individuals who did not receive treatment nor a placebo group who received sham acupuncture was included. Fourthly, without a follow-up evaluation it would be difficult to determine if the treatment produces only temporary improvement or more clinically relevant long-term sustainable effects. Nevertheless, the scientific methodological guidelines were followed strictly through the trial, and the outcomes still showed meaningful and effective treatment corresponding to other previous publications.

5. Conclusions

In summary it can be stated that the enormously important topic screen handling, eye diseases, and possible therapeutic aspects with the help of acupuncture or moxibustion has not yet been investigated adequately from a scientific perspective, although some work (mainly from China) already exists. The problem, however, is not only interesting for Asia, also in the Western world ametropia [11] caused by screen handling will increase, as the scientific search and research of this work illustrates.

Our transcontinental pilot study showed that both acupuncture and moxibustion can improve mild and/or moderate myopia of young patients (6–12 years). Acupuncture seems to be more effective than moxibustion in treating myopia however at the moment we do not have conclusive explanations concerning the underling mechanisms of needle and thermal stimulation on myopia from a neurophysiological perspective.

Author Contributions: X.S., L.C., G.L., Y.S., C.P., C.-Z.L., D.L. and L.W. created the study design, X.S. and L.C. performed the measurements, G.L., D.L. and L.W. performed the data analyzes, G.L. designed the manuscript, and all authors (X.S., L.C., G.L., Y.S., C.P., C.-Z.L., D.L. and L.W.) participated in the discussion section and read the final manuscript.

Acknowledgments: Lu Wang and Gerhard Litscher are also visiting professors at the Capital Medical University, Beijing, China and G. Litscher is also guest professor at the Beijing University of Chinese Medicine in Beijing, China.

References

1. Wu, L.J.; Wang, Y.X.; You, Q.S.; Duan, J.L.; Luo, Y.X.; Liu, L.J.; Li, X.; Gao, Q.; Zhu, H.P.; He, Y.; et al. Risk factors of myopic shift among primary school children in Beijing, China: A prospective study. *Int. J. Med. Sci.* **2015**, *12*, 633–638. [CrossRef] [PubMed]
2. Wu, L.J.; You, Q.S.; Duan, J.L.; Luo, Y.X.; Liu, L.J.; Li, X.; Gao, Q.; Zhu, H.P.; He, Y.; Xu, L.; et al. Prevalence and associated factors of myopia in high-school students in Beijing. *PLoS ONE* **2015**, *10*. [CrossRef] [PubMed]
3. Zorena, K.; Gladysiak, A.; Slezak, D. Early intervention and nonpharmacological therapy of myopia in young adults. *J. Ophthalmol.* **2018**, *2018*. [CrossRef] [PubMed]
4. Holden, B.A.; Fricke, T.R.; Wilson, D.A.; Jong, M.; Naidoo, K.S.; Sankaridury, P.; Wong, T.Y.; Naduvilath, T.J.; Resnikoff, S. Global prevalence of myopia and high myopia and temporal trends from 2000 through 2050. *J. Ophthalmol.* **2016**, *123*, 1036–1042. [CrossRef] [PubMed]
5. Czepita, M.; Czepita, D.; Lubiński, W. The influence of environmental factors on the prevalence of myopia in Poland. *J. Ophthalmol.* **2017**, *2017*. [CrossRef] [PubMed]
6. Eye Problems through Screen Work. Available online: http://vorarlberg.orf.at/news/stories/2726280/ (accessed on 13 August 2015).
7. Le, Q.; Zhou, X.; Ge, L.; Wu, L.; Hong, J.; Xu, J. Impact of dry eye syndrome on vision-related quality of life in a non-clinic-based general population. *BMC Ophthalmol.* **2012**, *12*. [CrossRef] [PubMed]
8. Wang, Y.; Gao, Y.X.; Sun, Q.; Bu, Q.; Shi, J.; Zhang, Y.N.; Xu, Q.; Ji, Y.; Tong, M.; Jiang, G.L. Acupuncture for adolescents with mild-to-moderate myopia: Study protocol for a randomized controlled trial. *Trials* **2014**, *15*. [CrossRef] [PubMed]
9. Acupuncture Breakthrough for Treating Eye Condition. Available online: http://www.chinadaily.com.cn/hkedition/2010-06/15/content_9977403.htm (accessed on 15 June 2010).
10. Brucker, K. *Augen-Akupunktur: Sehstörungen Natürlich Heilen*; Georg Thieme Verlag: Stuttgart, Germany, 2001.
11. Disease and Injury Country Estimates. Available online: http://www.who.int/healthinfo/global_burden_disease/estimates_country/en/ (accessed on 12 February 2012).

2

Children are Born to Dance! Pediatric Medical Dance/Movement Therapy: The View from Integrative Pediatric Oncology

Suzi Tortora [1,2]

[1] Memorial Sloan Kettering Cancer Center, New York, NY 10021, USA; tortoras@mskcc.org; Tel.: +1-845-265-1085

[2] The Andréa Rizzo Foundation, Charlestown, RI 02813, USA

Abstract: Children freely expressing themselves through spontaneous dance is a natural part of childhood. The healing powers of dance are universal in all cultures across history. Dance/movement therapy (DMT) in pediatric oncology is little known and underutilized. This article discusses DMT, specifically focusing on pediatric oncology. It defines and clarifies the difference between medical DMT as a psychotherapeutic modality aimed at addressing the patient's psychosocial needs, and dance and therapeutic dance used recreationally to engage patients during their hospital visits. A literature review of DMT with medically ill children in the United States and worldwide is provided. It culminates with a focus on advancements in the field, discussing the future of pediatric medical DMT. Grounded in a biopsychosocial perspective, the intrinsically nonverbal and embodied nature of pediatric medical DMT is uniquely positioned to be a strong component of integrative oncology services. The use of DMT to synthesize potentially traumatic aspects of the medical experience is proposed. It ends with a call for research posing the question: Can pediatric medical DMT support the patient to express feelings while in cancer treatment within the context of a psychotherapeutic milieu, enabling the patient to create an embodied coherent narrative that fosters expressivity and empowerment?

Keywords: pediatric cancer; integrative oncology; integrative medicine; dance/movement therapy; dance therapy; dance/movement psychotherapy; trauma and PTSD; complementary and alternative medicine; symptom management; creative arts therapy

---

1. Introduction

Children freely expressing themselves through spontaneous dance is an intrinsic part of childhood. As a child explores the world by actively engaging physically in it, a sense of self and empowerment in the world develops [1]. When children become ill with cancer, their ability to participate in playful childhood activities is frequently compromised. This loss is akin to the sense of disempowerment and loss of control of one's body and stress physiology when facing a threatening, traumatic life event [2–5]. These experiences create a wide variety of emotions difficult to understand and express through words. Dance/movement therapy (DMT), also known in Europe as dance movement psychotherapy (DMP), can help the pediatric oncology patient regain access to this natural innate aspect of childhood by providing psychosocial therapeutic support. DMT is a body- and movement-based psychotherapeutic field that utilizes the creative expressive elements of dance to enable the patient to express feelings and gain a deeper understanding of experiences that may be difficult to speak about [6]. By creating activities that consider the pediatric patient's emotional, social, cognitive, communicative, and motoric development, pediatric DMT provides a therapeutic holding environment in the Winnicottian sense [7,8], and reintroduces the child to her (pronouns are used interchangeably throughout the article). [Changing] body through creative dance and movement-based activities, supporting her emotional expression about her experience [9–11].

The generally innate pleasure in childhood of creative dance, with the sense of body control it fosters, can be especially therapeutic for pediatric oncology patients, who have the sense that their body and their disease are out of their control [11]. Nearly all treatments for traumatic stress include mastery and control over traumatic events [3,12–15]. These treatments offer solutions for the feelings of helplessness by helping the patient reimagine their body's potential for health and comfort. This article presents the concept that offering nonverbal body and dance/movement-based solutions for the feelings of helplessness for children with medical illness, opens the potential to create a nonverbal narrative that can prevent or heal the conceivably traumatic effects of the medical experience.

The use of DMT with children with medical illness is a little known yet growing application in the field. This review article summarizes DMT with pediatric medical illness specifically focusing on pediatric oncology. The author is the senior dance/movement therapist for the Dréa's Dream Dance Therapy Program at Memorial Sloan Kettering Cancer Center (MSKCC) within Integrative Medicine Service (IMS). The article discusses the role of DMT in pediatric oncology as an integral part of integrative medicine services. It begins with a definition of integrative oncology and shows how and why DMT fits into these services. The article clarifies the difference between DMT as a psychotherapeutic modality aimed at addressing the patient's psychosocial needs, and dance, therapeutic dance and other recreational activities, used to engage and entertain patients during their hospital visits. The article provides a description and literature review of the state of the science of DMT with medically ill children in the United States and around the world. A world view is included to make evident the global efforts of dance/movement therapists working within this specialization. As requested by the editors of this special issue of *Children*, the article culminates with a focus on advancements in the field, going beyond history and current practice, to discuss the future of pediatric DMT and integrative oncology in the United States and around the world.

Goals of This Article

The overarching goals of this article are to introduce pediatric medical DMT to a wider audience and demonstrate that it is an underutilized specialty, which can contribute a great deal to integrative oncology. Grounded in a biopsychosocial perspective, the intrinsically nonverbal and embodied nature of pediatric medical DMT is uniquely positioned to be a strong component of integrative oncology services.

2. Definitions

2.1. Integrative Oncology

Integrative oncology is defined as "... a patient-centered, evidence-informed field of cancer care that utilizes mind and body practices, natural products, and/or lifestyle modifications from different traditions alongside conventional cancer treatments. Integrative oncology aims to optimize health, quality of life, and clinical outcomes across the cancer care continuum, and to empower people to prevent cancer and become active participants before, during, and beyond cancer treatment" [16] (p. 3).

2.2. Dance/Movement Therapy (DMT)

Body and mind integration is the cornerstone of DMT. Primarily an embodied approach, DMT enables patients to express their nonverbal felt-experiences through sensorial emotionally-rich dance and movement-based activities developed around themes of creative self-expression. These individual and group explorations create deeper conscious and unconscious self-understandings, that can transform into verbalizations, cognitive understandings and behavioral changes in daily life [17,18]. The American Dance Movement Therapy Association (ADTA) defines DMT as "the psychotherapeutic use of movement to promote emotional, social, cognitive, and physical integration of the individual, for the purpose of improving health and well-being" [19]. DMT is conducted in group, family, dyadic and individual sessions to best support the needs of the patient and the condition being treated.

2.3. *The Orgins of "Dance" in Dance/Movement Therapy*

Dance, as the first word in the name of the profession has caused some misunderstanding about the breadth and depth of the services dance/movement therapists provide. As stated by Sherry Goodill, a prominent dance/movement therapist who has spent many years developing and researching the use of DMT with medical illness, "I think there is a still an assumption about needing the capacity to move fully that keeps people from imagining DMT in the hospital settings" [20]. This belief is especially evident when introducing DMT to a pediatric patient who is not ambulatory. The word dance in the professional name has many references. Dance activities are one of many active body-awareness activities employed in the method. The field evolved from modern dancers in the forties and fifties that recognized the emotional healing powers of expressive dance [6]. Dance/movement therapists emphasize the role of dance as a form of cultural identity and acknowledge that contemporary DMT is rooted in the universal healing powers of dance in all ancient cultures across history [21].

2.4. *Medical Dance/Movement Therapy*

Goodill has built upon the ADTA definition to include, "the application of dance/movement therapy services for people with primary medical illness, their caregivers and family members... in the medical realm, DMT functions primarily as a psychosocial support intervention, complementary to conventional and standard medical treatments" [22] (p. 17). Treatment goals focus on improving experiences and addressing concerns specifically related to having a medical illness. They include: improving stress management; improving quality of life; becoming skilled in pain management techniques; reducing anxiety and depression; improving body awareness and body-self-image; decreasing fatigue; increasing vitality and energy; building a sense of resilience and hope; increasing self-care; improving social support and the ability to receive social support; and learning to accept the unpredictability of life [9,18,23,24].

2.5. *Pediatric Medical DMT*

Pediatric medical DMT is distinct from DMT used for other childhood and adolescent disorders primarily psychiatric or behavioral such as: ADHD, mental disability, anxiety, depression, and disordered eating [22]. Pediatric medical DMT serves children and adolescents suffering from chronic, acute or life-threatening medical conditions including cancer, asthma, chronic pain, migraines, scoliosis, physical accidents, Tourette's syndrome and other neurological disorders, heart disease, and prematurity and medical complications at birth. DMT is practiced in both inpatient and outpatient hospital settings, pediatric intensive care units (PICU), and private practice clinics [11]. Adapting the definition of medical DMT to the pediatric population requires attending to additional aspects of the child's life including: developmental considerations; a greater focus on the nonverbal communication components of DMT for assessment and treatment; and considering the family and other systems in which the child is engaged, including school and peers [9–11].

2.6. *DMT in Pediatric Oncology*

Cancer is a series of conditions which start with the out of control growth of cells that over-crowd normal cells, causing hundreds of site-specific diseases, rather than one specific disease [22,25]. A cancer diagnosis typically takes a profound emotional toll on the patient and the whole family. When that patient is a child, emotional reactions are often extreme. There is an overwhelming impact on all developmental stages of growth; the physical body; body image; and body mind/biopsychosocial experience of the child patient. The diagnosis and treatment demands on the family system due to the life-threatening nature and long-term high-intensity treatment protocols of a cancer diagnosis greatly affect the quality of life of the whole system. The body, mind, and emotionally-integrative approach of DMT coupled with the primary use of nonverbal and dance and movement-based expressive methods of assessment and intervention make DMT in pediatric oncology a strong psychotherapeutic method of support for the patient and the whole family system as they process this overpowering experience not easily expressed verbally [10,22,23]. The adaptability of DMT conducted in group, dyadic, or individual sessions supports both the immediate and long-term needs of the patient and family, building strong relationships throughout the full course of the treatment.

In childhood a sense of self and body image is continually growing based on the interactive experiences between self and others. Navigating medical illness during this important time of self-formation, exploration and discovery can affect the child in profound ways felt but often difficult to understand and express in words. Verbalizing these experiences can be difficult for children because they may not yet have gained the verbal and intellectual competence to speak about the complex emotions related to their illness. The emotional pain and stress of parenting a medically ill child can also make it difficult for parents to talk with their child. The role of creative expression becomes an especially salient component of DMT sessions with the pediatric population. As stated by Madden et al., "By using creative expression, a child or adolescent with cancer can express feelings about the course of the disease and tumultuous treatment through dance/movement, music, and art. This outlet allows the patient to creatively and kinesthetically process the assaults of cancer and its treatment, and thus establish a stronger sense of self and improved quality of life" [23] (p. 133).

Susan Rizzo Vincent, the founder and president of The Andréa Rizzo Foundation, a prominent organization that funds many of the pediatric oncology DMT programs in the USA uses the acronym ART to describe DMT: "I have a nice simple way of describing what dance/movement therapy is: A—The dance/movement therapist ACCESSES emotions like fear, anxiety, anger that a child with cancer may be feeling, through dance and movement expression, usually with the child taking the lead. R—The emotions are RELEASED through this movement (we all know how good it might feel to dance out our frustrations). T—a TRANSFORMATION takes place physically and emotionally through the dance and movement. Giving the child new ways to express themselves and to cope" [26].

2.7. Pediatric Multisensory Dance Movement Psychotherapy (MSDMT)

This author has created a specific method of DMT to support pediatric patients through medical procedures they perceive as difficult or painful, called multisensory dance/movement psychotherapy (MSDMT) [9]. MSDMT is the application of DMT with an added emphasis on the role of the body and multisensory experience to support physiologic and psychological coping, specifically related to medical illness. It supports and encourages emotional expressivity for the patient using a systematic layering of multisensory input developmentally attuned to support the pediatric patient. This includes: dance/movement, play, live and recorded music, touch, breath awareness, imagery, mindfulness, and meditation to augment pain control. MSDMT is a non-invasive treatment that compliments pharmacological and medical treatments. It is an "embodied analgesic" supporting the patient to attune to somato-sensorial sensation to engage, soothe, and empower a sense of self and coping during medical procedures [27].

MSDMT treatment focuses on engaging the whole family to create a soothing holding environment that enables both the parents and the patient to feel safe and comfortable. MSDMT is based on the premise from attachment system theory that in a secure relationship the primary caregiver acts as a protective factor whom the child [patient] goes to, to share pleasurable moments and look towards, and receive comfort from, during times of perceived danger [28]. In MSDMT the dance/movement therapist creates a sensorially-rich environment to engage the patient, family, and even the nurses and other medical staff administering the treatment. This environment can be simultaneously playful and comforting since it is created by attuning to the interests and activity level of the patient and family members moment-by-moment during the treatment. The treatment tries to help the patient achieve a relaxed, meditative state by maintaining their focus of attention on the layered sensory sensations rather than the painful sensations.

The goal of the MSDMT pain management activities is to create a multisensory environment that shifts the child's focus away from pain, towards more pleasurable sensations. Through this process the child often drifts into a meditative or more peaceful state. This treatment includes the parents, optimizing the attachment system. Early in the development of the MSDMT activities, it became very apparent that if the parents experience their child as well cared for, they are more relaxed and available for their child, which enables the child to process his experiences with a sense of agency and control. The parents' sense of competence is also essential. When the child looks towards his parent for comfort, he can sense if the parent is available or pre-occupied by the stress the child is experiencing. The MSDMT activities give both the parents and the child a sense of agency over medical procedures that can strip them from feeling a sense of control.

3. Mind-Body, Body-Mind, Bodymind, and Body-Mind-Emotion

The common thread in integrative oncology, DMT, medical DMT and pediatric DMT is the focus on the body, mind, and emotional experience from a whole person and family perspective. Focusing on practices that integrate mind and body aligns with the prevalent abolition of Cartesian mind-body dualistic thinking across medical, psychological and philosophical fields [10,22,29,30]. Eliminating this dualistic thinking causes a dilemma in discussing the relationship between the mind and the body. Starting with the word "mind" in the "mind-body" phrase can imply a directional emphasis placing the mind and cognition as the primary entrance point into the body. Mind-body techniques, such as guided imagery or mindfulness, direct the mind to notice body sensation, as a way to sense somatic experience, influence the body, and most typically to quiet the body [31]. Switching the term to body-mind emphasizes the body's influence on the mind. In body-mind practices attention is first directed to body sensations, physical action patterns, and movements as they influence the whole body, and as an entrance point into mindful consciousness [31].

The term bodymind was first coined by Dychtwald in his book by the same name [32]. Dychtwald integrates ancient Eastern philosophy with ideas from the work of classic psychological and body-focused pioneers Wilhelm Reich, Fritz Perls, and Moshe Feldenkrais to describe the vital body mind relationship. Combining the two words as one emphasizes the body's influence but comes closer to addressing the union of body and mind.

3.1. *Biopsychosocial and Pediatric Palliative Care*

Current research in psychosomatic illness has abandoned the mind-body and body-mind terminology, aiming to eradicate the directionality of influence between the two terms, adapting the term biopsychosocial to better represent the nonexistent differentiation between mind and body [33]. The term biopsychosocial is also used in palliative care to delineate a more holistic care approach to symptom management [34]. Pediatric palliative care as defined by the American Academy of Pediatrics (AAP) describes an integrative model providing continual care starting at the outset of diagnosis and throughout the illness regardless of whether the outcome is curative or terminal [35]. AAP pain management "... includes the control of pain and other symptoms and addresses the psychological, social and spiritual problems of children and their families" [35] (p. 351). Biopsychosocial in palliative care emphasizes there is an interdependent relationship between all three dimensions of human experience: bio, relating to the physical; psychosocial, referencing the concept of self and interactive functioning; and an implied spiritual, existential understanding related "to the meaning the patient ascribes to the illness or injury" [34] (p. 245). This definition underscores that though each dimension may to be examined separately, all symptoms occur simultaneously within all dimensions and must be reintegrated to provide holistic patient care. In their work with pediatric cancer patients, Cohen and Walco also discuss the unique DMT concept "that psychological and somatic constructs are truly identical" noting that it is only the "point of entry" that distinguishes them [10] (p. 35).

3.2. Body-Mind-Emotion Continuum

This author has created the term "body-mind-emotion continuum" (Figure 1) to emphasis the continuous, circular connection between each aspect of the self [36,37]. The therapeutic process begins by entering into an exploration of self through any of these aspects of self, based on the patient's presenting focus. The dance/movement therapist may start the session with attention on the patient's felt-experience, sensations or energy level (body). A common opening line when beginning a DMT session with a pediatric patient is, "Are you in the mood to get your body up and going or calm and relaxed?" The session can begin with a discussion of the patient's thoughts, images and associations about their illness (mind). "How's your day going?" Or, the patient's emotional state may drive the intervention (emotion). "Hmm. I wonder how you are feeling today—what mood are you in today?" Each focused question is simply the starting point of the therapeutic exploration. It is not the specific point of entrance but the awareness and integration of each domain experienced through the exploration that creates true healing.

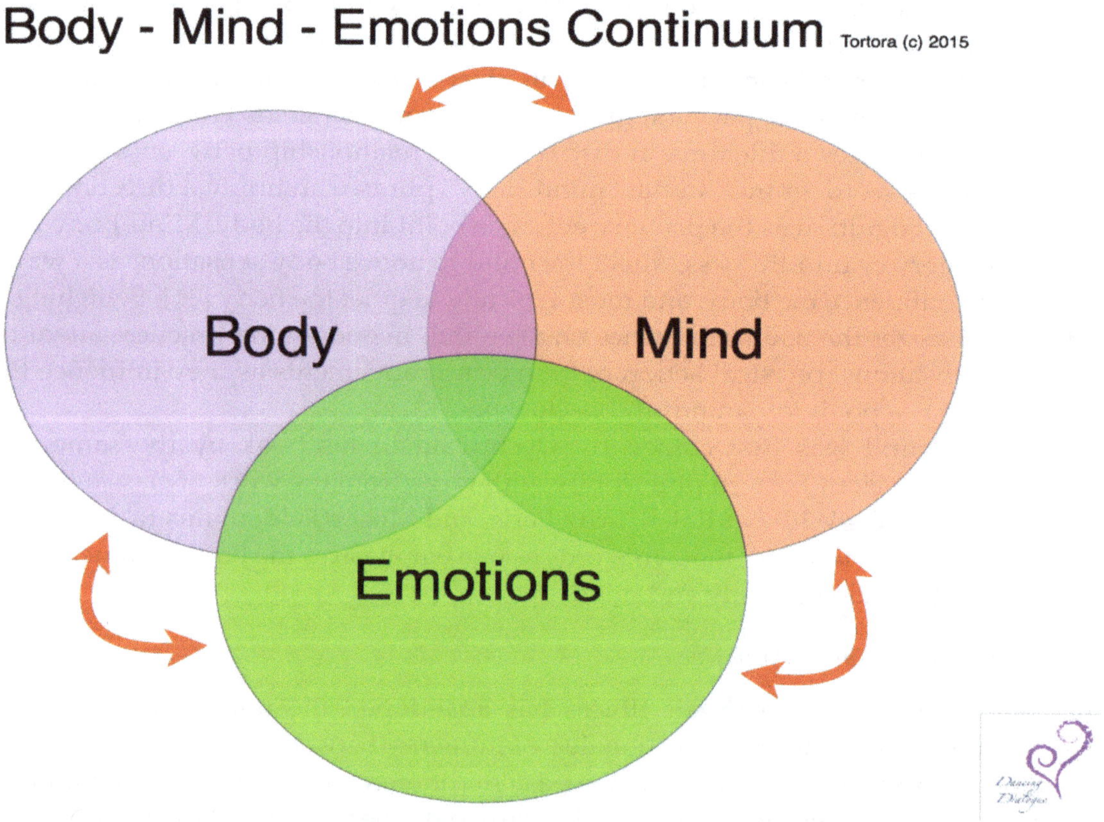

Figure 1. Tortora's image of the continuous, circular connection between each aspect of the self.

3.3. DMT within the Integrative Oncology Team: Cancer-WWW

Regardless of which term is used to depict the body, mind, and emotional continuum, this discussion highlights integration and includes the role of embodied experience from a whole person perspective. These methods aim to improve the quality of life for the individual, and family members and friends, creating a community of support with the health care team. Integrative oncology and pediatric medical DMT share may similar viewpoints. They both work from the perspective of integrating body and mind. They also focus on empowering both the patient and family members to be active participants in their cancer care, supporting the optimization of health and quality of life for the patient and family, across the cancer care continuum. This commitment requires team collaboration across disciplines in the medical staff.

At MSKCC, pediatric DMT is part of pediatric integrative medicine, which includes music therapy, mind-body and martial arts, yoga, and massage. The pediatric integrative medicine team works closely with child life, social work, psychiatry, nurses, doctors and the Pediatric Pain and Palliative Care Team (PACT), contributing to team meetings about patients and treatment plans bringing in psychosocial and developmental aspects of the patient's needs. Dance/movement therapists also engage in joint sessions with other integrative medicine practitioners as well as speech and language therapists, physical therapists and occupational therapists when a psychosocial approach supports the patient's engagement.

Both DMT and integrative medicine come from the perspective of a Whole child approach; looking at the child within the context of the experience of the Whole family system; creating a sense of community through a Whole staff collaboration—*Cancer-WWW* [27]. One goal of this article is to demonstrate why and how pediatric medical DMT is an essential member of the pediatric integrative *Cancer-WWW* team.

4. DMT, Child Development, and Embodied Experience

The intrinsically nonverbal and embodied approach of pediatric medical DMT embraces the body-mind-emotion continuum in a unique way that attunes, addresses and supports the [medically ill] child's primary modes of expression and experience. Infants and young children gain experience of self and social relatedness through their active physical experience of moving and engaging in the world around them [38]. They express their feelings and develop their sense of self through their felt-embodied experiences. Stern created the term "core self "to describe the infant's bodily experiential sense of self from birth [39] (p. 11). Core self is one of the four "sense of self" domains, from which the infant views and experiences the world from a place of reality and awareness. In this viewpoint Stern departs from the psychoanalytic view of psychic phenomena that describes this early developmental stage consisting of "delusions of merge or fusion, splitting, and defensive or paranoid fantasies" [39] (p. 11).

A more reality-based, bodily-felt experience is an essential viewpoint to take with the medically ill child of any age for it acknowledges that even young pediatric patients are present and deeply experiencing their cancer treatment. Recent research in infancy memory [40,41] substantiates the premise that even though infants and young children may not have the words to describe their experiences, these experiences can impact their development on many developmental levels later in life. Dance/movement therapists are specifically trained to attend to the patient's nonverbal expressions as a means of assessment, expression and intervention [1,9–11,42]. Through sensitive observation of the patient's nonverbal vocabulary dance/movement therapists create movement and dance activities—natural actions in the healthy child's explorations—that provide avenues of self-expression for the medically ill child.

5. Dance/Movement Therapist Differentiation from Dance Teacher

It is important to emphasis the phrase "psychotherapeutic use of movement" in the ADTA definition to clarify a frequent misunderstanding for those not familiar with or only observing DMT in action. Due to the physical nature of DMT, it is often confused with other movement and body-focused activities used to promote wellness and wellbeing such as yoga, mindfulness, martial arts, contemporary dance, improvisation, ballroom dance, Broadway theater, jazz dance and therapeutic dance. These programs are fun, creative and often provide physical skill training taught by a professional teacher in the specific field. Such activities include learning specific dance choreography, yoga postures, martial art moves, or meditation breathing techniques to focus one's attention. These are extremely useful skills supporting the cancer patient to feel a sense of competence and control of their body. Many dance/movement therapists are also trained in these techniques and include these activities as part of their therapeutic repertoire.

The core difference between the activities described above and DMT is that DMT is a form of psychotherapy with an added experiential physical creative arts focus. Using the body enables rich nonverbal psychic material to emerge supporting embodied discoveries along the body-mind-emotion continuum [36,37,43]. The creative arts dance and movement aspect of the work occurs within the psychotherapeutic container created by the therapist witnessing and moving with the patient. It is the psychotherapeutically supported personally aesthetic and deeply personal creative explorations, which uniquely distinguishes DMT from other mindfulness, body and dance forms. In DMT the patient uses physical activities to convey emotions creating psychological connections between their nonverbal and verbal expressions. Through DMT the patient explores how their body, mind and emotions work together to express their feelings, while gaining coping skills facilitated by the embodied explorations.

6. Dance/Movement Therapy Educational Training

Many dancers pursue further training to become dance/movement therapists due to their own experiences of the communicative emotionally empowering aspects of dance as dance performers and/or dance teachers. In the USA there are two tracks to becoming a dance/movement therapist. Dance/movement therapists can get a master's degree from a university program accredited by the ADTA. If they have a masters in an allied field such as mental health counseling, psychology, marriage and family counseling, social work, or dance they can pursue the alternate route track through the ADTA by taking specifically-required supplemental courses in DMT and psychology taught by ADTA approved dance/movement therapists and other professionals. Many dance/movement therapists have additional licensing in psychological fields including mental health counselors, marriage and family counselors or social workers. A growing number of dance/movement therapists have earned a doctorate in such fields as psychology, education, infant mental health or dance/movement therapy.

7. State of the Art of Pediatric Medical DMT—The Specifics

At MSKCC, DMT happens everywhere—in the inpatient room, outpatient play room, and even in the hallway. Sessions occur individually, with parents, family members, friends, and groups of patients. Even the nurses and doctors join. The goal is for the patient and whole family to feel that the dance/movement therapists are available and present anywhere at any time.

This author designed the MSKCC program to be all encompassing. It provides an avenue for the child to express his or her needs, concerns and experience with cancer treatment through the supportive creative and aesthetic medium of self-expressive dance, music, play, relaxation, and talking, by meeting the child wherever he is in the moment, along the emotional cancer continuum. Each session follows the child's lead. One day the child may want to gleefully dance exploring the joys of moving, while another day the same child may feel listless, needing to share a sense of quiet contemplation with the dance/movement therapist. These child-directed dance-play sessions build the pediatric patient's sense of competence, mastery, and autonomy on a very embodied level.

A core premise of the program comes from this author's understanding that all infants enter the world and accumulate experiences first and foremost through bodily sensations, reactions, expressions, and experiences, developing a "sense of body" that informs the development of a sense of self [1] (p. 31). Since these body experiences, define and continually inform the child about who he or she is, it is essential that the pediatric patient's felt-embodied experience is taken into account. It is critical that the dance/movement therapist tries to detect who the patient "is" beneath this layer of illness, determining how the medical experience may be coloring the patient's pre-existing sense of body, and subsequently influencing the patient's sense of self. The dance/movement therapist strives to help the patient experience themselves separate from the confines of the illness. Dance/movement therapists training in nonverbal analysis greatly informs how they analyze the movement actions to gain a deeper understanding of the patient's self-expression and felt-experience.

7.1. Pediatric Medical DMT and Nonverbal Analysis

As stated by Mendelsohn, "Dance/movement therapists believe that the body "speaks" and it is our task to decipher what the body behavior of hospitalized children is trying to communicate in order to help medically ill children cope better with their illnesses and hospitalization" [42] (p. 65). Deciphering nonverbal bodily expression is at the core of DMT practice used in both assessment and intervention [1,10,44–47].

Dance/movement therapists train in one or more nonverbal analysis systems, with Laban Movement Analysis (LMA) [44] and Kestenberg Movement Profile (KMP) being the most prominent. LMA is the original nonverbal analysis method, developed by the modern dancer, Rudolf Laban, in the 1960s [48]. It provides a way to analyze the qualitative and quantitative components of action and the processes involved in executing movements rather than simply describing the goal of the movement [44]. The KMP, developed by psychiatrist Judith Kestenberg, also in the 1960s, is "a Laban-derived method" to categorize actions that includes a development and psychological interpretation of the mover's movement repertoire [49] (p.5). Through these systems dance/movement therapists observe the qualitative aspects of the patient's movement patterns to gain understanding of how their body actions may reflect their coping style and emotional state [50]. Through nonverbal analysis the dance/movement therapist assesses the level of physical engagement the patient can sustain, the theme and symbolic nature of the creative expressive dance activities and the patient's intra- and interpersonal functioning [9,10,47].

7.2. Laban Nonverbal Movement Analysis: Short Description

This author is trained and certified in both LMA and KMP. A thorough description of each system and their categories goes beyond the scope of this article, so a simple explanation of the LMA system is explained to provide clarification for the case vignettes that follow.

The qualitative elements of Laban nonverbal movement analysis are described through five movement categories: Body, Shape, Effort, Space, and Phrasing [44,48,50]. The Body category includes what areas of the body are used most frequently to determine the sense of body coordination and sequential movement patterns. The Shape category reveals how the position and shape of the child's body reflects their experience in the moment of their own body, and how they position themselves in relationship to others. The feeling tone of the actions includes the use of weight, spatial directional focus, timing, and the tension and flow patterns of the movement, described as Efforts. Space reflects how one's body takes up space, and moves through space, including spatial levels and spatial pathways. Phrasing describes the rhythmic, arrhythmic, syncopated or melodic phrasing of the mover's actions.

7.3. Socially-, Religiously-, Culturally-, and Ethnically-Sensitive Practice

Attuning to nonverbal expression also enables the DMT to be sensitive to social, religious, cultural, and ethnic differences communicated through actions, gestures and rhythmic patterns of the individual patient and family member, as well as the group dynamics expressed nonverbally. This is especially important at MSKCC where the specialization in specific and rare childhood cancers such as retinoblastoma and neuroblastoma, bring families from all around the world for treatment. Observing, attuning, and responding to the qualitative differences expressed through nonverbal postures, actions and gestures enables the dance/movement therapist to learn about the pediatric patient while being sensitive to the family dynamics within their culture. The dance/movement therapist uses this information to create an environment that is supportive and familiar to the patient and family. Understanding social, religious, cultural, and ethnic difference is especially important to support the patient and family during palliative and end of life care.

7.4. Embodied Countertransference

Though the DMT strives to attune to and be sensitive to the unique characteristics and behaviors of the patient and his family, the therapist is viewing and interpreting these behaviors from her own lens of personal experiences. The term countertransference is used by psychoanalysts and psychodynamic therapists to describe thoughts, feelings, reactions and interpretations the therapist has that may be triggered by her own life. Dance/movement therapists consider their bodies and movement actions as essential tools in the treatment. Attention to their personal bodily-felt reactions, sensations and responses is a core process in the embodied countertransference experience. A thorough description of how dance/movement therapists explore countertransference goes beyond the scope of this article and can be found elsewhere [1,51,52]. Simply stated here, dance/movement therapists pay attention to their thoughts, images and associations within the context of their felt-sense reactions on a body and emotional level. Dance/movement therapists actively use their own bodies to sense the patient's nonverbal experience while observing and moving with the patient. Understanding the personal lens that may influence the therapist's responses plays an important role in how the session unfolds. The dance/movement therapists Plevin and Parteli describe their use of nonverbal analysis on the onco-hematology unit to determine how they structured their interventions and how they attended to their own embodied countertransference responses during the treatment [47].

8. What Does DMT Look Like?

To exemplify the elements of pediatric medical DMT, this section provides case study vignettes organized by age group, demonstrating the changing developmental considerations. The first vignette is the longest example that provides a full overview of the DMT experience. It presents a thorough description of the nonverbal LMA approach within the context of the dance/movement therapist's embodied countertransference and cultural considerations when working with a parent-infant dyad. The remaining shorter vignettes offer additional examples to portray other aspects of the work. Each vignette is a composite. All names and identifying specifics of patients, including details about family members or other social details, have been changed to protect their privacy.

8.1. Parent-Infancy Dyadic DMT—Four Session Description

As I enter the inpatient room of Jae-joon, a nine-month-old with choroid plexus carcinoma (this is a rare malignant brain tumor that occurs most often in children under the age of 2 years old) I am instantly struck by the emotional stillness I experience in the room. Jae-joon is sitting in a forward concave posture in his crib, staring motionless at his mother, who is sitting lower down on the other side of the crib, on the edge of the sleeper couch. She is also in a concave posture with her elbows on her knees, holding her head in her hands. As I come closer to the crib to introduce myself, Jae-joon immediately tenses his whole body, quickly folds his torso over his legs as he vigilantly attempts to reach his arms through the crib bars towards his mother, seeming to attempt to get away from me. He audibly whimpers with a strained cry. Mom does not move. In my own embodied countertransference, I sense my breath tighten as my stomach clenches and a feeling of deep sadness and isolation comes over me. "Does Mom not hear her baby's cry?" I wonder. I take a few long breaths to soften my own bodily stance and pause too. I review what I know in my mind. Mom conceived this baby at age forty, after waiting to conceive for five years, due to her previous birth of a baby who died of the same condition.

The emotional anguish in the room is palpable. Jae-joon, at age nine months is rightfully at the height of stranger-anxiety, which can only be amplified by his mother's obvious agony over the potential loss of him. During this first visit I speak softly to Jae-joon without moving closer, to respect his attempt to spatially distance himself from me, assuring him I am only here for play and comfort. I will perform no medical procedures on him. I slowly walk over and quietly stand next to Mom keeping my arms close to my torso without gesturing on respect her private contained spatial stance.

I gently explain my role as the dance/movement therapist. She does not look up, but softly moans and rocks her body forward and backward almost imperceivably. I crouch down, next to her while still maintain spatial distance, and am at eye level to Jae-joon without staring at him. I slowly rock my body and hum to the rhythm of her actions. Mom looks up at me and for a moment our eyes meet, tenderly. I delicately state I understand how hard this is and tell her I am here to help.

When I return for the next session Mom and Jae-joon are again in the same positions. Though, this time Mom looks up on her own when I come to her side. Jae-joon pays attention to this, giving me a quick glance when he sees his mother look towards me. I ask Mom how she and the patient are doing. Mom looks at me stating something in a heavy accent I cannot understand. I smile and show her my music selections attempting to indicate I want her to show me some Korean music they are familiar with. She does not understand, so I put on a classic Korean lullaby and softly sway to the rhythms. Jae-joon maintains his vigilant stance but watches as mom looks at me and smiles. She does not seem to notice Jae-joon looking at her. I am patient with this, for I know if I can make Mom feel more comfortable, she can be more present for her baby. She faintly nods to the musical beat and I mirror her actions. Jae-joon attentively watches this exchange with less vigilance, though he does not move. As our session ends I feel lighter and Mom, though still quiet, also appears more relaxed. Our shared dance has had a calming effect.

Though the medical records state that Mom understands English, I bring Juhee, a Korean colleague with me to the next session. I am wondering if the baby might feel more comfortable seeing me with Juhee and if Mom will open up in her native language. I also ask Juhee to give me the names of current popular Korean children's songs, which I download on my iPhone before the next session. When I enter Juhee takes the lead speaking in Korean to introduce herself. This time Jae-joon does not immediately avert his eyes towards his mother but looks directly up at Juhee. Mom stands up and softly welcomes Juhee. Juhee explains in Korean what DMT is. She asks Mom about music they like to listen to and fortunately I have that song downloaded. As I put the familiar song on, both Jae-joon and Mom look up and naturally sway to their familiar beat. In this way, we all dance, in our private spaces and the solemnness of the room dissolves. The session ends with Mom sharing more details about her feelings and her concerns and sadness about Jae-joon's illness. She specifically states that Jae-joon had been crawling and pulling up to standing but has dramatically regressed, not having the desire or capability to move.

When I return alone for the next session Jae-joon does not lean over to his Mom but greets me with an expression of curiosity. Mom stands up and comes over to me with a friendly sway to her step. I put on the same song and this time encourage Mom to hold Jae-joon as we dance together. I want Jae-joon to experience the warm body-to-body contact of his mom moving in a rhythmic manner to support their emotional relationship and to stimulate his own physical awareness. When the recorded music stops, Mom sings her own favorite song to Jae-joon, and Jae-joon softens even more in her arms as he looks up at her face with a smile. From this session on, we begin each session with Mom's singing to Jae-joon, who becomes more and more engaged both emotionally and physically. He pulls himself up in his crib reaching his arms out to be held. His physical, emotional and social skills improve simultaneously as Mom is more emotionally available to him. During these dance therapy sessions Mom also shares more of her feelings and becomes more responsive to receiving support from the whole staff.

8.2. Preschool-Age Individual DMT Session

James, age four is sitting in the outpatient playroom with his Mom when I see him. It is eleven o'clock in the morning and he has not had breakfast due to his upcoming procedure that requires general anesthesia. I know him well for James has been coming to MSKCC for retinoblastoma treatment (retinoblastoma is a rare childhood cancer that most often effects infants and young children, occurring in the retina of the eye. It may occur in one or both eyes), for over a year and the medical treatments have been difficult for him to handle. I am drawn to him today for I notice his restless body actions and mournful exclamations, despite Mom's efforts to read a book to him while awaiting his procedure. As I walk over Mom, looks up, with a pleading expression, indicating this has not been an easy morning. I ask James if he wants to dance and he jumps up readily. When I ask what music he wants to dance to he recites the words to the classic children's song, "We're going on a bear hunt" [53]. I put on an instrumental piece of music with a syncopated drumbeat and melodic strings creating a sense of suspense to support the adventurous tone of the storyline. I join James in reciting the first lines of the story, complete with the gestures miming the action words. "We're going on a bear hunt. We're going to catch a big one. What a beautiful day!" I mirror James widespread arms to depict catching "a big one" and then reach way up high to feel the beautiful day. This is followed by placing our hands on our hips and shaking our heads "No," to demonstrate our lack of fear, in response to "We're not scared!" But suddenly the danger sets in. "Uh! Oh! Grass, long wavy grass." Quickly our eyes open wide and our hands go to our mouth in mock surprise. "We can't go over it. We can't go under it. Oh no! We've got to go through it." We arc our arms up and over, then down and up, followed by a determined stretch forward as far as we can reach. We perform these gestures repeatedly, as this refrain repeats between each new obstacle that comes our way. We must pass through a deep cold river; step with conviction into thick oozy mud; stumble and trip within a big dark forest; and spin and sway through a swirling whirling snowstorm. Making ourselves small, we tip toe into the cave. We come face to face with the bear, which briskly sends us pantomiming back through each obstacle until we are safely under our covers in bed.

As we encounter each new hurdle, James' actions become more determined and stronger, taking up more space, as he recites the words of the refrain with increasing conviction. As I mirror his actions, matching his mood and tone, I am taken by the metaphor of the words. The message is clear ... "We're [trying to] not [be] scared! ... But... Uh! Oh! There is no choice.... We can't avoid it [the cancer experience]. We must go through it [and find a way to bravely approach it]." My heart beats with a quickened pace and I look up to see the dad of a teen I have also worked with, watching us. As our eyes meet, I see tears glistening in his eyes. I smile warmly, privately sensing my own emotions quietly welling up too. I know, he knows the journey we are dancing out through our embodied drama. James soldiers on with renewed strength evidenced in the clarity of his body actions and eagerness to repeat this song repeatedly. The details of each stanza pale in comparison to his enactment of the refrain, which become bolder with each repetition. His bravery surges as the bear hunt becomes a lion hunt. In my attuned felt-experience I understand the stakes are getting higher. I ask him if he wants to hear a lion roar and he eagerly agrees. I happen to have some recordings of a lion roaring. I put it on. James shudders, for just a moment and whispers, "That's scary!" "Yes" I say with compassion, "but what are we going to do?" James does not miss a beat and shouts as his actions get even stronger, "We're not scared! We can't go over it. We can't go under it. Oh no! We've got to go through it." Our dance continues. When I tell him this is our last round, he adds a tiger to our hunt, singing out even louder, with his gestures passionately matching his words. James is beaming, standing tall and proud when we finish our dancing pantomime. As I reflect upon my experience with James I am touched by his wise soul. He knows without knowing, just the right song he needs to add courage to his upcoming treatment. Beaming, Mom thanks me for the transformation that has taken place, as James snuggles cozily with her now.

I walk over to the dad watching. He takes my hand, thanking me for today, for the opportunity to experience the tender beauty of the moment. He thanks me for the courage and joy that dance/movement therapy awakens. He shares that watching our dance evoked his experience with his own son at that age, when he was getting his cancer treatment, from which he is now in remission. He knows the journey ahead for this boy and his family. At that moment his own teen son comes over with a bounce in his step and his loving gaze of gratitude and pride is palpable.

8.3. Music and Dance/Movement Therapy Group Session—Elementary Age

Every Monday morning Karen Popkin and I offer a music and dance therapy group in the pediatric ambulatory care center (PACC). The group is attended by children of all ages, their siblings and other family members. For many, it seems to ease the transition back to the hospital after the weekend break at home. Music and dance therapy, both part of the creative arts therapy field (along with art, drama and poetry therapy) are wonderfully complementary. Through Karen's intuitive live guitar improvisations and my attuned embodied actions in response to Karen and the participants spontaneous music making we can draw out each participant to access their emotions through music, dance and their imagination.

On this day we have seven participants. Three patients ranging in age from four to seven, two siblings approximately age five and eight and two patients' parents. At this point in the session each child is playing an instrument, choosing from Karen's assortment of tambourines, egg shakers, bells, rainsticks, and drums. One child starts an even paced beat and Karen strums along holding the rhythm steady. One by one each participant adds to this beat creating a rhythmic symphony. I notice Pierre, age seven stamping to the beat as he sways his body forward and backward in his chair. I mirror his actions with precision and ask him, "Let's go on a journey. Where are we going?" "We are in the ocean, there is a storm" he shouts! Immediately the pace picks up as the other participants excitedly join in. Clara, age five, jumps up, "I fell off the boat" she exclaims as she feigns falling. Two more children stand up, swaying to and fro, arms flailing, as if caught in the waves, while the remaining children add more vigor to the musical accompaniment. "A shark" someone calls out and instantaneously all the children begin to scutter around as sharks lunging zealously toward imaginary bait. I pull out a large blue sheer scarf and the parents help me hover it over the children, who dart and dive and dip, exploring this underwater scene, spurred on by the eager musicians, accelerating the beat. At some point the waves part as the rainstick and melodic guitar take over the percussive beat. The shark children slow their bodies as they begin to stretch out, "floating" above the surface of the water and then settle back on their boat-chairs. We discuss how powerful the sharks are, how brave they are, how they endure the storm to capture their prey and how good it feels to be safely back on shore. The concrete and the symbolic merge here as the children explore both the scariness and the potency the shark imagery evokes in them. The shark metaphor is a common image parents use with their children, to depict how the cancer treatment is attacking the bad cancer cells. Again, I marvel at how through this imagery created by the children they confront their fears, embodying both the aggressor and the warrior and then, savor in their success.

8.4. Adolescent DMT Individual Sessions—Summary

Dimitri, age 16, recently received a Hodgkin lymphoma diagnosis (this is a cancer that effects the lymphatic system and starts in the white blood cells). As a high school basketball player, he is referred by Child Life to DMT to provide support for his active lifestyle. He is surprised but welcoming, "Hey I'll try anything at least once!" he says with a warm smile. He visibly relaxes even more after I explain that DMT is more than dancing. We settle on having him show me some of his basketball warm-up activities. Once out of bed I look up at his tall lean yet muscular 6′2′ frame and take a breath. Through my own kinesthetic empathic countertransference, I experience his current physical strength and ponder about his potential vulnerability. I imagine the journey ahead and wonder what imagery will work best to keep him moving, even if on some days it is only figurative. I ask about music choices and to my surprise he is a "High School Musical" fan. We agree on "Get your head in the game!"—an apt choice for a basketball player. As Dimitri reaches his arms way up high arcing over to his left and then right, the high energy, upbeat rhythms and focused message of the song directs our pulsing actions.

Dimitri continues to take the lead, demonstrating his agility as he pumps his legs up one at a time and slaps his knees. As he becomes more limber, he also opens up about his recent experience with his illness. Between stretches, in which he seems to be unconsciously testing what his body could do, and what it can do now, he tells me he is the captain of his team. One of his jobs as captain is to lead the warm-ups. It was during such a warm-up that he suddenly felt weak and collapsed. He actually hadn't been feeling like himself for a while, but thought it was just the lack of sleep due to his heavy basketball schedule and trying to keep up with his homework. In my active following, I experience Dimitri leading his whole team, keeping them challenged to keep them going. I playfully ask him about this and he laughs in agreement. He discusses how much he enjoys physical challenges. He pauses and looks directly at me. We each take a deeper breath, spontaneously. This opens up a discussion about his cancer treatment plan. He wants to know what to expect; he wants to be included in decisions; and he wants to do everything he can to stay active. We plan for regular sessions and I explain there are many ways to keep him active, even when his body may not be as energetic as he is used to.

During his treatment, the team keeps Dimitri informed, and he stays true to his word with me. Even on days of active chemotherapy when his red blood cell count is low, he bruises easily, and he is feeling extreme nausea and fatigue, he welcomes me with a faint smile. Over the months of our work together we create a full playlist of songs to fit his different moods. Some uplifting and hopeful, some wordless tunes that induce quiet contemplation. Some days he is chatty, some days we can do a version of his stretches, other days, his fatigue takes over and he participates through guided visualizations we created during our sessions over time. Throughout our work, Dimitri rises to the challenges his cancer treatment present, as he learns how to attune and dialogue with his mind, body and emotional messages.

8.5. Pediatric Medical DMT and the Caregiver-Infant/Child Relationship

As stated in Section 3.3, an intricate part of the Dréa's Dream Dance Therapy Program as practiced at MSKCC is to support the whole family as they navigate their experience of cancer treatment. Providing support for family members and other significant caregivers takes many forms depending on the age of the patient, the needs of the caregivers and the patient's stage of treatment. At the most primary level, caregivers of patients of all ages experience great pleasure and relief in seeing their child participate in an active, joyful and creative physical activity that is such a typical part of childhood. This enjoyment turns to gratitude quickly as most caregivers see the underlying emotional expression that the DMT activities foster. They frequently request the presence of a dance/movement therapist to support the patient before, during or after a difficult procedure.

Though the child treated for cancer is the designated patient the dance/movement therapist pays keen attention to the needs of the caregivers focusing on the significant role they play in the patient's overall wellbeing. Psychosocial supports for the caregiver include verbal therapy specifically addressing the caregiver's immediate concerns, sorrows, experiences, and personal associations that arise from their child's illness. Dance/movement and mindfulness activities are created to also support the caregiver's nonverbal expression. Psychoeducational information focusing on infant, child and adolescent development is an integral part of the treatment as well. These sessions can occur separate from the patient or within the context of a patient session.

Caring for the caregiver in the context of the patient's treatment also strengthens the child-caregiver relationship [54]. With infants and toddlers, the caregiver is encouraged to participate in activities fostering the patient's felt-experience of their parent, literally and symbolically providing a secure emotional base. Caregivers are often hesitation and fearful to physically engage in playful ways with their medically ill babies. Creating safe activities together that foster a natural body-to-body connection filled with loving touch rather than anxious tense touch re-connects baby and parent on a deeply emotional level. Building activities that support interactive engagement strengthens the primary attachment system. In this growing era of even the youngest patients showing intense interest in electronic devises and visual media, preserving the emotional embodied live parent-child relationship as the primary source for pleasure and comfort is essential.

Minde and other infant mental health researchers provide evidence that interventions directed at supporting the parent–infant relationship during an infant's early hospitalizations build the parent-infant interactional patterns and psychological functioning of the infant [14]. Minde highlights the importance of interventions that allow the infant to direct and modulate the intensity of the free play with the caregiver. This promotes a sense of interactive agency, security, and competence that the child does not always have within the context of his medical treatment relationships.

As the pediatric patient reaches pre-school and elementary age, caregivers become both active participants and audience members, depending on the child's requests. During this stage of growing independence, the child's sense of agency blossoms as they direct their own dance-play or choose to include their caregivers or even the nursing or medical team. Themes of these storylines enable the patient to enact a sense of control over their bodies and their medical experience, in marked contrast to the adult-driven medical procedures they actually go through. The medical team's willingness to participate becomes another way to strengthen their rapport with the patient. This playfulness and sense of trust carries over during subsequence medical procedures. At this age, parents also take pleasure in seeing their child build multiple secure relationships.

During adolescence, the dance/movement therapist has both a separate and joint relationship with the patients and their caregivers. At times the whole family engages in activities and verbal conversations. Often caregivers at some point leave the room to give the patient private time with the dance/movement therapist. Interests and concerns, including ways to support the patient's perspective that may be different than the family's views are addressed.

Supporting the whole family system is especially important during end of life care. Activities are created to both sooth the patient's experience and help the caregiver's cope with this next stage. Rituals are created, building upon the rapport developed between the dance/movement therapist, the patient and family members through their work together. Memories of favorite songs and activities are incorporated into these sessions, providing family members with the opportunity to express their emotions, while holding the patient's needs as well, to support a peaceful transition.

With all age groups the overarching goal of the DMT treatment is to provide a safe place for each patient's expression of their embodied experiences within the context of supporting the whole family. These experiences may be felt and known or felt and unknown on an emotionally conscious level. Providing support with awareness of the dynamics of the whole family can greatly augment the whole cancer treatment.

8.6. Pediatric Medical DMT within the Context of the Medical Team

The dance/movement therapists at MSKCC work closely with many members of the medical team, participating in meetings to plan treatment goals and pre and post-operative care, writing chart notes and working side-by-side during treatments. A dance/movement therapist attends weekly inpatient pain and palliative care (PACT) meetings participating in discussions about how to support the patients to cope with their medical experience; increase engagement and activity level; or transition to end of life care. The nonverbal aspects of support DMT provides is especially integral in helping patients who are too young, or reticent to talk about their experience; exhibit resistance or anxiety during treatments; or are overly reactive and sensitive to routine procedures such as dressing changes, taking medicine, getting shots or finger pricks. In these situations, the dance/movement therapist typically meets with the medical team to learn details about the case. She presents her ideas about the psychological themes that might be underlying the behaviors, which can include information gleaned from previous sessions with the patient. She has a session with the patient, writes-up the session in the patient's medical files and follows up with the medical team to share any important shifts that occurred during the treatment.

The dance/movement therapists work very closely with the child life team providing group dance therapy sessions that support the many year-round themes and events the child life staff organize such as sibling day, the prom dance and many holiday celebrations. Each member of the child life team is also assigned to work directly with patients with specific diagnoses. The dance/movement therapists often organize treatment goals and work in tandem with specific child life specialists to create continuity in the patient's psychosocial care. This author has used her expertise in infant mental health to help child life staff create charts for the patient's room outlining age appropriate developmental activities to support the infant or toddler's social/emotional engagement.

The MSDMT activities discussed in Section 2.7 were created specifically to support the family and nursing staff during the administration of an antibody treatment for high-risk neuroblastoma [9]. MSDMT is used as a nonpharmacological support alongside of the pharmacological supports, to help reduce the patient's anxiety and side effects of the treatment, which include pain [55]. The MSDMT activities evolved the first year this author was working at MSKCC when she was asked by a nurse administering the antibody treatment, to assist her with a toddler that was exhibiting extreme stress. Upon entering the room, the dance/movement therapist surmised that if she could create a soothing environment to easy the toddler, and by natural association the parent's distress, the nurse would be able to administer the treatment more efficiently. The success of this partnership between the nurse and the dance/movement therapist is evidenced in its continuation over fifteen years later. Nurses and parents request the support of the dance/movement therapy team during the administration of the antibody treatment, each dance/movement therapy intern learns the activities and other integrative medicine and child life staff have incorporated the activities into their support activities as well.

9. Prevalence of DMT in Pediatric Oncology and Other Medical Illnesses

To prepare for this article, the author reached out through phone calls and emails to the ADTA and European Association Dance Movement Therapy (EADMT) email listserves; colleagues and leaders of DMT organizations; and DMT researchers to gather information about past and present pediatric oncology and other medical DMT programs. She also conducted a literature search about DMT in pediatric medicine from 2007–2018. Creative arts therapy programs not including a dance/movement therapist on staff were excluded from the search, to delineate DMT programs and dance/movement therapists employed in pediatric medical DMT. Since this was not an exhaustive or systematic search based on a research protocol, there may be unintentional omissions. It is complete only within the author's knowledge and responses received.

Despite the natural fit of DMT with the pediatric population, the underutilization of DMT in medical settings is profound [56]. Of the 120 citations in PubMed, Embase, CINAHL, and PsycINFO with search strategies using variations on dance therapy with infants, children, and adolescents only three articles are specifically about medical DMT. Of those only two are specifically about pediatric oncology [9,23,56]. This author's own library of medical DMT literature spanning 1993–2018 adds seven literature sources, with only two specifically about DMT in pediatric oncology [10,11,18,22,34,42,57].

Research in pediatric DMT oncology is even more sparse, though this is not surprising because research in all DMT populations is lacking due to several factors. The obstacles for DMT research include: the lack of manualized treatment methods due to the creative improvisational and patient-driven nature of the clinical work; the lack of consistent, valid standardized outcome measures; verbal intervention tools do not accurately measure the nonverbal body-oriented interventions; many of the studies are pilot studies with small sample sizes without larger follow-up studies; and there are very few research faculty positions for DMT worldwide [11,18,24]

The dance/movement therapists, Sherry Goodill, Robin Cruz, and Jennifer Frank Tantia in the USA; Sabine Koch, Marianne Eberhard-Kaechele, Helen Payne, Iris Braeuninger, Vicky Karkou, Bonnie Meekums, and Rosemarie Samaritter in Europe; and Elizabeth Loughlin and Kim Dunphy in Australia have helped to address this research dilemma by developing new research strategies to encourage colleagues and masters and doctorial DMT students to undertake research. This list of dance/movement therapy researchers is based on this author's current knowledge and may not be complete. Any omissions are accidental.

In a recent investigation for specific research about DMT using the search terms cancer, psycho-oncology, and oncology from 1960–2017, Goodill found ten studies, with only one in pediatrics—pediatric brain tumor patients receiving outpatient chemotherapy [18,23]. A common factor in all the studies Goodill found, which include participants both actively and finished with treatment, is a low dropout rate of participation, suggesting that patients experienced benefits that included improvements supporting quality of life. A meta-analysis by Koch et al. found similar results [24]. The study states that participants experienced a decrease in depressive symptoms and anxiety leading to stress reduction. The participants had a greater sense of vitality and a sense of self-efficacy, predicting higher-levels of adaption and symptom management. The creative expressive process, which included affirmative images, metaphors, and symbols enabled the participants to find inner resources and experience personal strengths.

9.1. Pediatric Medical DMT in the USA

One of the earliest articles published in 1993 about pediatric medical DMT is written by Goodill and Morningstar [11]. The article outlines the principles of DMT including the use of movement as our primary communication, the importance of the creative process and symbolic expression and the dynamic aspects of body image. A list of the psychosocial goals of DMT, include: decreasing anxiety related to the hospital experience and medical procedure; help the pediatric patient adjust to functional changes in the body and body image; support the patient's active experience of their body; and supporting the child's expression of their illness and hospital experience, rather than focusing on their dysfunctions caused by the disease. Goodill focused her doctorate on medical DMT with all illnesses of all age groups. This became the basis of her 2005 book [22]. She is now a primary researcher in the field striving to build the efficacy of DMT [18,58]. Her 1993 article and her book are key references used in all subsequent publications about medical DMT.

The recent growth of DMT oncology in pediatrics is largely due to the generous support of The Andréa Rizzo Foundation [59]. The Andréa Rizzo Foundation is a 501c3 non-profit that funds Dréa's Dream Dance Therapy Program for children with cancer and special needs in hospitals and schools nationwide [60]. Susan Rizzo Vincent, the founder and president of the foundation, began The Andréa Rizzo Foundation after the tragic loss of her daughter, Andréa, at age 24, who was struck by a drunk driver [61]. Andréa, a cancer survivor herself, cured from neuroblastoma at MSKCC as a baby, had the dream of starting a pediatric DMT program in MSKCC. She was taking preliminary DMT courses at the time of her death in 2002. Through the tireless support of her mother and friends, The Andréa Rizzo Foundation was founded, with MSKCC as the inaugural Dréa's Dream Dance Therapy Program in 2003. Starting with three hours a week, it quickly grew to a thirty hour a week schedule including two part-time dance/movement therapists and an internship program. In addition to the DMT school programs, The Andréa Rizzo Foundation now supports pediatric hospital programs in eight hospitals ranging from monthly visits to our thirty-hour a week program. At the time of this writing the hospital programs include: Children's Hospital Los Angeles; Connecticut Children's Medical Center; SSM Cardinal Glennon Children's Medical Center in Missouri; Levine Children's Hospital in North Carolina; Hasbro Children's Hospital in Providence, RI; MSKCC in New York; Ronald McDonald House of New York and St Mary's Hospital for Children also in New York.

The following hospitals also have pediatric medical DMT programs for acute and chronic medical conditions. These are added based on responses to the email inquiry: a part-time DMT internship program at RWJBarnabas Health, in New Jersey; a full time DMT program in the Child Life and Expressive Therapies Department of Children's Hospital of Wisconsin [62]; a part-time dance/movement therapists and internship program at Children's Hospital of Philadelphia (CHOP); and a DMT internship program at St. Christopher's Hospital in Philadelphia.

Once a thriving medical DMT program for pediatric oncology-hematology, the child life/creative arts therapy program at the Joseph M. Sanzari Children's Hospital, at Children's Cancer Institute, Hackensack University Medical Center in New Jersey (formerly The Tomorrows Children's Institute) is omitted on this list for [to the best of this author's knowledge] it has no dance/movement therapist on staff. This program which began 1987, was first supervised by an art therapist. In 1995, Orkand (formally Cohen), became the first dance/movement therapist to become the supervisor. She also became a certified child life specialist. Orkand supervised this program, which included and extensive DMT internship program from 1995–2007. In 2007 she was hired by the pediatric pain and palliative medicine department to bring her DMT skills in attending to the nuances of communication to this aspect of patient care. In this position, she became "... a weaver, taking a wholistic approach to listening to patients and their family's stories attuning to help the medical team attune to their style of communication and decision making" [63]. Orkand's writings (written with the surname, Cohen) about the role of medical DMT in pediatric oncology-hematology and pain and palliative care are also widely read [10,34].

9.2. Inaugural Pediatric Creative Arts Therapy Conference at CHOP

This past April 20–21, 2018, The Creative Art Therapy Department at CHOP organized its inaugural Pediatric Creative Arts Therapy Conference. A call for proposals was distributed nationwide. Of the eighteen presentations three were about pediatric medical DMT. Of those three, one was presented by Erin Gallagher, the dance/movement therapist at CHOP, discussing the benefits of DMT with a range of acute and chronically ill pediatric illnesses. The second was by Jocelyn Shaw, a DMT and psychologist working at The Ronald McDonald House of New York, funded by The Andréa Rizzo Foundation. With Jessica Horn, a research nurse at CHOP, they discussed collaborative care between DMT and nursing. The third presentation, also representing a program funded by The Andréa Rizzo Foundation was by this author and DMT colleague Jennifer Whitley at MSKCC, discussing the core elements of our MSKCC pediatric medical DMT program, to best support cancer patients and their families.

9.3. Pediatric Medical DMT Worldwide

At this time to the best of this author's knowledge, based on email inquiries, there are no current pediatric medical DMT programs in hospital settings in other parts of the world. This author has recently received inquiries about providing support for future pediatric medical DMT program in a few countries, including China, Canada and Sweden. In 2016, three members of the MSKCC pediatric integrative medicine team, this author, music therapist Karen Popkin and yoga instructor Catherine Genzler were invited by the Italian Psycho-Oncology Society in Brescia, Italy to present our work at their congress titled, Complementary Therapies in Oncology: Dance, Yoga, Music, Art. Are There Evidences of Efficacy?

The programs that did existed took several forms with many DMTs holding degrees in allied professions such as social work, counseling, psychology, nursing or psychiatry with post graduate training in DMT. Despite the apparent patient interest and satisfaction with these programs, the main reason these programs no longer exist seems to relate to loss of funding, the short-term group special workshop nature of their design, the dance/movement therapist moving, the DMT activities getting absorbed into other general, other arts-based, child life, or recreational [therapeutic] activities offered at the hospital.

9.4. Pediatric Medical DMT—Australia

Elizabeth Loughlin, a dance movement therapist in Australia, has worked extensively with the pediatric population in several contexts. Loughlin offers therapeutic playgroups and individual DMT for depressed and anxious mothers and their infants in the hospital outpatient and psychiatric inpatient settings [64]. She also worked in medical DMT within her social work role in a pediatric hospital setting for over 20 years providing DMT programs for children and adolescents with medical conditions [57,65,66]. The initial dance program was supported by the director who "... saw that expressive dance may address a gap in treating the psychosocial problems in specific life-long chromosomal or hormonal heath conditions" [67] (p. 13). A video *Just Go* created in 1990 about her Turner syndrome (TS) dance group was presented at a European international health conference and was written about in a 1993 issue of the American Journal of Dance Therapy. This video provides evidence of how the dance program she offered for young and midlife women from the TS Support group with this health condition provided them with new ways to think about their condition [57,65].

In a recent article for the Dance Therapy Association Australia Loughlin describes DMT in Australia in the following way "... DMT in Australia is outside the current industrial award and often must rely on serendipity, health staff that know and love the arts, and the availability of funding" [67] (p. 13). This article presents Loughlin's research about how to creatively sustain and communicate the effectiveness of dance arts programs within settings that employ allied health and education professionals. Loughlin found it was more helpful for a dance/movement program, even a short one, to be situated—embedded—in the particular medical department/clinic/ward so one knew of the medical features of the broad diagnosis that the patients shared, and also a working understanding of the nuances in the hospital workplace that affect the day to day experience of young patients with that pediatric health condition and their families [68].

9.5. Pediatric Medical DMT—Israel

Judith Mendelsohn also ran a well-respected pediatric medical DMT starting in 1991, known at the time as the Hadassah School at Hadassah Medical Center in Jerusalem, Israel. Her 1999 article about DMT with hospitalized children, for the American Journal of Dance Therapy is a commonly referenced article in the field. Though the program still exists as an educational school for children with serious medical illness, the recreational activities listed do not include DMT.

From 1981–1998 Ety Shachar Siman-Tov worked at a Therapeutic Center in Tirat-Ha-Carmel organized under the Ministry of Education. It was not a medical setting but serviced children with medical issues including neurological, cerebral palsy (CP), and orthopedic conditions and children with learning disabilities, development disabilities, sensory integration issues, and emotional and behavioral difficulties. There were two dance/movement therapists on staff, along with an art therapist, drama therapist and a consulting medical pediatric doctor. Treatment programming was for ages 4–17 years old and included individual, groups and parents. Siman-Tov states, "During these years children with medical issues were referred to me for DMT treatment. They referred them to me because of my medical knowledge as a Registered Occupational Therapist. They received DMT treatment from me" [69].

9.6. Pediatric Medical DMT—Italy

From 2006–2013, Marcia Plevin ran a DMT program on the oncology-hematology unit of the pediatric hospital Bambino Gesù (known as the Vatican Hospital), in Rome. She worked with children going bed-to-bed during their hospitalizations. During that period, she also supervised three dance/movement therapy interns. There were dance/movement therapist's interested in continuing this program, but it was closed due to lack of funding [70].

Lorena Candini, worked with congenital heart disease from 2008–2012 through the Piccoli Grandi Cuori Association in cooperation with the Unit of Pediatric (Developmental) Cardiology and Cardiac Surgery (U.O. Cardiologia e Cardiochirurgia Pediatrica e dell'età evolutiva) at the Azienda Ospedaliero-Universitaria Policlinico Sant'Orsola-Malpighi in Bologna. Hired as a psychologist, her "... daily work was always led by DMT principles and techniques as if I were in DMT session... [using] touch, movements, relaxing techniques, bodily awareness and attunement, body mirroring, somatic countertransference... as a way of better understanding the patient's feelings..." [69]. She also supervised dance/movement therapy interns. The initial outpatient program design was ten weekly sessions divided into three age groups (7–8; 9–11; 13–15). It became two groups for ages 8–10 and 13–17. These children and adolescents with congenital heart disease, had been hospitalized, and had experienced heart surgery or other invasive procedures. Families were involved at the beginning of the groups to be introduced to the program and collect information about the children. Parents met in groups regularly with Candini and her team to share about the children's experiences, progresses and difficulties [69]. At the end of the first year of this program a conference was organized to present the successful results, which were also published in an in-hospital publication [71,72].

10. Advances in Pediatric Medical DMT within Integrative Oncology—Future Steps

The last section addresses the next steps for pediatric medical DMT highlighting why and how it is an essential therapeutic modality within the integrative oncology team. The focus considers our need to support the psychological health of the growing number of survivors of pediatric cancers; the role of trauma in the body; DMT as an embodied psychotherapeutic modality for trauma prevention; supporting young pediatric patients to regain lost stages of development; educating professionals, patients and families about pediatric medical DMT; and the need for further research.

As this discussion turns to more difficult topics related to potentially painful traumatic reactions and developmental considerations children with medical illness may experience, it is done with utmost respect to the medical professionals deeply committed to healing children without causing harm. The care, kindness and dedication of the medical professionals working with the pediatric population is unprecedented. But many factors contribute to a family and child's reaction to the medical experience that are out of our control. This section aims to emphasize how the whole medical team, and the integrative oncology team specifically, play an essential role in supporting the quality of life of our patients. The biopsychosocial and patient-centered approach both DMT and integrative oncology effectively addresses, creates an environment to optimize health and empower the patient throughout their cancer care.

10.1. Pediatric Cancer Survivor Rates

The National Institute of Health (NIH) National Cancer Institute reports that the survival rate of children with cancer has steadily improved since 1975, when just over 50% of children with cancer under age twenty survived at least five years [73]. Survival rates improved to 83% for this population in a study looking at the years 2007–2013 [74]. The success rate of treatment, though promising, for the child with cancer requires medical professionals to consider how the child's experience having cancer, and the memories associated with this experience, may affect their later health and well-being.

Counter to the still popular belief commonly stated during medical treatments that the infant or young child is "too young to remember" the medical experience; the long-term psychological influences of the disease must be considered, even if there are no visible disabilities after completing the treatment course [10,23,42]. How much of this attitude may also be related to the difficulty in both recognizing and reconciling that a child, especially a very young one, might be experiencing pain or even trauma, and remembering it? Similarly, the phrase, "he is so resilient", often discussed with older children and adolescents may belie the complex emotions about the medical experience the pediatric patient may not understand, know how to process, or express. In addition, children and adolescents are actually very good at sensing their parent's vulnerabilities. Resilient acts can be as much a product of the child's attempt to support the parent's feeling of helplessness as the child's efforts to manage the incomprehensible aspects of the medical experience.

10.2. Trauma in the Body-Infancy Memory

Taking the viewpoint that integrating the body and mind creates a body-mind-emotional continuum that begins at or even prior to birth, and informs the infant's core self from a reality-based perception, leads to the understanding that our bodies hold our experiences [45]. Some experiences are felt and stay in our awareness, but there are also experiences, especially difficult or traumatic ones that are held out of awareness and stored deeply in the body. Gaensbauer, an infancy memory researcher, studying early childhood trauma, documents how sensory experiences and motor actions are linked, and become imprinted. These experiences are organized and represented through "perceptual-cognitive-affective-sensory-motor schemata" [41] (p. 29). These emotional and somatic experiences create a preverbal and sensory-based memory system and can manifest through later clinical symptoms and atypical behaviors including: nightmares; hyperarousal; phobias; anxiety; distress at reminders acting as triggers of the experience; and avoidance of the stimuli related to the traumatic event.

Through his clinical work Gaensbauer demonstrates how [preverbal] trauma is represented in the behavior and traumatic reenactment play schemes of infants, toddlers and children. Gaensbauer states, "... the intimate coupling between sensory experiences and motoric actions that replicate these experiences provides important depth to our understanding of the representations that underlie reenactment behavior" [41] (p. 29). The child's verbal and nonverbal understanding is separate from their conscious and unconscious expressions of their traumas [75]. Children's play is more representative of traumatic recall than their ability to verbally discuss their traumatic experiences. Through therapeutic symbolic play, children explore their traumatic reactions creating a coherent autobiographic narrative leading to understanding and healing. Creating a coherent verbal narrative of the traumatic experience enables the young child to make sense of the internalized memory facilitating coping.

10.3. Preverbal Trauma and Later Verbal Accessibility

A study about children's verbal memories related to retinoblastoma treatment specifically before 24 months of age or after 24 months of age and treated before 5 years old, sheds light on the need to use nonverbal methods to access early childhood memories [76]. This age distinction highlights the transition between pre-verbal and verbal language and was used in this study to "understand the relationship between age and verbal accessibility of traumatic memories" [76] (p. 566). Infants' abilities for verbal recall of events prior to language continues to be a contested debate. The results demonstrate that though both age ranges initiated verbal recall of the medical event, the older children were more able to access their memories of the experience verbally and through the props provided in the free-play task. The researchers conclude that children undergoing retinoblastoma treatment in the first year of life may experience "misconceptions or gaps of knowledge" which may affect their later quality of life, for they "have limited access to a dialogue about these events in their early life" [76] (p. 576).

Susan Coates, a psychoanalyst well known for her work with young children and trauma, discusses whether early traumas experienced by preverbal children are available for symbolic interpretation later in treatment [77]. She concludes that toddlers, infants and neonates experience pain and demonstrate traumatic symptoms. These events can be stored in memory, can be symbolically represented and can affect later behavior and learning. Coates states that resolving the trauma is definitively affected by the quality and function of the attachment system.

10.4. Trauma in the Body—Implications Later in Life

Recent research about adult chronic pain, medically unexplained symptoms (MUS) and somatization spectrum disorders (SSD) state that children that have undergone painful or traumatic early medical experiences are more vulnerable to later chronic pain conditions as adults [12,13,78]. Current research and literature in trauma also confirms that trauma is stored in the body causing physiological changes [12,13,15]. Healing methods that enable a reintegration of body, mind, and emotions include therapies that incorporate body and movement-oriented activities.

10.5. Pediatric Medical DMT and Trauma Prevention

The intrinsically body and movement-focused aspects of pediatric medical DMT align with these suggested methods. The in-depth nonverbal foundation of DMT coupled with children's natural propensity for creative expressive dance and movement uniquely position DMT as a treatment method that can support a child to synthesize potentially traumatic aspects of their medical experience while they are actively undergoing treatment. Might this ability to express feelings while in treatment, within the context of an embodied psychotherapeutic milieu create perceptual-cognitive-affective-sensory-motor schemata that foster expressivity and empowerment rather than internalized representations of trauma?

10.6. Why Pediatric Medical DMT is an Essential Part of the CANCER-WWW Team?

Pediatric medical DMT and MSDMT enables the patient and family to explore their experience of their illness while it is occurring. The embodied focus, attention to subtle nonverbal cues and approach coming from the perspective of the body-mind-emotion continuum provides an immediate and safe psychological environment that is meaningful and enjoyable. The physical act of playful dancing literally mobilizes feelings and revives the pediatric patient's natural avenue of expression. Utilizing this innate form of expression during the treatment may prevent the unspoken [traumatic] aspect of the medical experience from being held in the body. This author proposes that pediatric medical DMT can be a form of trauma prevention. This is clinically confirmed, each time a patient returns for their yearly check-up and speaks with warm reverie about their playful dancing experiences delightfully recounting specific details of our dance activities, seemly without awareness of the difficult treatment experience going on simultaneously. A parent shared that one afternoon while the family was in a music store her child pointed to a rainstick—an instrument frequently used during MSDMT to create a soothing auditory sensation—and told her sister it was a toy for relaxation.

10.7. Strengthening the Presence of Pediatric Medical DMT—What it Will Take?

Though we can never know fully, the profound biopsychosocial experience of the pediatric patient and family's cancer journey, as [mental] health care providers we strive to make that passage smooth, and painless, embracing the patient and family with love, care and respect. Through DMT we can address the wordless experience, creating an *embodied coherent narrative* to support the patient and family's cancer voyage. A specific path must be taken to strengthen this role for dance/movement therapists working with the pediatric population.

First, a strong understanding of infant mental health is necessary. This training enables the dance/movement therapist to recognize and identify how the attachment system can best support the specific presenting family dynamics. Understanding the role of the parents and supporting their experience so they can be effectively available for their child is vital.

It is essential to know the influence the felt-body experience has at all levels of development starting in infancy and continuing throughout childhood and adolescence. This includes awareness of multi-sensory sensitivities that can develop and greatly affect the child's ability to maintain emotional and physiological regulation. This affects the child's social/emotional presentation, behavioral state and coping during their treatment, enabling the dance/movement therapist to sensitively attune to the amount of sensation and input that best supports the patient's engagement. In-depth comprehension of infant and early childhood mental health also provides an understanding of the metaphoric and symbolic levels of nonverbal expression specific to the developmental stages of childhood that also influence adolescence.

The role of early life experiences as it effects behaviors and later life stages is important. Starting with infancy development leads to childhood and adolescent development. A strong understanding of the social/emotional, physical and cognitive themes as they manifest in verbal and nonverbal behaviors is essential for the dance/movement therapist working in pediatric medical illness. Crucial to this training is an understanding of how children and adolescents at different stages of growth comprehend, experience and symbolically represent life and death both verbally and nonverbally. Cultural, religious and ethnic differences related to end of life beliefs must be considered.

Next, is educating the medical team, patients and families about DMT. The psychotherapeutic aspects of DMT must be explained to enable dance/movement therapists to implement the full breadth and depth of their skills, differentiating DMT from other complimentary yet distinct dance and movement-based programming. This will enable more appropriate referrals and effective participation in the Cancer-WWW team.

Increased awareness about the significant contribution pediatric medical DMT has in the integrative oncology team will facilitate dance/movement therapists being hired specifically as dance/movement therapists. This will expose the unique and salient contributions that a dance/movement therapist can make, rather than adding this perspective through the lens of an allied profession such as social work, psychologist, child life specialist, or recreational therapist.

The last imperative is research. With the increasing need for evidence-based practice developing research tools that effectively analyze both the art and science of pediatric medical DMT is essential. Goodill, Koch, Cruz, and others in the field advocate for a research paradigm that synthesizes both quantitative and qualitative methods [18,24,58,79]. Examining its efficacy can wait no longer. Each pediatric medical DMT article discussed in this paper starting in 1993 has stated the need for research. Madden et al.'s research on the creative arts therapies used to improve the quality of life of pediatric brain tumor patients is the only research to date that includes pediatric medical DMT in their study design [23].

1993 was twenty-five years ago. It is time for a call for action. Disallowing treatment protocols due to a lack of evidence-based research is a growing reality. Pediatric medical DMT cannot take an influential place on the integrative oncology team with only clinical narratives as its evidence.

11. Conclusions

Pediatric medical DMT is a body-mind-emotion psychotherapeutic approach that supports the patient and the whole family enabling them to express thoughts and feelings about their medical experience using many dance, movement, music, play, and mindfulness techniques. Through this method patients can explore all their emotions along the spectrum from joyful to fearful and rage, creating a sense of empowerment, while attuning to their bodies. DMT also supports body awareness, increases mobility, flexibility, and range of motion, and supports regaining skills in all areas of development. The emotional, felt-body focus supports all stages of the cancer experience from treatment to palliative and end-of-life care.

With the current understanding of the integral relationship between the body-mind-emotions, the psychotherapeutic perspective and the intrinsically nonverbal and embodied nature of pediatric medical DMT, it is uniquely positioned to be a strong member of the integrative oncology team. The extensive definition of terms, literature and research review, and discussion about the national and international state of pediatric medical DMT aims to clarify and define the field, placing it as a central psychotherapeutic treatment modality in integrative oncology that supports the biopsychosocial experience of the pediatric oncology patient and family members. As stated by a parent of a pediatric patient that extensively used pediatric medical DMT and specifically MSDMT methods, along with other integrative medicine services at MSKCC, *"Integrative medicine didn't change the outcome for us, but it did change the story"* [80].

This paper ends by reiterating a central question: Can pediatric medical DMT support the patient to express feelings while in cancer treatment within the context of a psychotherapeutic milieu, enabling the patient to create an embodied coherent narrative that fosters expressivity and empowerment rather than internalized representations of trauma? If this clinical hypothesis is true, postponing the research to prove this theory is denying services that can greatly contribute to the quality of life for all pediatric cancer patient and family members.

Acknowledgments: This material was made possible in part by a grant from The Andréa Rizzo Foundation, which funds the Dréa's Dream dance therapy program in hospitals and schools throughout the country. This work was supported by funding from the NIH/NCI Cancer Center Support Grant P30 CA008748." Tortora is grateful for the support of Susan Rizzo Vincent, president and founder of The Andréa Rizzo Foundation, and all of the dance/movement therapists who provide DMT through The Andréa Rizzo Foundation: Leslie Armeniox, Lori Baudino, Katie Bohn, Andee Dooley, Toni Freni, Sharon O'Neill Mulcahy, Melissa Sabatini, Jocelyn Shaw, and Jennifer Whitley. Thanks to the dance/movement therapists who assisted in accurately depicting past and present DMT programs across multiple national and international time zones. USA: Jennifer Whitley (DMT at

MSKCC and eNewletter editor, fundraiser, and advocate for The Andréa Rizzo Foundation), Sherry Goodill, Elizabeth Veltrie, Jessica Young, Jenna Mao. Europe: Sabine Koch, Rosamaria Govoni, Lorena Candini, Marcia Plevin, Hilda Wengrower, Ety Shachar Siman-Tov. Australia: Kim Dunphy, Elizabeth Loughlin. Tortora is also grateful for the support of MSKCC, Department of Pediatrics and Integrative Medicine Service with special thanks to: Jun Mao—Chief Attending; Gary Deng—Medical Director; and Eva Pendleton—Associate Director. Thanks also goes to the staff of *Children*, with particular gratitude to Goran Lisic for his kind and diligent editing.

Bio: Tortora is a New York State Licensed Creative Arts Therapist (LCAT); Licensed Mental Health Counselor (LCAT); Board Certified Dance/Movement Therapist (BC-DMT); and Certified Laban Movement Analyst (CMA). She is the International Medical Creative Arts Spokesperson for the Andréa Rizzo Foundation, having created and continuing to be the senior dance/movement therapist since its inception in 2003 at Integrative Medicine Service, Memorial Sloan-Kettering Cancer CenterNYC,. She is the founder and director of Dancing Dialogue LCAT LMHC PLLC. Dr Tortora has numerous publications about her work and teaches in Europe, South America, New Zealand, the Middle East, and Asia.

References

1. Tortora, S. *The Dancing Dialogue: Using the Communicative Power of Movement with Young Children*; Paul H. Brookes Publishing Company: Baltimore, MD, USA, 2006.
2. Schechter, D.S. Traumatically skewed intersubjectivity. *Psychoanal. Inq.* **2017**, *37*, 251–264. [CrossRef]
3. Cloitre, M.; Stolbach, B.; Herman, J.; van de Kolk, B.; Pynoos, R.; Want, J.; Petkova, E. A Developmental Approach to Complex PTSD: Childhood and Adult Cumulative Trauma as Predictors of Symptom Complexity. *J. Trauma. Stress* **2009**, *22*, 399–408. [CrossRef] [PubMed]
4. Nir, Y. Post-truamatic stress disorder in children with cancer. In *Post-Truamatic Stress Disorder in Children*; Eth, S., Pynoos, R., Eds.; American Psychatric Association Publishing: Washington, DC, USA, 1985; pp. 123–132.
5. Terr, L. *Too Scared to Cry: How Trauma Affects Children... and Ultimately Us All*; Basic Books: New York, NY, USA, 1992.
6. Levy, F. *Dance and Other Expressive Art Therapies: When Words Are Not Enough*; Routledge: New York, NY, USA, 1995.
7. Winnicott, D.W. Basis for self in body. *Int. J. Child Psychother.* **1972**, *1*, 7–16.
8. Winnicott, D.W. *Playing and Reality*; Penguin Books: London, UK, 1985.
9. Tortora, S. Dance/movement psychotherapy in early childhood treatment and pediatric oncology. In *The Art and Science of Dance/Movement Therapy: Life is Dance*; Chaiklin, S., Wengrower, H., Eds.; Routledge: New York, NY, USA, 2015.
10. Cohen, S.; Walco, G. Dance/movement therapy for children and adolescents with cancer. *Cancer Pract.* **1999**, *7*, 34–42. [CrossRef]
11. Goodill, S.; Morningstar, D. The role of dance/movement therapy with medically ill children. *Int. J. Arts Med.* **1993**, *2*, 24–27.
12. Levine, P.; Kline, M. *Trauma-Proofing Your Kids: A Parent's Guide for Instilling Confidence, Joy and Resilience*; North Atlantic Books: Berkeley, CA, USA, 2008.
13. Levine, P. *An Unspoken Voice: How the Body Releases Trauma*; North Atlantic Books: Berkeley, CA, USA, 2012.
14. Minde, K. Prematurilty and serious medical conditions in infancy: Implications for development, behavior, and intervention. In *Handbook of Infant Mental Health*, 2nd ed.; Zeanah, C., Ed.; The Guildford Press: New York, NY, USA, 2000; pp. 176–194.
15. Van der Kolk, B. *The Body Keeps the Score: Brain, Mind and Body in the Healing of Trauma*; Penguin Books: New York, NY, USA, 2015.
16. Witt, C.; Balneaves, L.; Cardoso, M.; Cohen, L.; Greenlee, H.; Johnstone, P.; Kucuk, O.; Mailman, J.; Mao, J. A comprehensive definition for integrative oncology. *J. Natl. Cancer Inst. Monogr.* **2017**, *52*, 3–8. [CrossRef]
17. Koch, S.; Fischman, D. Embodied enactive dance/movement therapy. *Am. J. Dance Ther.* **2011**, *33*, 57–32. [CrossRef]
18. Goodill, S. Accumulating evidence for dance/movement therapy in cancer care. *Front. Psychol.* **2018**, *9*, 1778. [CrossRef]
19. American Dance Therapy Association. Available online: https://adta.org/2014/11/08/what-is-dancemovement-therapy/ (accessed on 28 October 2018).

20. Goodill, S.; Chairperson, Department of Creative Arts Therapies, Drexel University, USA. Personal communication, 6 November 2018.
21. Bernstein, P. *Eight Theoretical Approaches in Dance—Movement Therapy*; Kendall/Hunt Publishing Company: Dubuque, IA, USA, 1979.
22. Goodill, S. *An Introduction to Medical Dance/Movement Therapy*; Jessica Kingsley Publishers: Philadephia, PA, USA, 2005.
23. Madden, J.; Mowry, P.; Gao, D.; Cullen, P.; Foreman, N. Creative arts therapy improves quality of life for pediatric brain tumor patients receiving outpatient chemotherapy. *J. Pediatr. Oncol. Nurs.* **2010**, *27*, 133–145. [CrossRef]
24. Koch, S.; Kunz, T.; Lykou, S.; Cruz, R. Effects of dance movement therapy and dance on psychological outcomes: A meta-analysis. *Arts Psychother.* **2014**, *41*, 46–64. [CrossRef]
25. American Cancer Society: What is Cancer? Available online: https://www.cancer.org/treatment/understanding-your-diagnosis/after-diagnosis/what-is-cancer.html?_ga=2.67345239.711542427.1541340649-333493092.1541340649 (accessed on 4 November 2018).
26. Vincent, S.R.; President, The Andréa Rizzo Foundation. Personal communication, 27 October 2018.
27. Tortora, S. Dance/movement therapy in psycho-oncology: Are there evidences of its efficacy? In Proceedings of the Complimentary Therapies in Oncology: Dance, Yoga, Music, Art, Brescia, Italy, 6–7 October 2016.
28. Bowlby, J. *Attachment and Loss: Attachment*, 2nd ed.; Basic Books: New York, NY, USA, 1999; Volume I.
29. Landa, A.; Bossis, A.; Boylan, L.; Wong, P. Beyond the unexplainable pain: Relational world of patients with somatization syndromes. *J. Nerv. Ment. Dis.* **2012**, *200*, 413–422. [PubMed]
30. Sheets-Johnstone, M. *The Primacy of Movement*, 2nd ed.; John Benjamin's Publishing Company: Philadelphia, PA, USA, 2011.
31. Eddy, M. *Mindful Movement: The Evolution of the Somatic Arts and Conscious Action*; Intellect, The University of Chicago Press: Chicago, IL, USA, 2016.
32. Dychtwald, K. *Bodymind*; Pantheon books: New York, NY, USA, 1977.
33. Landa, A. Principles of psychosomatic integrative care: Towards a neuroscience-based paradigm shift in medicine. In *4th Columbia Psychosomatics Conference: Healing "Unexplainable" Pain*; New York State Psychiatric Institute at Columbia University Medical Center: New York, NY, USA, 2018.
34. Hain, R.; Zeltzer, L.; Hellsten, M.; Cohen, S.; Orloff, S.; Gray, D. Holistic management of symptoms. In *Palliative Care of Infants, Children and Adolescents: A Practical Handbook*, 2nd ed.; Carter, B., Levetown, M., Friebert, S., Eds.; The Johns Hopkins University Press: Baltimore, MD, USA, 2011; pp. 244–274.
35. American Academy of Pediatrics. *Pediatrics*; American Academy of Pediatrics: Elk Grove Village, IL, USA, 2000; Volume 106, pp. 351–352.
36. Tortora, S. Mindfulness and movement. In *Teaching Mindfulness Skills to Kids and Teens*; Willard, C.S.A., Ed.; Guildford Press: New York, NY, USA, 2015.
37. Tortora, S. *Stories our bodies tell. The American Psychoanalyst*; Spring/Summer: Boston, MA, USA, 2017; pp. 16–18.
38. Thelen, E. The improvising infant: Learning about learning to move. In *The Developmental Psychologists: Research Adventures across the Life Span*; Merrens, M., Brannigan, G., Eds.; McGraw-Hill Co. Inc.: New York, NY, USA, 1996.
39. Stern, D. *The Interpersonal World of The Infant*; Basic Books, Inc.: New York, NY, USA, 1985.
40. Gaensbauer, T. Trauma in the preverbal period. Symptoms, memories, and developmental impact. *Psychoanal. Study Child* **1995**, *50*, 122–149. [CrossRef]
41. Gaensbauer, T. Telling their stories: Representation and reenactment of traumatic experiences occurring in the first year of life. *Zero Three* **2004**, *24*, 25–31.
42. Mendelsohn, J. Dance/Movement therapy with hospitalized Children. *Am. J. Dance Mov. Ther.* **1999**, *21*, 65–80. [CrossRef]
43. Tortora, S. The importance of being seen—Winnicott, Dance Movement Psychotherapy and the embodied experience. In *The Winnicott Tradition: Lines of Development—Evolution of Theory and Practice over the Decades*; Spelman, M., Thomson-Salo, F., Eds.; Karnac: London, UK, 2015.
44. Bartenieff, I.; Lewis, D. *Body Movements: Coping with the Environment*; Gordon and Breach Science Publishers: New York, NY, USA, 1980.
45. Tortora, S. Our moving bodies tell stories, which speak of our experiences. *Zero Three* **2004**, *24*, 4–12.

46. Tortora, S. Ways of Seeing: An early childhood integrated therapeutic approach for parents and babies. *Clin. Soc. Work J.* **2010**, *38*, 37–50. [CrossRef]
47. Plevin, M.; Parteli, L. Time out of time: Dance/movement therapy on the onco-hemotology unit of a pediatric hospital. *Am. J. Dance Ther.* **2014**, *36*, 229–246. [CrossRef]
48. Laban, R. *The Mastery of Movement*; MacDonald and Evans: London, UK, 1980.
49. Kestenberg Amighi, J.; Loman, S.; Sossin, K.M. *The Meaning of Movement: Embodied Development, Clinical and Cultural Perspectives of the Kestenberg Movement Profile*, 2nd ed.; Routledge: New York, NY, USA, 2018.
50. Tortora, S. Join my dance: The unique movement style of each infant and toddler can invite communication, expression and intervention. *Zero Three* **1994**, *15*, 1–12.
51. Bloom, K. *The Embodied Self: Movement and Psychoanalysis*; Karnac: London, UK, 2006.
52. Pallaro, P. *Authentic Movement: Essays by Mary Starks Whitehouse, Janet Adler and Joan Chodorow*; Jessica Kingsley Press: Philadelphia, PA, USA, 1999.
53. Rosen, M.; Oxenbury, H. *We're Going on a Bear Hunt*; Little Simon: New York, NY, USA, 1997.
54. Keren, M.; Hopp, D.; Tyano, S. *Does Time Heal? Exploring Mental Health in the First 3 Years*; Zero to Three: Washington, DC, USA, 2018.
55. Ahmed, M.; Modak, S.; Sequeira, S. Acute Pain Relief After Mantram Meditation in Children With Neuroblastoma Undergoing Anti-GD2 Monoclonal Antibody Therapy. *J. Pediatr. Hematol. Oncol.* **2014**, *36*, 152–155. [CrossRef]
56. Zilius, M. Dance movement therapy in pediatrics: An overview. *Altern. Compliment. Ther.* **2010**, *16*, 87–92. [CrossRef]
57. Loughlin, E. Why was I born among mirrors? Therapeutic dance with teenage girls and women with Turner syndrome. *Am. J. Dance Ther.* **1993**, *15*, 107–124. [CrossRef]
58. Bradt, J.; Shim, M.; Goodill, S.W. Dance/movement therapy for improving psychological and physical outcomes in cancer patients. *Cochrane Database Syst. Rev.* **2015**, *1*, CD007103. [CrossRef] [PubMed]
59. Vincent, S.R.; Tortora, S.; Shaw, J.; Basiner, J.; Devereaux, C.; Mulcahy, S.; Ponsini, M.S. Collaborating with a mission: The Andrea Rizzo Foundation spreads the gift of dance/movement therapy. *Am. J. Dance Ther.* **2007**, *29*, 51–58. [CrossRef]
60. The Andréa Rizzo Foundation. Available online: www.dreasdream.org (accessed on 25 October 2018).
61. The Andréa Rizzo Foundation: About Andréa. Available online: www.dreasdream.org/about-andrea/ (accessed on 5 November 2018).
62. Dickinson, H. Dance/movement Therapy promotes mobility while lifting spirits 2017. Available online: https://medium.com/@childrenshospitalwi/childrens-hospital-of-wisconsin-patients-express-themselves-through-dance-movement-therapy-951bea3a1bb1 (accessed on 5 November 2018).
63. Orkand, S.; Ease Stress Holistically, USA. Personal communication, 2 November 2018.
64. Ericksen, J.; Loughlin, E.; Holt, C.; Rose, N.; Hartley, E.; Buultjens, M.; Gemmill, A.W.; Milgrom, J. A therapeutic playgroup for depressed mothers and their infants: Reasibility study and pilot randomized trial of community HUGS. *Infant Ment. Health J.* **2018**, *39*, 396–409. [CrossRef] [PubMed]
65. Loughlin, E.; Werther, G. A Phenomenological approach to Turner Syndrome. In *Proceedings: 5th International Turner Symposium, Optimising Care for the Turner Patient in the 21st Century*; Saenger, P., Pasquino, A., Eds.; International Congress series No. 1212; Elsevier Science B.V.: Naples, Italy, 2000; pp. 105–111.
66. Loughlin, E. Infertility, An unspoken presence in the lives of teens and young women with Turner syndrome. In *Sexuality and Fertility Issues in Ill health and Disability, Balen, R.C.M., Ed.*; Jessica Kingsley: London, UK, 2006; pp. 159–176.
67. Loughlin, E. The Arts, in Liminal Space, and the Visible Outcomes Dance Therapy Collections No. 4. 2017, pp. 12–26. Available online: https://dtaa.org.au/category/dtc4/ (accessed on 4 November 2018).
68. Loughlin, E.; Private practice, Australia. Personal communication, 11 November 2018.
69. Candini, L.; Private practice, Italy. Personal communication, 28 October 2018.
70. Pelvin, M.; Private practice, Italy. Personal communication, 23 October 2018.
71. Candini, L. *Il gruppo in cardiologia e cardiochirurgia pediatrica e dell"età evolutiva*; Report aziendale; Cardiologia e Cardiochirurgia Pediatrica e dell'età evolutive: Bologna, Italy, 2008.
72. Candini, L.; Cortesi, A. Corpo ri-trovato, corpo ri-mosso: Percorsi di danzamovimento terapia. In *Giornata di.studio "nuove opportunità di supporto alla cura e all"assistenza delle.cardiopatie.congenite*; Cardiologia e Cardiochirurgia Pediatrica e dell'età evolutive: Bologna, Italy, 2009.

73. Ries, L.A.G.; Smith, M.A.; Gurney, J.G.; Linet, M.; Tamra, T.; Young, J.L.; Bunin, G.R. *Cancer Incidence and Survival among Children and Adolescents: United States SEER Program 1975–1995*; National Cancer Institute, SEER Program; NIH Pub: Bethesda, MD, USA, 1999; No. 99–4649.
74. NIH, Childhood cancer rates calculated using the Incidence SEER18 Research Database, November 2016 submission (Katrina/Rita Population Adjustment). All cancer site rates are based on the SEER site codes with the exception of medulloblastoma, which used site code C71.6 and International Classification Code of Diseases for Oncology, Third Edition (ICD-O-3) malignant histologic codes 9470/3, 9471/3, and 9474/3.
75. Gaensbauer, T. Personal communication, 7 November 2018.
76. Norgate, S.; Littleton, K. Children's memories for events relating to treatment for eye cancer: Influence of age at loss of eye. *Infant Ment. Health J.* **2011**, *32*, 563–577. [CrossRef] [PubMed]
77. Coates, S. Can Babies Remember Trauma? Symbolic Forms of Representation in Traumatized Infants. *J. Am. Psychoanal. Assoc.* **2016**, *64*, 751–776. [CrossRef]
78. Anderson, F.S. It was not safe to feel angry: Disruptive early attachment and the development of chronic pain in later life. *Attach. New Dir. Psychother. Relat. Psychoanal.* **2017**, *11*, 223–241.
79. Cruz, R. Evaluation and assessment in dance/movement therapy. In *The Art and Science of Evaluation in the Arts Therapies: How Do You Know What Is Working?* Cruz, R., Feder, F., Eds.; Charles C. Thomas Publisher: Springfield, IL, USA, 2013.
80. Goldberg, W. Personal communication, 2 November 2018.

3

Integrative Approaches in Pediatric Palliative Care

Kate Shafto [1], Suzanne Gouda [2], Kris Catrine [3] and Melanie L. Brown [3,4,*]

[1] Department of Internal Medicine and Pediatrics, University of Minnesota, Minneapolis, MN 55455, USA; kshafto@umn.edu

[2] Department of Pediatrics, University of Chicago, Chicago, IL 60637, USA; suzanne.gouda@uchospitals.edu

[3] Department of Pain Medicine, Palliative Care and Integrative Medicine, Children's Hospitals and Clinics of Minnesota, Minneapolis, MN 55404, USA; kris.catrine@childrensmn.org

[4] Department of Pediatrics, University of Minnesota, Minneapolis, MN 55455, USA

[*] Correspondence: melanie.brown@childrensmn.org

Abstract: Pediatric palliative care is a field which focuses on caring for and treating the symptoms and distress typically associated with life-limiting illness. Integrative medicine is supported by evidence and aims to heal the whole person, including all aspects of one's lifestyle. Therapies offered by integrative medicine often empower patients and families, allowing for a sense of control. This review addresses the merging of integrative medicine philosophy and modalities with the care given to children with life-limiting illness. We review an introduction to integrative medicine, trends in its incorporation in the healthcare setting, application to patients receiving palliative care and the management of specific symptoms. A case study is offered to illustrate these principles.

Keywords: pediatrics; palliative care; integrative medicine; symptom management; mind-body medicine; pain management; acupuncture; yoga

---

1. Introduction: Integrative Medicine

Integrative medicine is not a new concept, though in recent decades the terminology has become solidified and more widely used. Dating back to early human history, there are writings describing how humans are composed of body, mind and spirit, with healers addressing these realms together when illness occurred [1]. The current definitions of integrative medicine center around a goal of healing, the patient's lifestyle, environment, history, and a patient-provider partnership which considers lifestyle, allopathic diagnosis and treatment, environmental factors, emotional/spiritual factors and the role of other healing systems when caring for the patient. The University of Arizona's Center for Integrative Medicine, USA, a leader in training and research around integrative medicine for several decades, defines integrative medicine as: "healing-oriented medicine that takes account of the whole person, including all aspects of lifestyle. It emphasizes the therapeutic relationship between practitioner and patient, is informed by evidence, and makes use of all appropriate therapies" [2].

Integrative medicine is distinct from complementary and alternative medicine (CAM), which refers to a practice or treatment that differs from the conventional approach, or therapies which complement the conventional model. Integrative medicine, as its name suggests, intentionally integrates too-often separate approaches to healing, with an additional emphasis on empowering the patient with skills for self-care, promotion of wellbeing and self-management (at times with even prevention or reversal) of disease.

2. Integrative Medicine Trends in US Healthcare

Modern western medicine is based on a reductionist approach to the body and disease, dating back to the 1600s, out of which grew the current system of medical specialization and compartmentalization of organs and body systems [1]. This model has come at a great cost financially, and, in many cases, led to disempowerment of patients, a fragmented healthcare system, and patient dependence on healthcare providers for treatment and management of disease. Chronic diseases, due to their multi-organ pathophysiology and high correlation with lifestyle, are often not adequately addressed using a reductionist model. Additionally, the locus of control in an allopathic model is frequently external to the patient, being the healthcare provider and their prescribed treatment. A study examining the health locus of control for youths with chronic illnesses found that those with an external locus of control had poorer health outcomes than those with an internal locus of control [3]. Integrative medicine seeks to leverage a combination between the internal and external, which in turn shifts the locus of control to include a patient's own capacity to influence their health or disease in addition to the provider.

There is clear and rising interest among patients as well as providers in a whole-person care model. Fellowships in integrative medicine are providing evidence-informed knowledge and tools for practice [4]; additionally, a myriad of conferences in integrative medicine [5], restorative medicine [6], lifestyle medicine [7], mind-body medicine [8] and nutrition [9] are offering continuing medical education for clinicians. The internet and social media are making consumers/patients more aware of options in addition to medications and surgeries often offered by traditional allopathic healthcare delivery systems.

In the most recent survey from the National Institutes of Health's Center for Complementary and Integrative Health on the use of complementary health approaches, several trends are evident. This 2012 survey collected information on the use of various approaches, including dietary supplements, chiropractic or osteopathic manipulation, yoga, massage, and mind-body practices such as meditation. Findings from this survey demonstrated about 33% of adults and 11.4% of children use some form of complementary health approaches. The survey also found that roughly 59 million Americans spend money out-of-pocket on complementary health approaches, with total spending around \$30.2 billion/year. Pain was one of the main reasons people sought out complementary therapies, and the most utilized mind-body approaches were chiropractic manipulation, meditation, massage and yoga. Interestingly, yoga has become more popular among children as well in the last 15 years: 3.1% of US children practiced yoga in 2012, compared to 2.3% in 2007. These are samples of a large set of data illustrating the increase in interest, use and willingness to pay for integrative (here described as complementary) therapies [10].

The growing demand and value recognition of such therapies and practices has led many healthcare systems to incorporate integrative medicine's modalities, practitioners and practices in service to their patients and families. A 2010 survey by Samueli Institute and the American Hospital Association's Health Forum was conducted to study these trends, entitled Complementary and Alternative Medicine Survey of Hospitals [11]. Out of almost 6000 hospitals receiving the 42-question survey, 714 responded (12%), and 299 of respondents (42%) offered one or more complementary and alternative medicine (CAM) therapies. There was significant regional variation, with the largest number of respondents offering CAM being in the East-North-Central region (23%; Illinois, Indiana, Michigan, Ohio, Wisconsin) and the fewest being in the East-South-Central region (3%; Alabama, Kentucky, Mississippi, Tennessee). Almost half of the respondent institutions offering CAM were academic medical centers, or teaching hospitals, and 72% were urban. The most commonly offered inpatient CAM therapies included pet therapy, massage therapy, music therapy, guided imagery and relaxation training, and Reiki or therapeutic touch. Outpatient modalities were most commonly massage therapy, acupuncture, guided imagery, meditation, relaxation and biofeedback [12].

Despite growing interest and demand for an integrative approach in healthcare, acceptance and adoption of these modalities into mainstream healthcare systems remains limited, and thus inaccessible for many patients and families. Contributing factors to this lack of access include inadequate numbers of trained practitioners, lack of insurance reimbursement for interventions, billing or productivity structures which do not support the time needed to do significant patient counseling and education, and other financial or ideological limitations of healthcare institutions and individual providers alike [13,14]. Medical education at all levels remains limited in training physicians with integrative medicine tools and non-pharmacologic alternatives to symptom management or disease treatment and modification. There are, however, increasing efforts among some medical schools to incorporate lifestyle medicine curricula [15], an integrative medicine elective, or some exposure to CAM therapies in their curriculum. According to the Association of American Medical Colleges, 43% of medical schools offered CAM in their curricula as of 2010. In addition, a survey of University of California medical students' perceptions about CAM, 75% felt that "western medicine would benefit from incorporation of CAM therapies and ideas" [11]. At the Graduate Medical Education level, programs such as Integrative Medicine in Residency (IMR), an online curriculum, is now utilized in 63 residency programs nationally and internationally at the time of this writing [16]. In 2014 the American Board of Physician Specialties began offering a national integrative medicine board exam, for physicians who have completed a two-year fellowship in integrative medicine [17], adding further recognition and standardization to the field of integrative medicine.

One common example of a complex, multi-faceted problem seen from primary care to palliative care is anxiety. Children and teens are experiencing anxiety at unprecedented rates, and according to Kessler et al. in a National Comorbidity Survey of adolescents, the lifetime prevalence of any anxiety disorder was 31.9% between the ages of 13–18 years [18], with females (38%) being affected more than males (26%). Although this does not separate adolescents with comorbidities, it is well known that this population group often suffers from anxiety at higher rates [19,20].

Our understanding of anxiety grows by the week, with more studies detailing the connection between gut health and its role in anxiety [21], depression [22,23], pain, obesity, diabetes [24], autoimmune diseases, and the list goes on. Additionally, a history of adverse childhood experiences (ACEs) such as trauma, neglect or abuse predisposes one to an increased risk of developing anxiety over their lifetime [25]. Social media use, sleep deprivation and social isolation have all been associated with higher rates of anxiety [26]. Genetics, diet [27,28], family history and environmental exposures also have significant bearing on an individual's mental health. Given the numerous etiological influences, and individual variation in life experiences and exposures, it is not reasonable to expect that a single drug or treatment would be adequate for such a multidimensional condition.

Numerous studies, as well as centuries of tradition in eastern medicine, support the efficacy of mind-body techniques for management of anxiety, chronic pain, illness and stress. Examples include various types of meditation [29]; hypnosis and self-hypnosis [30,31], mindfulness-based stress reduction (MBSR) [32], and yoga [33]. Despite the evidence-supported efficacy and cost-savings, providers are not routinely trained in these treatments over a pharmaceutical approach. Integrative medicine interventions carry a low risk of harm, making them an attractive adjunct or when appropriate, alternative to pharmaceuticals, which are not without adverse risks. An additional benefit of integrative therapies is the active participation required by the patient in the regulation of their own nervous system or mind when addressing problems, allowing the patient to feel in control. These approaches are highly empowering and without significant cost once the technique has been adequately taught to the patient and family to employ when desired. Integrative medicine combines all appropriate therapies using an evidence-based approach with consideration to safety, tolerability and efficacy. Studies have shown that combining mind-body techniques with pharmacologic interventions can reduce distress. For example, pediatric leukemia patients undergoing painful procedures in a study comparing a combined intervention (CI) with pharmacologic only (PO) demonstrated significant reduction in distress associated with the procedure in the CI arm, compared to the PO group [34].

This example illustrates how complex and multifaceted many of today's medical issues are, and ways in which integrative medicine can address that complexity using a myriad of tools and modalities suited for a variety of settings and preferences. Many such techniques can be employed in the outpatient, inpatient or community health care setting, with little to no cost and are adaptable to a variety of cultures, backgrounds, ages, disease-states and patient preferences.

3. Overview of Integrative Medicine Modalities

Specific domains in which integrative medicine providers offer care, interventions and education for patients may include nutrition, mind-body techniques, regulation of stress physiology, sleep support, therapeutic movement, Reiki and other energy work techniques, use of herbs and supplements, aromatherapy, mental health support and identification/modification of environmental factors contributing to disease. Knowledge of other healing systems, such as traditional Chinese medicine, Ayurveda, naturopathy, chiropractic and homeopathy, allows integrative medicine providers from an allopathic background to appreciate the role these fields play in healing, and appropriately counsel patients seeking care.

We will briefly describe the following common, well-tolerated integrative modalities that can be used to support patients receiving hospice and palliative care: acupuncture/acupressure, relaxation and stress-physiology regulation techniques, essential oils, botanicals and supplements and reiki.

3.1. Acupuncture/Acupressure

Acupuncture is an ancient tradition in which the practitioner inserts thin needles in the body to manipulate specific points. It is a key component of traditional Chinese medicine and is also used for the management of distressing symptoms such as pain and nausea. Acupuncture points can also be stimulated noninvasively with the use of low level lasers or microcurrent. Acupuncture is safe when performed by qualified professionals and is well tolerated by children [35,36]. Acupressure uses firm, steady pressure at these same points. Depending on the location of the acupressure points, and the indications, patients are sometimes able to perform this on themselves. Shonishin is another needleless acupuncture technique that uses pressure and massage along the meridians to influence the flow of energy.

3.2. Relaxation Techniques and Stress-Physiology Regulation

The ancient practices of meditation, yoga, tai chi and qi gong are making their way into western culture, as well as being utilized to address a range of present day health problems. In each of these practices, the activation of the parasympathetic nervous system, through intentional, regulated breathing, has been shown to improve autonomic nervous system balance, heart-rate variability, chronic pain, fibromyalgia, anxiety, depression, post-traumatic stress disorder and promote overall well-being [37–40]. The activation of the parasympathetic nervous system in what has been termed the "relaxation response", as described above, counters the often overactive sympathetic nervous system stress response, triggered by numerous stimuli that occurs during illness, pain and threatening circumstances. The ability for a person to regulate the stress response and elicit the relaxation response is empowering, and often shifts the locus of control for patients during illness, anxiety, pain and especially at the end-of-life. The use of these physiologic principles in healthcare settings includes modalities such as breathing practices, guided imagery, self-hypnosis and progressive muscle relaxation (PMR). All of these practices have the potential to elicit the relaxation response and can be tailored to individual preferences, functional limitations, age, experiences and culture [41].

3.3. Essential Oils

Aromatherapy is the use of aerosolized or inhaled essential oils, the potent extracts of roots, plants or herbs, for therapeutic purposes. Topical application of essential oils diluted in a carrier oil, with or without massage, is also a route by which therapeutic effects may be obtained. The parts of the plant used, the species, and the quality of the extract all bear on the quality of the essential oil and thus its therapeutic effect [42].

Essential oils have been used for centuries in many cultures and have also made their way into western healing practices and alongside allopathic medicine in many places. Examples of these uses will follow, related to specific symptoms commonly encountered in patients who are receiving palliative care services.

3.4. Botanicals and Supplements

For some patients, due to the burden of polypharmacy, additional supplements are not desired. In others, taking supplements may improve symptoms and allow them to feel a greater sense of self-management over their treatment. Supplements can be taken orally, sublingually or absorbed through the skin. It is critical that any health care provider ask patients about their use of supplements and botanicals, with consideration to any possible side effects as well as drug interactions. An extensive treatment of this topic is beyond the scope of this paper; several specific supplements are covered below in the section on symptom management.

3.5. Reiki

Reiki is an ancient healing art which involves the gentle laying on of hands with the intent to connect the universal life-force energy with the person's own innate power to heal. This treatment is individualized, can be empowering to the patient, and generally has no adverse effects or harm.

4. Integrative Medicine for Distressing Symptoms in Critical Illness and Palliative Care

Below we discuss the integrative approach to several common distressing symptoms to those receiving palliative care: nausea and vomiting, pain and neuropathic pain, stress, and dyspnea.

4.1. Nausea and Vomiting

Nausea and/or vomiting are common symptoms that develop in serious illness related to a wide range of disorders and/or the treatments used to address them. Traditional pharmacologic treatments, such as ondansetron and metoclopramide, do not come without side effects and limitations. Integrative therapies have been shown to provide significant relief as both primary and adjunct therapies in the management of nausea/vomiting with few side effects or adverse reactions. Herbal supplements, such as oral ginger, have long been regarded as a natural antiemetic, but its demonstrated effectiveness in scientific studies remains inconclusive. Currently, ginger has been used to address nausea/vomiting related to motion sickness, pregnancy, post-surgical and chemotherapy [43–45]. In a systematic review of randomized control trials studying the efficacy of ginger for post-operative nausea and vomiting, Ernst et al. concluded that ginger was superior to placebo and demonstrated equal effectiveness compared to metoclopramide [46]. There are few trials related to chemotherapy induced nausea and vomiting, a common problem plaguing many pediatric palliative care patients with cancer. Although the availability of literature yields mixed results, some studies have shown statistically significant benefit. One of the largest randomized control trials to date involved 576 patients undergoing chemotherapy cycles demonstrated a significant decrease in nausea when using ginger compared with placebo [47].

Acupuncture and acupressure have also been utilized to address nausea and vomiting. Specific to pediatrics, there is a rising popularity of acupuncture, with now over one-third of pediatric pain treatment programs offering services [48]. Studies have demonstrated many significant benefits for a myriad of systems, with the strongest evidence demonstrated in the post-operative period. For example, a 2015 systematic review of randomized trials utilizing wrist acupuncture for postoperative nausea and vomiting in both children and adults found a significant reduction in symptoms and need for rescue antiemetics compared to sham treatment [49]. Studies involving exclusively pediatric patients remain limited, although a meta-analysis of clinical studies investigating acupuncture for postoperative nausea/vomiting in children following tonsillectomy further supported these findings [50]. Of note, acupuncture has proven to be well tolerated and safe in the pediatric population. One systematic review involving over 140 randomized clinical trials and 12,000 pediatric patients found acupuncture to be safe for when performed by trained practitioners, with over 90% of adverse events being mild [51].

Aromatherapy, via direct application or inhalation, may also provide benefit in the management of nausea and vomiting. For example, the use of peppermint oil has been recognized as an effective treatment for controlling nausea [52]. Other products, such as ginger oil, have also been utilized in aromatherapy application, with the most updated Cochrane review concluding that participants who received aromatherapy may require less antiemetic medications, although the strength of this evidence was lacking [52]. It is important to state that direct application of peppermint oil, specifically products diluted with methanol, to the nares or chest of infants is not recommended due to the documented risk of apnea, laryngeal and bronchial spasms, and acute respiratory distress [53,54].

4.2. Pain

In chronic disease, throughout the continuum of care and at the end-of-life, many patients struggle with uncontrolled pain. The balance between comfort and over sedation can be difficult for caretakers and families. The most common pharmacologic approach to pain management currently relies heavily on opioid medications, which may have unintended side effects. The Support study, which included more than 4000 hospitalized patients at the end-of-life, demonstrated that over 50% of patients suffered from moderate to severe pain in the days before their death [55]. Integrative modalities can be an effective adjunct to traditional pharmacologic approaches to pain.

In recent years, various relaxation techniques in the management of pain have been studied. These include progressive muscle relaxation, guided imagery, and autogenic training, with the goal of inducing one's own natural relaxation response, described above. For example, a meta-analysis of randomized clinical trials utilizing guided imagery for pain control demonstrated a significant reduction in non-musculoskeletal pain in 11 out of 15 trials reviewed [56]. Studies involving pediatric patients remain limited, but the same principles can be extended to this population with adjustments for age and developmental capabilities.

Acupuncture has become increasingly recognized in western medicine for the management of both acute and chronic pain, making it a viable adjunct for patients suffering with pain at the end-of-life. One Cochrane review concluded that acupuncture demonstrated effectiveness as a treatment for pain associated with migraines, headaches, neck pain, arthritis, and low back pain, all of which often plague those in the end-of-life [57]. A majority of research specific to the field of hospice and palliative medicine focuses on cancer patients, with many positive results shown with the use of acupuncture not only in pain relief, but also decreased use of traditional analgesics [58–60]. For example, one case series of 29 cancer patients at the end-of-life with severe pain demonstrated significant relief and discontinuation of injection analgesics (i.e., morphine, hydromorphone, fentanyl) in 62% of patients, and decreased use in an additional 27% [61].

As one of its many benefits, aromatherapy has been used for pain relief, especially when combined with therapeutic massage, and is another modality to be considered in the management of pain, as well as anxiety and stress. A meta-analysis of literature examining the effectiveness of aromatherapy in treating multiple types of pain found a significant positive effect in reducing pain, typically reported on a visual analog scale [62]. Specific to the pediatric population, one study demonstrated a 40% reduction of acetaminophen usage in children recovering from tonsillectomy who were treated with lavender aromatherapy [63]. Although there are no known studies in the pediatric palliative population, given proven benefits in other population groups, further research of the use of aromatherapy should be pursued.

4.3. Neuropathic Pain

Neuropathic pain can be a significant cause of discomfort and distress to those receiving palliative care and at the end-of-life. Neuropathy can result from multiple etiologies, but the mechanism of pain remains the same, with nerve damage and resultant hyperexcitability of peripheral nerves. Traditional therapy modalities for neuropathic pain, such as neuroleptic drugs, antidepressants, and opioids, have variable success and frequent unwanted side effects. Topical capsaicin is a treatment modality that may be considered for neuropathic pain. Produced from chili peppers, capsaicin binds nociceptors in the skin, leading to initial stimulation and release of substance P. Research has shown that repeat applications of capsaicin can deplete substance P, ultimately resulting in nerve desensitization [64]. Several studies have demonstrated symptom relief in comparison to placebo with the use of topical capsaicin, including Mason et al.'s review of randomized, controlled trials examining the use of capsaicin for chronic neuropathic and musculoskeletal pain in adults [65]. In addition, a recent Cochrane review examined the use of high concentration capsaicin (8% capsaicin patch) for treatment of neuropathic pain, finding moderate to substantial pain relief in patients with several types of neuropathic pain. Additional improvements in sleep, fatigue, depression, and quality of life were also demonstrated. The most common adverse effect to be noted is initial burning at the application site, which decreases with continued use [66].

4.4. Stress Response Regulation, Depression, Anxiety and Insomnia

Any clinician caring for a patient who is receiving palliative care must be prepared to address the psychological symptoms common at the end-of-life in addition to the physical ones. Furthermore, the psychological and the physical are physiologically interconnected. Depression and anxiety may plague patients and non-pharmacologic treatments have long been utilized in the management of depression and anxiety.

Mind-body and relaxation techniques, previously detailed for pain relief, have been shown to provide significant relief of depression, anxiety, and stress. A Cochrane meta-analysis of 15 randomized controlled studies of relaxation techniques with patients diagnosed with depression showed improvement compared to no or minimal traditional treatment. It is important to note, the most significant positive outcome was demonstrated when combined with psychological therapies, such as cognitive behavioral therapy [67]. Furthermore, mindfulness meditation has been demonstrated to provide significant improvements in overall mood and well-being, including stress-reduction, anxiety reduction, alleviating depression, and improved sleep cycles [68]. Specific to pediatrics, one study of 13 adolescents suffering from cancer underwent eight weekly meditation sessions (8 of the 13 enrolled). After completion of the course, investigators analyzed differences in overall mood, depression, sleep, and quality-of-life compared to pre-trial participant responses via questionnaire. Those in the treatment group compared to the control group showed a significant improvement in all areas [69].

As noted, aromatherapy and/or massage have also demonstrated benefit in overall well-being, mood, and sleep patterns. A randomized control trial of aromatherapy massage in the hospice setting found statistically significant improvements in sleep scores and depression reduction [70].

Reiki has been shown to have benefits of relaxation, decreased pain perception, anxiety reduction, overall sense of well-being, and quality-of-life in the palliative patient population [71]. Similar to reiki, therapeutic touch has also demonstrated significant benefits [72].

4.5. Dyspnea

Patients often experience shortness of breath, or dyspnea, related to their underlying disease process and this can worsen during the last six months of life and at the end-of-life. Beyond the physical discomfort, dyspnea can also be anxiety-provoking for many patients and caregivers who have to watch their loved ones suffer. Although the most effective management is to modify the underlying etiology, often in the terminally ill this is not possible. Traditional therapies such as opioids, steroids, nebulizers, and supplemental oxygen can be effective, but not always sufficient [73]. Complementary methods and therapies can provide significant relief as an adjunct therapy. For example, Acupuncture and acupressure have proven beneficial in the chronic-obstructive pulmonary disease (COPD) and asthma patient populations. Jobst et al. conducted a single-blind randomized control trial of 24 COPD patients with disabling shortness of breath who underwent 13 sessions of acupuncture over a three-week period compared to sham acupuncture. Patients in the treatment group reported less subjective breathlessness [74]. Although studies remain limited, and more research is needed in the pediatric population, these benefits could be extended to the palliative care population in pediatrics as well.

Below we provide a case illustration to demonstrate how integrative medicine can be used in practice to improve quality of life.

5. Case Illustration

Janey was a 16-year-old who presented to her general practitioner with complaints of abdominal pain and was found to have angiosarcoma of the spleen with metastasis to the liver, spine and portal venous system. She was being raised by her grandparents due to parental substance abuse. Following the diagnosis, she underwent first line therapy with chemotherapy and radiation. Unfortunately, the social disconnection from her peers created by her medical therapies and the psychological distress of her diagnoses led to a mental health crisis that resulted in a suicide attempt by overdose. While Janey recovered medically in the hospital, the Integrative Medicine team was consulted in the hopes that they might offer a more holistic approach to the impacts of cancer on Janey's life.

The integrative medicine practitioner worked intensively with Janey around the use of guided imagery to relieve anxiety and fears related to her diagnosis and uncertain future. Specifically, they chose to focus on scenes in which Janey traveled to Bora Bora, which she had seen in a travel magazine and viewed as the most relaxing location she could imagine. This technique combined with diaphragmatic breathing and aromatherapy was particularly helpful during times of heightened anxiety when waiting for results of imaging studies to evaluate the effectiveness of her ongoing treatment.

Computed tomography (CT) scans early in the second year of her treatment showed progression of the hepatic portion of her cancer. Discussions about the possibility that she may not be cured became more frequent with her medical team. While she proceeded with a new chemotherapy regimen, she also began planning a Make-A-Wish trip to Bora Bora. Planning her trip motivated her to intensify her practice of integrative strategies and she began a daily meditation practice and engaged in biofeedback. With minimal medications, she had excellent symptom management and was able to enjoy the trip and add more depth to her subsequent imagery work.

By the third year of her cancer journey, her tumor was again growing more quickly, and Janey struggled with progressive abdominal pain. She was very reluctant to use opioid pain medications due to fears about addiction raised by her parents' substance abuse histories. She was motivated to maintain as normal a life as possible despite her medical condition and prioritized having a job babysitting for the neighbors' children each afternoon. Her palliative care physician and integrative medicine practitioner worked with her to design a plan involving long- and short-acting pain medications, as well as mind-body practices, to enable her to maintain function, acceptable pain control and still attend to her responsibilities and relationships.

This plan was quite effective for many months before the cancer progressed. At that time, she had processed many of her fears about addiction with psychology support and was able to accept increased medication for pain control when integrative techniques alone could not manage her symptoms. Janey was aware that she was approaching the end of her life and worked with a child life specialist to participate in legacy activities.

Janey spent many weeks planning for a wedding to her longtime boyfriend and utilized her arsenal of imagery, breathing, aromatherapy and techniques learned in biofeedback to minimize medications used during the ceremony and reception. As her liver failure progressed, nausea became a prominent symptom and she sought new strategies for treatment. She found a combination of lorazepam and acupressure wrist bands with peppermint aromatherapy and imagery to be most effective. Near the end of her life, she became minimally wakeful and less able to utilize strategies herself. However, her husband and grandparents were able to perform massage with her lavender essential oil and use home music therapy provided through hospice to keep her relaxed as she died.

Family participation in integrative strategies made loved ones feel empowered to help Janey through the last stage of her life and has provided crucial legacy memories to help them through their grief.

This case illustrates the numerous ways that integrative medicine modalities were employed alongside, and at times in place of, pharmaceutical and conventional treatments, equipping Janey and her family to manage her disease and symptoms. The shared locus of control (both internal and external) concept is also demonstrated in the combination of integrative therapies as well as medication management, which provided Janey with the ability to live out her life in meaningful ways.

6. Summary

Integrative medicine is the multimodal approach to improved quality of life and patient care that respects and builds upon the strengths of the patient in combination with appropriate medical management. In the setting of palliative and end-of-life care an integrative approach can serve to reduce symptom burden and empower patients and their families.

Author Contributions: M.L.B., S.G. and K.S. are primarily responsible for the conception and design of this article. S.G. and K.S. are co- first authors and share the first author position equally. M.L.B. is the senior author. M.L.B., K.S., S.G., and K.C. drafted the text. All authors provided evaluation and revision of the manuscript and have given final approval of the manuscript.

Acknowledgments: Thank you to Janey (name has been changed for patient privacy) and her family for giving permission for her story to be shared as a part of her legacy project.

References

1. Rakel, D. *Integrative Medicine*, 4th ed.; Elsevier: Philadelphia, PA, USA, 2017.
2. Arizona Center for Integrative Medicine. What is IM/IH? Available online: https://integrativemedicine.arizona.edu/about/definition.html (accessed on 3 March 2018).
3. Nazareth, M.; Richards, J.; Javalkar, K.; Haberman, C.; Zhong, Y.; Rak, E.; Jain, N.; Ferris, M.; van Tilburg, M.A. Relating health locus of control to health care use, adherence, and transition readiness among youths with chronic conditions, North Carolina, 2015. *Prev. Chronic Dis.* **2016**, *13*. [CrossRef] [PubMed]
4. Arizona Center for Integrative Medicine. Fellowship in Integrative Medicine. Available online: https://integrativemedicine.arizona.edu/education/fellowship/index.html (accessed on 3 March 2018).
5. Upcoming Integrative Medicine & Health Events. Available online: https://www.imconsortium.org/events/upcoming-conferences/conferences.cfm (accessed on 3 March 2018).
6. AARM. 2018 Annual Conference. Available online: https://restorativemedicine.org/conferences/2018-annual-conference/ (accessed on 3 March 2018).
7. American Collage of Lifestyle Medicine. Bringing Together Medical Professionals Committed to Lifestyle Medicine As a First Treatment Option. Available online: https://www.lifestylemedicine.org/Lifestyle-Medicine-Conference (accessed on 3 March 2018).
8. The Center for Mind-Body Medicine. Teaching Thousands to Heal Millions. Available online: https://cmbm.org/ (accessed on 3 March 2018).
9. Nutrition & Health. Available online: https://nutritionandhealthconf.org/ (accessed on 3 March 2018).
10. National Center for Complementary and Integrative Health. Use of Complementary Health Approaches in the U.S. Available online: https://nccih.nih.gov/research/statistics/NHIS/2012/key-findings (accessed on 25 March 2018).
11. 2010 Survey of Complementary and Alternative Medicine in Hospitals: Summary of Results. Available online: http://www.samueliinstitute.org/File%20Library/Our%20Research/OHE/CAM_Survey_2010_oct6.pdf (accessed on 25 March 2018).

12. Barnes, P.M.; Bloom, B.; Nahin, R.L. Complementary and alternative medicine use among adults and children: United States, 2007. *CDC Natl. Health Stat. Report.* **2008**, *10*, 1–23.
13. Ross, C.L. Integral healthcare: The benefits and challenges of integrating complementary and alternative medicine with a conventional healthcare practice. *Integr. Med. Insights* **2009**, *4*, 13–20. [CrossRef] [PubMed]
14. Willison, K. Integrating complementary and alternative medicine into primary health care in Canada: Barriers and opportunities. *J. Cancer Integr. Med.* **2005**, *3*, 71–74. [CrossRef]
15. The Institute of Lifestyle Medicine. Medical School Education. Available online: http://www.instituteoflifestylemedicine.org/education-2/medical-school-education/ (accessed on 3 March 2018).
16. Integrative Medicine in Residency. Available online: https://integrativemedicine.arizona.edu/education/imr.html#Sites (accessed on 3 March 2018).
17. American Board of Integrative Medicine. Available online: http://www.abpsus.org/integrative-medicine (accessed on 25 March 2018).
18. Kessler, R.C.; Chiu, W.T.; Demler, O.; Merikangas, K.R.; Walters, E.E. Prevalence, severity, and comorbidity of 12-month DSM-IV disorders in the National Comorbidity Survey Replication. *Arch. Gen. Psychiatr.* **2005**, *62*, 617–627. [CrossRef] [PubMed]
19. Angold, A.; Costello, E.J.; Erkanli, A. Comorbidity. *J. Child Psychol. Psychiatr.* **1999**, *40*, 57–87. [CrossRef]
20. Thapar, P.A.; Collishaw, S.; Pine, D.S.; Thapar, A.K. Depression in adolescence. *Lancet* **2012**, *379*, 1056–1067. [CrossRef]
21. Cryan, J.P.; O'Mahoney, S. The microbiome-gut-brain axis: From bowel to behavior. *Neurogastroenterol. Motil.* **2011**, *23*, 187–192. [CrossRef] [PubMed]
22. Deans, E. Microbiome and mental health in the modern environment. *J. Physiol. Anthropol.* **2017**, *36*, 1–4. [CrossRef] [PubMed]
23. Rogers, G.B.; Keating, D.J.; Young, R.L.; Wong, M.L.; Licinio, J.; Wesselingh, S. From gut dysbiosis to altered brain function and mental illness: Mechanisms and pathways. *Mol. Psychiatr.* **2016**, *21*, 738–748. [CrossRef] [PubMed]
24. Cani, P.D.; Osto, M.; Geurts, L.; Everard, A. Involvement of gut microbiota in the development of low-grade inflammation and type 2 diabetes associated with obesity. *Gut Microbes* **2012**, *3*, 279–288. [CrossRef] [PubMed]
25. Karatekin, C. Adverse Childhood Experiences (ACEs), stress and mental health in college students. *Stress Health* **2018**, *34*, 36–45. [CrossRef] [PubMed]
26. O'Keeffe, G.S.; Clarke-Pearson, K.; Council on Communications and Media. The impact of social media on children, adolescents, and families. *Pediatrics* **2011**, *127*, 800–804.
27. Rahe, C.; Unrath, M.; Berger, K. Dietary patterns and the risk of depression in adults: A systematic review of observational studies. *Eur. J. Nutr.* **2014**, *53*, 997–1013. [CrossRef] [PubMed]
28. O'Neil, A.; Quirk, S.E.; Housden, S.; Brennan, S.L.; Williams, L.J.; Pasco, J.A.; Berk, M.; Jacka, F.N. Relationship between diet and mental health in children and adolescents: A systematic review. *Am. J. Public Health* **2014**, *104*, e31–e42. [CrossRef] [PubMed]
29. Goyal, M.; Singh, S.; Sibinga, E.M.S.; Gould, N.F.; Rowland-Seymour, A.; Sharma, R.; Berger, Z.; Sleicher, D.; Maron, D.D.; Shihab, H.M.; et al. Meditation programs for psychological stress and well-being: A systematic review and meta-analysis. *JAMA Intern. Med.* **2014**, *174*, 357–368. [CrossRef] [PubMed]
30. Liossi, C.; Hatira, P. Clinical hypnosis versus cognitive behavioral training for pain management with pediatric cancer patients undergoing bone marrow aspirations. *Int. J. Clin. Exp. Hypn.* **1999**, *47*, 104–116. [CrossRef] [PubMed]
31. Deng, G.; Cassileth, B.R. Integrative oncology: Complementary therapies for pain, anxiety, and mood disturbance. *CA Cancer J. Clin.* **2005**, *55*, 109–116. [CrossRef] [PubMed]
32. Reibel, D.K.; Greeson, J.M.; Brainard, G.C.; Rosenzweig, S. Mindfulness-based stress reduction and health-related quality of life in a heterogeneous patient population. *Gen. Hosp. Psychiatr.* **2001**, *23*, 183–192. [CrossRef]
33. Tilbrook, H.E.; Cox, H.; Hewitt, C.E.; Kang'ombe, A.R.; Chuang, L.; Jayakody, S.; Aplin, J.D.; Semlyen, A.; Trewhela, A.; Watt, I.; et al. Yoga for chronic low back pain: A randomized trial. *Ann. Intern. Med.* **2011**, *155*, 569–578. [CrossRef] [PubMed]
34. Kazak, A.; Penati, B.; Brophy, P.; Himelstein, B. Pharmacologic and psychologic interventions for procedural pain. *Pediatrics* **1998**, *102*, 59–66. [CrossRef] [PubMed]

35. Brown, M.L.; Rojas, E.; Gouda, S. A mind–body approach to pediatric pain management. *Children* **2017**, *4*, 50. [CrossRef] [PubMed]
36. Jindal, V.; Ge, A.; Mansky, P.J. Safety and efficacy of acupuncture in children a review of the evidence. *J. Pediatr. Hematol. Oncol.* **2008**, *30*, 431–442. [CrossRef] [PubMed]
37. Vohra, S.; McClafferty, H.; Becker, D.; Bethell, C.; Culbert, T.; King-Jones, S.; Rosen, L.; Sibinga, E.; Bailey, M.; Weydert, J.; et al. Mind-body therapies in children and youth. *Pediatrics* **2016**, *138*, 1896. [CrossRef]
38. Pittig, A.; Arch, J.J.; Lam, C.W.; Craske, M.G. Heart rate and heart rate variability in panic, social anxiety, obsessive-compulsive, and generalized anxiety disorders at baseline and in response to relaxation and hyperventilation. *Int. J. Psychophysiol.* **2013**, *87*, 19–27. [CrossRef] [PubMed]
39. Hassett, A.L.; Radvanski, D.C.; Vaschillo, E.G.; Vaschillo, B.; Sigal, L.H.; Karavidas, M.K.; Buyske, S.; Lehrer, P.M. A pilot study of the efficacy of heart rate variability (HRV) biofeedback in patients with fibromyalgia. *Appl. Psychophysiol. Biofeedback* **2007**, *32*, 1–10. [CrossRef] [PubMed]
40. Karavidas, M.K.; Lehrer, P.M.; Vaschillo, E.; Vaschillo, B.; Marin, H.; Buyske, S.; Malinovsky, I.; Radvanski, D.; Hassett, A. Preliminary results of an open label study of heart rate variability biofeedback for the treatment of major depression. *Appl. Psychophysiol. Biofeedback* **2007**, *32*, 19–30. [CrossRef] [PubMed]
41. Lazar, S.W.; Bush, G.; Gollub, R.L.; Fricchione, G.L.; Khalsa, G.; Benson, H. Functional brain mapping of the relaxation response and meditation. *Neuroreport* **2000**, *11*, 1581–1585. [CrossRef] [PubMed]
42. American Cancer Society Aromatherapy. *American Cancer Society Complete Guide to Complementary and Alternative Cancer Therapies*, 2nd ed.; American Cancer Society: Atlanta, GA, USA, 2009; pp. 57–60. ISBN 978-0-944235-71-3.
43. Bode, A.M.; Dong, Z. The amazing and mighty ginger. In *Herbal Medicine: Biomolecular and Clinical Aspects*, 2nd ed.; Benzie, I.F.F., Wachtel-Galor, S., Eds.; CRC Press/Taylor & Francis: Boca Raton, FL, USA, 2011.
44. Dupuis, L.L.; Nathan, P.C. Options for the prevention and management of acute chemotherapy-induced nausea and vomiting in children. *Paediatric Drugs* **2003**, *5*, 597–613. [CrossRef] [PubMed]
45. Quimby, E.L. The use of herbal therapies in pediatric oncology patients: Treating symptoms of cancer and side effects of standard therapies. *J. Pediatr. Oncol. Nurs.* **2007**, *24*, 35–40. [CrossRef] [PubMed]
46. Ernst, E.; Pittler, M.H. Efficacy of ginger for nausea and vomiting: A systematic review of randomized clinical trials. *Br. J. Anaesth.* **2000**, *84*, 367–371. [CrossRef] [PubMed]
47. Ryan, L.J.; Heckler, C.E.; Roscoe, J.A.; Dakhil, S.R.; Kirshner, J.; Flynn, P.J.; Hickok, J.T.; Morrow, G.R. Ginger (*Zingiber officinale*) Reduces Acute Chemotherapy-Induced Nausea: A URCC CCOP Study of 576 Patients. *Support. Care Cancer* **2012**, *20*, 1479–1489. [CrossRef] [PubMed]
48. Lin, Y.C.; Lee, A.C.; Kemper, K.J.; Berde, C.B. Use of complementary and alternative medicine in pediatric pain management service: A survey. *Pain Med.* **2005**, *6*, 452–458. [CrossRef] [PubMed]
49. Lee, A.; Chan, S.K.; Fan, L.T. Stimulation of the wrist acupuncture point PC6 for preventing postoperative nausea and vomiting. *Cochrane Database Syst. Rev.* **2015**, *2*, CD003281. [CrossRef] [PubMed]
50. Shin, H.C.; Kim, J.S.; Lee, S.K.; Kwon, S.H.; Kim, M.S.; Lee, E.J.; Yoon, Y.J. The effect of acupuncture on postoperative nausea and vomiting after pediatric tonsillectomy: A meta-analysis and systematic review. *Laryngoscope* **2016**, *126*, 1761–1767. [CrossRef] [PubMed]
51. Adams, D.; Cheng, F.; Jou, H.; Aung, S.; Yasui, Y.; Vohra, S. The safety of pediatric acupuncture: A systematic review. *Pediatrics* **2011**, *128*, e1575–e1587. [CrossRef] [PubMed]
52. Hines, S.; Steels, E.; Chang, A.; Gibbons, K. Aromatherapy for treatment of postoperative nausea and vomiting. *Cochrane Database Syst. Rev.* **2012**, *18*. [CrossRef] [PubMed]
53. Javorka, K.; Tomori, Z.; Zavarska, L. Protective and defensive airway reflexes in premature infants. *Physiol. Bohemoslov.* **1980**, *29*, 29–35. [PubMed]
54. Blake, K.D.; Fertleman, C.R.; Meates, M.A. Dangers of common cold treatments in children. *Lancet* **1993**, *341*. [CrossRef]
55. A controlled trial to improve care for seriously ill hospitalized patients. The study to understand prognoses and preferences for outcomes and risks of treatments (SUPPORT). The SUPPORT principal investigators. *JAMA* **1995**, *274*, 1591–1598.
56. Paul, P.; Lewandowski, W.; Terry, R.; Ernst, E.; Stearns, A. Guided imagery for non-musculoskeletal pain: A systematic review of randomized clinical trials. *J. Pain Symp. Manag.* **2012**, *44*, 95–104.
57. Lee, M.S.; Emst, E. Acupuncture for pain: An overview of Cochrane reviews. *Chin. J. Integr. Med.* **2011**, *17*, 187–189. [CrossRef] [PubMed]

58. Gadsby, J.G.; Franks, A.; Jarvis, P.; Dewhurst, F. Acupuncture like transcutaneous electrical nerve stimulation within palliative care: A pilot study. *Complement. Ther. Med.* **1997**, *5*, 13–18. [CrossRef]
59. Avellanosa, A.M.; West, C.R. Experience with transcutaneous electrical nerve stimulation for relief of intractable pain in cancer patients. *J. Med.* **1982**, *13*, 203–213. [CrossRef]
60. Ostrowski, M.J. Pain control in advanced malignant disease using transcutaneous nerve stimulation. *Br. J. Clin. Pract.* **1979**, *33*, 157–162. [PubMed]
61. Wen, H.L. Cancer pain treated with acupuncture and electrical stimulation. *Mod. Med. Asia* **1977**, *13*, 12–16.
62. Lakhan, E.S.; Sheafer, H.; Tepper, D. The effectiveness of aromatherapy in reducing pain: A systematic review and meta-analysis. *Pain Res. Treat.* **2016**. [CrossRef] [PubMed]
63. Rasool, S.; Soheilipour, S.; Hajhashemi, V.; Asghari, G.; Bagheri, M.; Molavi, M. Evaluation of the effect of aromatherapy with lavender essential oil on post-tonsillectomy pain in pediatric patients: A randomized controlled trial. *Int. J. Pediatr. Otorhinolaryngol.* **2013**, *77*, 1579–1581.
64. Rains, C.; Bryson, H.M. Topical capsaicin. A review of its pharmacological properties and therapeutic potential in post-herpetic neuralgia, diabetic neuropathy and osteoarthritis. *Drugs Aging* **1995**, *7*, 317–328. [CrossRef] [PubMed]
65. Mason, L.; Moore, R.A.; Derry, S.; Edwards, J.E.; McQuay, H.J. Systematic review of topical capsaicin for the treatment of chronic pain. *BMJ* **2004**, *328*. [CrossRef] [PubMed]
66. Derry, S.; Sven-Rice, A.; Cole, P.; Tan, T.; Moore, R.A. Topical capsaicin (high concentration) for chronic neuropathic pain in adults. *Cochrane Database Syst. Rev.* **2013**, *28*. [CrossRef]
67. Jorm, F.A.; Morgan, A.J.; Hetrick, S.E. Relaxation for depression. *Cochrane Database Syst. Rev.* **2008**, *4*. [CrossRef] [PubMed]
68. Latorraca, C.O.C.; Martimbianco, A.L.C.; Pachito, D.V.; Pacheco, R.L.; Riera, R. Mindfulness for palliative care patients. Systematic review. *Int. J. Clin. Pract.* **2017**, *71*. [CrossRef] [PubMed]
69. Malboeuf-Hurtubise, C.; Achille, M.; Muise, L.; Beauregard-Lacroix, R.; Vadnais, M.; Lacourse, É. A mindfulness-based meditation pilot study: Lessons learned on acceptability and feasibility in adolescents with cancer. *J. Child Fam. Stud.* **2015**, *25*, 1168–1177. [CrossRef]
70. Soden, K.; Vincent, K.; Craske, S.; Lucas, C.; Ashley, S. A randomized controlled trial of aromatherapy massage in a hospice setting. *Palliat. Med.* **2004**, *18*, 87–92. [CrossRef] [PubMed]
71. Burden, B.; Herron-Marx, S.; Clifford, C. The increasing use of reiki as a complementary therapy in specialist palliative care. *Int. J. Palliat. Nurs.* **2005**, *11*, 248–253. [CrossRef] [PubMed]
72. Tabatabaee, A.; Tafreshi, M.Z.; Rassouli, M.; Aledavood, S.A.; AlaviMajd, H.; Farahmand, S.K. Effect of therapeutic touch in patients with cancer: A literature review. *Med. Arch.* **2016**, *70*. [CrossRef] [PubMed]
73. Rome, R.B.; Hillary, H.L.; Deborah, A.B.; Christopher, M.B. The role of palliative care at the end of life. *Ochsner J.* **2011**, *11*, 348–352. [PubMed]
74. Jobst, K.; Chen, J.H.; McPherson, K.; Arrowsmith, J.; Brown, V.; Efthimiou, J.; Fletcher, H.J.; Maciocia, G.; Mole, P.; Shifrin, K.; et al. Controlled trial of acupuncture for disabling breathlessness. *Lancet* **1986**, *2*, 1416–1419. [CrossRef]

4

A Mind–Body Approach to Pediatric Pain Management

Melanie L. Brown [1,2,*], Enrique Rojas [1] and Suzanne Gouda [1]

1 Department of Pediatrics, The University of Chicago, Chicago, IL 60637, USA
erojas@peds.bsd.uchicago.edu (E.R.); Suzanne.Gouda@uchospitals.edu (S.G.)

2 Department of Pain, Palliative Care and Integrative Medicine, Children's Hospitals and Clinics of Minnesota, Minneapolis, MN 55404, USA

* Correspondence: melanie.brown@childrensmn.org

Abstract: Pain is a significant public health problem that affects all populations and has significant financial, physical and psychological impact. Opioid medications, once the mainstay of pain therapy across the spectrum, can be associated with significant morbidity and mortality. Centers for Disease and Control (CDC) guidelines recommend that non-opioid pain medications are preferred for chronic pain outside of certain indications (cancer, palliative and end of life care). Mindfulness, hypnosis, acupuncture and yoga are four examples of mind–body techniques that are often used in the adult population for pain and symptom management. In addition to providing significant pain relief, several studies have reported reduced use of opioid medications when mind–body therapies are implemented. Mind–body medicine is another approach that can be used in children with both acute and chronic pain to improve pain management and quality of life.

Keywords: mind–body medicine; pain management; pediatrics; acupuncture; yoga; meditation; hypnosis

---

1. Introduction

Pain is a significant public health problem leading to lost days of school and increased use of the healthcare system. Pain affects all populations and can significantly impact quality of life [1]. Over 11 million children have special health care needs and about 60% of them have difficulty participating in any activity [2]. In one cross-sectional study of pain prevalence in a pediatric hospital, the authors found that out of 241 patients, 27% had pain at the time of admission and 77% experienced pain at some point during their admission; what is more, pain medication was found to be single-agent and administered irregularly [3].

In recent years, opioid diversion, as well as the overuse and over prescription of opioid medications, have come to the forefront as a significant public health concern. Integrative medicine uses a patient centered approach to combine conventional medicine with evidence-based complementary approaches. Integrative therapies such as mind–body medicine can provide a non-opioid and nontoxic approach to pain management across the spectrum. Even in the case of end-of-life care [4,5], integrative and mind–body therapies are recommended [4,5]. For example, the Hospice and Palliative Nurses Association's most recent position statement supports and encourages the competent practice of complementary therapies for the purpose of promoting holistic end-of-life-care.

2. The Problem

2.1. What Is Pain

Pain can be defined as an unpleasant sensation. In some cases, pain is a warning sign of actual or potential tissue damage. However, dysregulation of the nervous system can also lead to a pain sensation when there is no present danger [6,7]. In addition to the physical sensation, pain behaviors are also influenced by pain perception. In a recent randomized control trial, pain sensitivity was assessed in over 700 adult patients with major depression. It was found that those suffering from major depression had higher pain sensitivity even after adjusting for factors such as poor sleep and physical inactivity [8]. Severity of anxiety also predicted decreased pain threshold.

Chronic pain is known to be associated with changes in not only brain function, but also in brain structure. In 2013, researchers demonstrated that the brain areas that were activated in acute low back pain for example were limited to regions involving acute pain; in the chronic pain group, activity was found in the emotion-related circuitry of the brain [9].

Pain perception and experience in the pediatric population is complex and multi-faceted, including but not limited to the nidus of pain itself, the fear of pain, previously developed pain memories, and familial influence. Acute pain is usually classified as pain lasting less than three months with a sudden onset that is often related to tissue damage. When considering the development of chronic pain in pediatrics, typically defined as pain persisting beyond three months or beyond the expected duration of healing, a fear-avoidance response can emerge, leading to a self-fulfilling cycle made up of pain, emotional distress, and functional disability [10]. In pediatrics, there is also an added complexity when considering developmental stage and parental influence. Not only do parents often have to serve as the surrogate communicator for the patient, parents own magnification, rumination, and anxiety surrounding pain influences the child and vice versa, leading to increased pain sensitivity and fear-avoidance behaviors [11]. It is clear that pain is not as simple as a noxious stimulus to an extremity that sends a danger signal to the brain.

2.2. The Opioid Crisis

Increases in opioid prescriptions have been noted over the past decade [12–14]. The opioid overdose and death rates have also been noted to increase [15–20]. 2016 Centers for Disease and Control (CDC) guidelines state that that non-opioid therapy is preferred for chronic pain outside of active cancer, palliative and end-of-life care in patients over the age of 18 years. Inappropriate medication use and dosing can lead to death and disability [15–20]. At times, significant morbidity can result even when recommended dosage ranges are used [15–20]. For example, deaths have been described with the use of codeine despite dosages prescribed in the recommended range. In the case of codeine, the prodrug must be converted into morphine in the liver via the cytochrome P450 2D6 system and drug over or under conversion may be the result of genetic variation [21]. Furthermore, tolerance, withdrawal, and dependence present a problem even in the pediatric population and the neuropsychological effects of opioids may also be a cause for concern [22–25]. Opioid medications can play an important role in the treatment of pain; however, a pain management plan is not complete without including mind–body therapies.

2.3. Pain in Pediatrics

In pediatrics, pain, both acute and chronic, is often under-recognized and under-treated [26]. Studies have shown that up to 40% of children experience pain at least weekly, and conservative estimates say chronic pain affects 20% to 35% of children and adolescents around the globe [27]. Despite this significant prevalence, pain often goes under-addressed. A large-scale study involving eight pediatric hospitals observed inadequate pain assessment and management for patients undergoing painful procedures, reporting that less than one-third of patients had documentation of one or more pain management interventions [28]. When pain becomes chronic, significant physical and psychological tolls are experienced by both the patient and their families. Often the pain itself continues into adulthood, with 17% of adult chronic pain patients reporting a history of chronic pain in childhood/adolescence [29]. In addition, patients with chronic pain are at increased risk for several comorbidities, including many psychiatric disorders, hyperactivity disorders, social disability, and educational/occupational disability [10]. This patient population also has increased use of medical services, with healthcare costs for children with moderate to severe chronic pain averaging 19.5 billion annually [30]. Despite approximately 1.7 million children affected by chronic pain in the US alone with approximately 20% of cases having developed from acute post-operative pain, assessment and management of pain in pediatrics continues to be a challenge [26,31]. Mind–body medicine can provide a different approach. The mind–body approach is one in which the strengths of the patient and family are considered. In addition, this approach focuses on designing a treatment plan that is efficacious and minimizes the need for opioid medications. Mind–body remains a relatively novel approach in medicine. Although most of the current literature focuses on adult populations and on the more conventional psychological therapies (e.g.; cognitive behavioral therapy and dialectical behavioral therapy) that share similar inherent characteristics with mind–body approaches [32–34], there is a growing body of evidence that supports other mind–body therapies as effective and practical treatment approaches in pediatrics [35–39], particularly in the symptomatic treatment of cancer [4,40–45].

3. The Mind–Body Approach to Pain

3.1. The Use of Mind–Body Medicine in Pain Management

The American Academy of Pediatrics' clinical report on Mind–Body Therapies in Children and Youth describes mind–body therapies as those that focus on the interaction between the mind and the body, with the intent to use the mind to influence physical functions and directly affect health [46]. Mind–body therapies show promise as adjunct and at times primary treatment for pain in children and adults, and can be used across the spectrum. For example, diaphragmatic breathing stimulates the vagus nerve and promotes the relaxation response. The vagus nerve, an essential component of the autonomic nervous system, affects many of the body's internal organs including: the heart, lungs, liver, spleen, kidneys and gastrointestinal tract. As with many therapies, a development-based approach is essential. Teens can use complex imagery, while younger children can be taught diaphragmatic breathing techniques with simple imagery, such as blowing a balloon or blowing out candles. A toddler can be encouraged to engage in diaphragmatic breathing with the use of bubbles or pin wheels. For infants or children with severe cognitive disabilities, rocking and rhythmic womb or heartbeat sounds are techniques that can encourage diaphragmatic breathing.

These techniques are well tolerated in children [36,44,47,48] and can be used in a developmentally appropriate manner to serve as adjunct or primary pain management [47,48]. Furthermore, a reduction in opioid use may be seen. One study demonstrated a greater than 60% reduction of opioid-like medication usage following routine surgery when acupuncture was used [49–51]. Although more research is needed in the pediatric population, given the low risk and low cost of many of these techniques [52–54] for patients and potentially for insurance companies as well, their use is encouraged to enhance symptom management whenever feasible. In the next section, we give an overview of selected mind–body therapies and their function and applications in the management of pain in the pediatric population.

3.2. Selected Mind–Body Approaches

3.2.1. Meditation and Mindfulness

Over the past few decades, mindfulness has emerged as a fundamental component of numerous therapies and interventions for a wide spectrum of clinical aliments [55]. Mindfulness, described as "the awareness that emerges through paying attention on purpose, in the present moment, and non-judgmentally to the unfolding of experience moment by moment", is a meditation practice with ancient Buddhist origins that focuses on experiencing the present moment unobstructed by bias or judgmental thinking in an effort to improve cognitive and emotional well-being [56]. One such application of mindfulness is Kabat Zinn's Mindfulness-Based Stress Reduction (MBSR), a group intervention first introduced in 1990 that focuses on mindfulness meditation training as a complimentary therapy to the standard medical treatment of chronic pain and illness [57–64]. Research has suggested that mindfulness can improve symptoms associated with medical illnesses and increase quality of life [65]. From a neuroscientific perspective, magnetic resonance imaging (MRI) and functional magnetic resonance imaging (fMRI) studies have been conducted in hopes of identifying the neural mechanisms that are responsible for the efficacy of mindfulness meditation in pain relief [66–73]. In one study, thirteen skilled Zen mediators, each having had a minimum of 1000 hours of meditation experience, were recruited and experimentally exposed to pain via thermal stimuli while in an MRI [70]. During exposure to pain, the meditators exhibited increased brain activation in the insula, thalamus, and midcingulate cortex; areas associated with the sensory aspect of pain. Additionally, decreases in brain activity were observed within the hippocampus, amygdala, and caudate; areas responsible for the recollection, emotion, and appraisal components of pain, respectively. The authors concluded that the participants were completely aware of the sensation of pain but were able to inhibit the appraisal and emotional responses of pain. In other words, changes in the perception of pain were facilitated through the cognitive and affective components of the pain matrix rather than through the sensory properties of pain. Furthermore, the differences in brain activity were found to be inversely proportional to meditation skill level, establishing a correlation that supports the authors' hypothesis in regards to meditation's therapeutic effect on pain. As for neurophysiological findings, structural MRI results overlapped with the fMRI results: meditators were found to have thicker grey-matter in the same pain-related regions of the brain where changes in functional activity were observed [66,68,69].

In terms of overall clinical outcome research, controlled trials of adults suffering from various forms of chronic pain (chronic low back pain, chronic headache/migraine, chronic neck pain, arthritis, cancer, and fibromyalgia) have indeed demonstrated improved pain ratings in regards to multiple dimensions of pain including intensity, acceptance, functional limitations, quality of life, and psychological well-being [62]. Nonetheless, mindfulness as it relates to pain in children has not been extensively studied and although mindfulness meditation has shown to be beneficial in classroom and school settings for improving psychological distress [74–77], more research is required in order to determine whether the same effects can be translated in children and pediatric medicine.

3.2.2. Hypnosis

Hypnosis as a form of therapy has a long history and has been widely used across various disciplines of health care. While the current research establishes hypnosis as a beneficial treatment for the management of pain in regards to both acute medical conditions, such as trauma and post-operative care, and chronic medical conditions, such as cancer and sickle cell anemia [78–80]; it is only since the 1980s that it has been meaningfully applied to pediatric care [81,82].

In general, hypnosis includes three phases: induction, suggestion, and emergence [82]. During induction, the provider encourages patient relaxation by asking them to imagine a calm and serene setting on which they can focus all of their attention. Next, the patient is given therapeutic suggestions to achieve the desired effect. Lastly, the patient is asked to leave their imagined setting and to return to normal consciousness. Hypnosis for pain management follows this same protocol with a focus on suggestions that either turn down or decrease pain perception or increase pain thresholds [83].

Given the significance of the suggestion stage of hypnosis, an important factor in clinical outcomes is the degree to which an individual is responsive or susceptible to hypnotic suggestions—a trait that is often referred to as hypnotizability. Of note, studies that have attempted to measure hypnotizability among children via the Children's Hypnotic Susceptibility Scale and the Stanford Hypnotic Scale for Children have shown a positive correlation between hypnotizability [84,85] and age, thus suggesting that hypnosis may be an especially viable form of therapy for pain management in the pediatric population [82].

Taking a neuroscientific approach, neuro-imaging studies have attempted to measure the effects of hypnosis on the neuroanatomy and the neuro-cognitive functions of the brain in the context of pain [85–88]. In other words, many researchers have set out to investigate how hypnosis affects the brain's neural-networks and physiology that in turn, are responsible for the perception of pain within an individual. This "pain matrix", as it has been described, is comprised of specific areas of the brain that collectively produce the experience of pain. In the simplest summary of the current literature, the components of the pain matrix include: the prefrontal cortex, frontal lobes, anterior cingulate cortex, primary and secondary somatosensory cortices, thalamus and insula. The cerebellum, though not technically a component of the pain matrix, also plays a role. Using fMRIs to measure brain activity during hypnosis, researchers have concluded that by influencing activity in the various components of the pain matrix, hypnosis is indeed able to have a collective therapeutic effect on pain.

Research focusing on clinical and experimental outcomes has also yielded positive results. A meta-analysis performed in 2000 of 18 studies found hypnosis to have a moderate to large analgesic effect [78]. When compared to groups receiving standard treatment and groups receiving no treatment, 75% of participants receiving hypnotic suggestion experienced a greater analgesic effect. Furthermore, the effect was seen with both clinical and experimental pain with no significant difference between the two settings.

Hypnosis is a tool that carries minimal risk when used appropriately for pain management. It can be used by patients as well as practitioners. The goal is often to instruct the patient on the hypnotic technique so that hypnosis will become a tool of empowerment that the patient is able to use themselves at appropriate times for symptom management. It is important to note that hypnosis should only be performed by an appropriately trained practitioner and only to treat conditions that the practitioner is competent to treat.

3.2.3. Yoga

Yoga is another mind–body modality that should be considered in the management of pain. In brief, the ancient practice of yoga aims to unite the mind, body, and spirit through different isometric exercises, body poses, and mindful breathing. The goal is to optimize body functioning and reconditioning, skeletal realignment, and blood/lymph flow to the tissues [89]. Beyond the biophysical benefits, yoga is also inexpensive, can be practiced by people of any age and physical skill level, and can be performed almost anywhere. The side effects are minimal, with the most common being musculoskeletal injury, often resulting from inappropriate supervision and/or technique [90].

Growing research has shown yoga to be an effective therapy for chronic pain among adults, but studies remain limited for the pediatric population [91]. In a 2006 meta-analysis, when yoga was incorporated into school curricula, improvements in academic performance, behavior, concentration, emotional balance, and self-esteem were all seen [92]. Regular practice of yoga has been associated with improvement in mood and function in patients suffering from depression [93].

These same techniques can be of great benefit in the management of chronic pain in particular. One pilot study of a yoga program in pediatric patients with Irritable Bowel Syndrome (IBS) and functional abdominal pain, demonstrated significant decreases in pain frequency and intensity, as well as improved quality of life per parents report [94]. A study of 30 children, aged 11–18, with amplified pain syndromes enrolled in an intensive interdisciplinary pain rehabilitation program incorporating 5–6 h of yoga weekly demonstrated improved pain and functioning without the use of pharmacology therapy [95]. Positive effects have also been shown in pediatric patients with rheumatoid arthritis [96]. Current evidence is encouraging, but more large-scale research is still needed to determine the efficacy of yoga in the treatment of pediatric chronic pain [39].

3.2.4. Acupuncture

Acupuncture has been a focus of Traditional Chinese Medicine (TCM) for thousands of years and since its introduction into western medicine, it has become one of the most popular complementary and alternative medical (CAM) therapies in the US [97]. First acknowledged as a medical therapy by the National Institute of Health (NIH) in 1997, the number of licensed acupuncturists in the US has grown exponentially over the decades with over 27,000 licensed acupuncturists in 2013—a one hundred percent increase from 2000—and an estimated one million annual American consumers. In 2001, Battlefield Acupuncture, an auricular acupuncture procedure, was developed by Richard Niemtzow as a simple and effective method for rapid pain relief that can be performed with minimal training by non-licensed acupuncturists [98–100]. Since then, it has since been utilized in emergency rooms and has been taught to US military and North Atlantic Treaty Organization (NATO) personnel for use in both medical and battlefield environments [99,101].

Research into the efficacy of the therapy has also increased over the years with many studies demonstrating acupuncture to be more effective at treating chronic pain than placebo, standard care, and no care [102–112]. Acupuncture is a viable alternative for the treatment and management of acute and chronic pain across various illnesses [22,103,113–115]. One overview of Cochrane reviews concluded that acupuncture demonstrates effectiveness as a treatment for pain associated with migraines, tension headaches, neck disorders, arthritis, and low back pain [104].

Research studies aiming at understanding the physiological and neurological mechanisms that make acupuncture an effective therapy have produced interesting results that have served as the basis for several potential hypotheses [107,116–129]. Many researchers believe that acupuncture stimulates nerves and muscles located within the acupuncture points and trigger a release of neurochemicals endorphins such as serotonin, oxytocin, and endogenous opioid peptides and therefore result in an analgesic effect [117,123,127]. However, while substantial research has shown acupuncture to be an effective therapy for pain among the adult population, there is limited research on acupuncture in regards to the treatment of pain among pediatric patients. Nonetheless, what little research does exist concludes that acupuncture is an effective and feasible therapy option for pain in pediatric populations [48,103,130–134]. One study in the pediatric intensive care unit (PICU) that used acupuncture for acute post-operative pain in children showed that acupuncture was highly accepted and well tolerated without morbidity. In addition, the majority (70%) of patients and families surveyed believed that acupuncture helped their pain. This particular study used the Japanese form of acupuncture with fine needles for older children and Shonishin (a non-needling technique using special tools) for those who were younger than two years of age [135]. A number of other articles have also shown some perceived pain relief without significant adverse effects due to acupuncture. [136,137]

Though acupuncture is safe when administered by appropriately trained and credentialed practitioners, there are some children who have a fear of needles or for medical reasons such as low platelet count or immunodeficiency that may not be recommended to receive acupuncture. For those patients, other techniques such as Shonishin or acupressure can be employed.

4. Discussion: H.O.P.E, A New Paradigm

The use of mind–body techniques in pediatrics can be a powerful adjunct to empower patients and their families and to give them hope for a brighter future with improved quality of life. In partnership with their physicians, families can begin to uncover what is in their tool box for pain and symptom management. One such framework developed by us is the pneumonic: H.O.P.E. We have used H.O.P.E. with success in clinical practice with families as a strategy for approaching pain management. H.O.P.E. addresses four essential components in the evaluation of pain and of the treatment plan. It is described in more detail below.

- H: **How** has the pain affected you and impacted your quality of life? **How** have they addressed the pain in the past and what therapies have been used?

- O: **Observations** about previous management approaches. What have they **observed**? What worked and what did not? What makes the pain perception worse?
- P: **Plan** for the future, set goals and determine the treatment plan.
- E: **Evaluate** the **efficacy** of the plan and manage **expectations.**

In addition to understanding what pharmacologic, non-pharmacological and integrative options are available; it is also important for all parties involved to discuss goals of care. In fully unpacking the child and family's needs, appropriate recommendations for pain management can be made. Recommendations will be different based on the clinical condition and goals of care.

5. Conclusions

Mind–body medicine provides an important approach to the management of both acute and chronic pain in the pediatric population. There are many modalities that are underutilized in pediatrics including mindfulness, hypnosis, yoga and acupuncture. It is important to note that these can be of significant benefit with minimal risk. Mind–body approaches can be used alongside conventional treatment or in some cases as the primary treatment for pain. Though more research is needed; the mind–body approaches discussed are recommended for patients who have no underlying contraindications. As our understanding of pediatric pain and pain management continues to mature, mind–body medicine is an area that is ripe for future studies and investigations.

Acknowledgments: Special thank you to Brian Steiner for sharing the paper that he published in The Atlantic on treating chronic pain with meditation and for his input during the initial planning of this article.

Author Contributions: M.B. is primarily responsible for the conception and design of this article. M.B.; S.G. and E.R. drafted the text. All authors provided evaluation and revision of the manuscript and have given final approval of the manuscript.

References

1. Goldberg, D.S.; McGee, S.J. Pain as a global public health priority. *BMC Public Health* **2011**, *11*, 770. [CrossRef] [PubMed]
2. National Hospice and Palliative Care Organisation. *NHPCO's Facts and Figures: Hospice Care in America*; National Hospice and Palliative Care Organization: Alexandria, VA, USA, 2015.
3. Taylor, E.M.; Boyer, K.; Campbell, F.A. Pain in hospitalized children: A prospective cross-sectional survey of pain prevalence, intensity, assessment and management in a Canadian pediatric teaching hospital. *Pain Res. Manag.* **2008**, *13*, 25–32. [CrossRef] [PubMed]
4. Carlson, L.E.; Bultz, B.D. Mind-body interventions in oncology. *Curr. Treat. Options Oncol.* **2008**, *9*, 127–134. [CrossRef] [PubMed]
5. Lafferty, W.E.; Downey, L.; McCarty, R.L.; Standish, L.J.; Patrick, D.L. Evaluating CAM treatment at the end of life: A review of clinical trials for massage and meditation. *Complement. Ther. Med.* **2006**, *14*, 100–102. [CrossRef] [PubMed]
6. Elvey, R.L. Physical evaluation of the peripheral nervous system in disorders of pain and dysfunction. *J. Hand Ther.* **1997**, *10*, 122–129. [CrossRef]
7. Woolf, C.J. What is this thing called pain? *J. Clin. Invest.* **2010**, *120*, 3742–3744. [CrossRef] [PubMed]
8. Hermesdorf, M.; Berger, K.; Baune, B.T.; Wellmann, J.; Ruscheweyh, R.; Wersching, H. Pain Sensitivity in Patients With Major Depression: Differential Effect of Pain Sensitivity Measures, Somatic Cofactors, and Disease Characteristics. *J. Pain* **2016**, *17*, 606–616. [CrossRef] [PubMed]
9. Hashmi, J.A.; Baliki, M.N.; Huang, L.; Baria, A.T.; Torbey, S.; Hermann, K.M.; Schnitzer, T.J.; Apkarian, A.V. Shape shifting pain: Chronification of back pain shifts brain representation from nociceptive to emotional circuits. *Brain* **2013**, *136*, 2751–2768. [CrossRef] [PubMed]

10. Asmundson, G.J.; Noel, M.; Petter, M.; Parkerson, H.A. Pediatric fear-avoidance model of chronic pain: Foundation, application and future directions. *Pain Res. Manag.* **2012**, *17*, 397–405. [CrossRef] [PubMed]
11. Friedrichsdorf, S.; Giordano, J.; Dakoji, K.D.; Warmuth, A.; Daughtry, C.; Schulz, C. Chronic Pain in Children and Adolescents: Diagnosis and Treatment of Primary Pain Disorders in Head, Abdomen, Muscles and Joints. *Children* **2016**, *3*, 42. [CrossRef] [PubMed]
12. Dunn, K.M. Opioid prescriptions for chronic pain and overdose: A cohort study. *Ann. Intern. Med.* **2010**, *152*, 85–92. [CrossRef] [PubMed]
13. Kuehn, B.M. Opioid prescriptions soar: Increase in legitimate use as well as abuse. *JAMA* **2007**, *297*, 249–251. [CrossRef] [PubMed]
14. Volkow, N.D.; McLellan, T.A. Characteristics of opioid prescriptions in 2009. *JAMA* **2011**, *305*, 1299–1301. [CrossRef] [PubMed]
15. Bohnert, A.S.; Valenstein, M.; Bair, M.J.; Ganoczy, D.; McCarthy, J.F.; Ilgen, M.A.; Blow, F.C. Association between opioid prescribing patterns and opioid overdose-related deaths. *JAMA* **2011**, *305*, 1315–1321. [CrossRef] [PubMed]
16. McLellan, A.; Turner, B. Prescription opioids, overdose deaths, and physician responsibility. *JAMA* **2008**, *300*, 2672–2673. [CrossRef] [PubMed]
17. International Association for the Study of Pain: Unrelieved Pain Is a Major Global Healthcare Problem. Available online: http://www.iasp-pain.org/AM/Template.cfm?Section=Home&Template=/CM/ContentDisplay.cfm&ContentID=2908 (accessed on 20 June 2017).
18. Okie, S. A flood of opioids, a rising tide of deaths. *N. Engl. J. Med.* **2010**, *363*, 1981–1985. [CrossRef] [PubMed]
19. Dhalla, I.A.; Mamdani, M.M.; Sivilotti, M.L.A.; Kopp, A.; Qureshi, O.; Juurlink, D.N. Prescribing of opioid analgesics and related mortality before and after the introduction of long-acting oxycodone. *CMAJ* **2009**, *181*, 891–896. [CrossRef] [PubMed]
20. Manchikanti, L.; Damron, K.S.; Pampati, V.; Fellows, B. Increasing deaths from opioid analgesics in the United States: An evaluation in an interventional pain management practice. *J. Opioid Manag.* **2008**, *4*, 271–283. [PubMed]
21. Friedrichsdorf, S.J.; Nugent, A.P.; Strobl, A.Q. Codeine-associated pediatric deaths despite using recommended dosing guidelines: Three case reports. *J. Opioid Manag.* **2013**, *9*, 151–155. [CrossRef] [PubMed]
22. Anand, K.J.; Arnold, J.H. Opioid tolerance and dependence in infants and children. *Crit. Care Med.* **1994**, *22*, 334–342. [CrossRef] [PubMed]
23. Anand, K.J.S.; Willson, D.F.; Berger, J.; Harrison, R.; Meert, K.L.; Zimmerman, J.; Carcillo, J.; Newth, C.J.L.; Prodhan, N.P.; Dean, J.M.; et al. Tolerance and withdrawal from prolonged opioid use in critically ill children. *Pediatrics* **2010**, *125*, 1208–1225. [CrossRef] [PubMed]
24. Yaster, M.; Kost-Byerly, S.; Berde, C.; Billet, C. The management of opioid and benzodiazepine dependence in infants, children, and adolescents. *Pediatrics* **1996**, *98*, 135–140. [PubMed]
25. Jain, G.; Mahendra, V.; Singhal, S.; Dzara, K.; Pilla, T.; Manworren, R. Long-term neuropsychological effects of opioid use in children: A descriptive literature review. *Pain Physician* **2014**, *17*, 109–118. [CrossRef] [PubMed]
26. Mathews, L. Pain in children: Neglected, unaddressed and mismanaged. *Indian J. Palliat. Care* **2011**, *17*, S70–S73. [CrossRef] [PubMed]
27. King, S.; Chambers, C.T.; Huguet, A.; MacNevin, R.C.; McGrath, P.J.; Parker, L.; MacDonald, A.J. The epidemiology of chronic pain in children and adolescents revisited: A systematic review. *Pain* **2011**, *152*, 2729–2738. [CrossRef] [PubMed]
28. Stevens, B.J.; Abbott, L.K.; Yamada, J.; Harrison, D.; Stinson, J.; Taddio, A.; Barwick, M.; Latimer, M.; Scott, SD.; Rashotte, J.; et al. Epidemiology and management of painful procedures in children in Canadian hospitals. *CMAJ* **2011**, *183*, 403–410. [CrossRef] [PubMed]
29. Hassett, A.L.; Hilliard, P.E.; Goesling, J.; Clauw, D.J.; Harte, S.E.; Brummett, C.M. Reports of chronic pain in childhood and adolescence among patients at a tertiary care pain clinic. *J. Pain* **2013**, *14*, 1390–1397. [CrossRef] [PubMed]
30. Groenewald, C.B.; Essner, B.S.; Wright, D.; Fesinmeyer, M.D.; Palermo, T.M. The economic costs of chronic pain among a cohort of treatment-seeking adolescents in the United States. *J. Pain* **2014**, *15*, 925–933. [CrossRef] [PubMed]

31. Simons, L.E.; Smith, A.; Ibagon, C.; Coakley, R.; Logan, D.E.; Schechter, N.; Borsook, D.; Hill, J.C. Pediatric Pain Screening Tool: Rapid identification of risk in youth with pain complaints. *Pain* **2015**, *156*, 1511–1518. [CrossRef] [PubMed]
32. Robins, C.J. Zen principles and mindfulness practice in dialectical behavior therapy. *Cogn. Behav. Pract.* **2002**, *9*, 50–57. [CrossRef]
33. McCracken, L.M.; Gauntlett-Gilbert, J.; Vowles, K.E. The role of mindfulness in a contextual cognitive-behavioral analysis of chronic pain-related suffering and disability. *Pain* **2007**, *131*, 63–69. [CrossRef] [PubMed]
34. Morgan, D. Mindfulness-based cognitive therapy for depression: A new approach to preventing relapse. *Psychother. Res.* **2003**, *13*, 123–125. [CrossRef] [PubMed]
35. Ball, T.M.; Shapiro, D.E.; Monheim, C.J.; Weydert, J.A. A pilot study of the use of guided imagery for the treatment of recurrent abdominal pain in children. *Clin. Pediatr.* **2003**, *42*, 527–532. [CrossRef] [PubMed]
36. Burke, C.A. Mindfulness-Based Approaches with Children and Adolescents: A Preliminary Review of Current Research in an Emergent Field. *J. Child. Fam. Stud.* **2009**, *19*, 133–144. [CrossRef]
37. Barnes, P.M.; Bloom, B.; Nahin, R.L. Complementary and alternative medicine use among adults and children: United States, 2007. *Natl. Health Stat. Rep.* **2008**, *10*, 1–23.
38. Gerik, S.M. Pain management in children: Developmental considerations and mind-body therapies. *South. Med. J.* **2005**, *98*, 295–302. [CrossRef] [PubMed]
39. Galantino, M.L.; Galbavy, R.; Quinn, L. Therapeutic effects of yoga for children: A systematic review of the literature. *Pediatr. Phys. Ther.* **2008**, *20*, 66–80. [CrossRef] [PubMed]
40. Post-White, J.; Hawks, R.G. Complementary and Alternative Medicine in Pediatric Oncology. *Semin. Oncol. Nurs.* **2005**, *21*, 107–114. [CrossRef] [PubMed]
41. Zeltzer, L.; LeBaron, S. Hypnosis and nonhypnotic techniques for reduction of pain and anxiety during painful procedures in children and adolescents with cancer. *J. Pediatr.* **1982**, *101*, 1032–1035. [PubMed]
42. Kelly, K.M. Complementary and alternative medical therapies for children with cancer. *Eur. J. Cancer* **2004**, *40*, 2041–2046. [CrossRef] [PubMed]
43. Laengler, A.; Spix, C.; Seifert, G.; Gottschling, S.; Graf, N.; Kaatsch, P. Complementary and alternative treatment methods in children with cancer: A population-based retrospective survey on the prevalence of use in Germany. *Eur. J. Cancer* **2008**, *44*, 2233–2240. [CrossRef] [PubMed]
44. Molassiotis, A.; Cubbin, D. 'Thinking outside the box': Complementary and alternative therapies use in paediatric oncology patients. *Eur. J. Oncol. Nurs.* **2004**, *8*, 50–60. [CrossRef]
45. Favara-Scacco, C.; Smirne, G.; Schilirò, G.; Cataldo, A.D. Art therapy as support for children with leukemia during painful procedures. *Med. Pediatr. Oncol.* **2001**, *36*, 474–480. [CrossRef] [PubMed]
46. Section On Integrative Medicine. Mind-Body Therapies in Children and Youth. *Pediatrics* **2016**, *138*, e20161896.
47. Lee, A.A.; Renee, L. Treatment of children in an acupuncture setting: A survey of clinical observations. *J. Chin. Med.* **2006**, *82*, 21–27.
48. Jindal, V.; Ge, A.; Mansky, P.J. Safety and efficacy of acupuncture in children: A review of the evidence. *J. Pediatr. Hematol. Oncol.* **2008**, *30*, 431–442. [CrossRef] [PubMed]
49. Lin, J.; Lo, M.; Wen, Y.; Hsieh, C.; Tsai, S.; Sun, W. The effect of high and low frequency electroacupuncture in pain after lower abdominal surgery. *Pain* **2002**, *99*, 509–514. [CrossRef]
50. Wang, B.; Tang, J.; White, P.F.; Naruse, R.; Sloninsky, A.; Kariger, R.; Gold, J.; Wender, R.H. Effect of the intensity of transcutaneous acupoint electrical stimulation on the postoperative analgesic requirement. *Anesth. Analg.* **1997**, *85*, 406–413. [CrossRef] [PubMed]
51. Zheng, Z.; Guo, R.J.; Helme, R.D.; Muir, A.; Costa, C.; Xue, C.C. The effect of electroacupuncture on opioid-like medication consumption by chronic pain patients: A pilot randomized controlled clinical trial. *Eur. J. Pain* **2008**, *12*, 671–676. [CrossRef] [PubMed]
52. Friedman, R.; Sobel, D.; Myers, P.; Caudill, M.; Al, E. Behavioral medicine, clinical health psychology, and cost offset. *Health Psychol.* **1995**, *14*, 509–518. [CrossRef] [PubMed]
53. Sobel, D.S. The cost-effectiveness of mind-body medicine interventions. *Prog. Brain Res.* **2000**, *122*, 393–412. [PubMed]
54. Sobel, D.S. MSJAMA: Mind matters, money matters: The cost-effectiveness of mind/body medicine. *JAMA* **2000**, *284*, 1705. [CrossRef] [PubMed]

55. Ludwig, D.S.; Kabat-Zinn, J. Mindfulness in medicine. *JAMA* **2008**, *300*, 1350–1352. [CrossRef] [PubMed]
56. Thera, N. *The Heart of Buddhist Meditation*; Rider Co.: London, UK, 1962.
57. Grossman, P.; Niemann, L.; Schmidt, S.; Walach, H. Mindfulness-based stress reduction and health benefits. *J. Psychosom. Res.* **2004**, *57*, 35–43. [CrossRef]
58. Miller, J.J.; Fletcher, K.; Kabat-Zinn, J. Three-year follow-up and clinical implications of a mindfulness meditation-based stress reduction intervention in the treatment of anxiety disorders. *Gen. Hosp. Psychiatry* **1995**, *17*, 192–200. [CrossRef]
59. Kabat-Zinn, J.; Lipworth, L.; Burney, R. The clinical use of mindfulness meditation for the self-regulation of chronic pain. *J. Behav. Med.* **1985**, *8*, 163–190. [CrossRef] [PubMed]
60. Morone, N.E.; Greco, C.M.; Weiner, D.K. Mindfulness meditation for the treatment of chronic low back pain in older adults: A randomized controlled pilot study. *Pain* **2008**, *134*, 310–319. [CrossRef] [PubMed]
61. Kabat-Zinn, J. An outpatient program in behavioral medicine for chronic pain patients based on the practice of mindfulness meditation: Theoretical considerations and preliminary results. *Gen. Hosp. Psychiatry* **1982**, *4*, 33–47. [CrossRef]
62. Rosenzweig, S.; Greeson, J.M.; Reibel, D.K.; Green, J.S.; Jasser, S.A.; Beasley, D. Mindfulness-based stress reduction for chronic pain conditions: Variation in treatment outcomes and role of home meditation practice. *J. Psychosom. Res.* **2010**, *68*, 29–36. [CrossRef] [PubMed]
63. Kabat-Zinn, J.; Massion, A.O.; Kristeller, J.; Peterson, L.G.; Fletcher, K.E.; Pbert, L.; Lenderking, W.R.; Santorelli, S.F. Effectiveness of a meditation-based stress reduction program in the treatment of anxiety disorders. *Am. J. Psychiatry.* **1992**, *149*, 936–943. [PubMed]
64. Edenfield, T.M.; Saeed, S.A. An update on mindfulness meditation as a self-help treatment for anxiety and depression. *Psychol. Res. Behav. Manag.* **2012**, *5*, 131–141. [CrossRef] [PubMed]
65. Jastrowski Mano, K.E.; Salamon, K.S.; Hainsworth, K.R.; Anderson Khan, K.J.; Ladwig, R.J.; Davies, W.H.; Weisman, S.J. A randomized, controlled pilot study of mindfulness-based stress reduction for pediatric chronic pain. *Altern. Ther. Health Med.* **2013**, *19*, 8–14. [PubMed]
66. Grant, J.A.; Courtemanche, J.; Duerden, E.G.; Duncan, G.H.; Rainville, P. Cortical thickness and pain sensitivity in zen meditators. *Emotion* **2010**, *10*, 43–53. [CrossRef] [PubMed]
67. Hölzel, B.K.; Lazar, S.W.; Gard, T.; Schuman-Olivier, Z.; Vago, D.R.; Ott, U. How does mindfulness meditation work? Proposing mechanisms of action from a conceptual and neural perspective. *Perspect. Psychol. Sci.* **2011**, *6*, 537–559. [CrossRef] [PubMed]
68. Lazar, S.W.; Kerr, C.E.; Wasserman, R.H.; Gray, J.R.; Greve, D.N.; Treadway, M.T.; McGarvey, M.; Quinn, B.T.; Dusek, J.A.; Benson, H.; et al. Meditation experience is associated with increased cortical thickness. *Neuroreport* **2005**, *16*, 1893–1897. [CrossRef] [PubMed]
69. Hölzel, B.K.; Ott, U.; Gard, T.; Hempel, H.; Weygandt, M.; Morgen, K.; Vaitl, D. Investigation of mindfulness meditation practitioners with voxel-based morphometry. *Soc. Cogn. Affect. Neurosci.* **2008**, *3*, 55–61. [CrossRef] [PubMed]
70. Grant, J.A.; Courtemanche, J.; Rainville, P. A non-elaborative mental stance and decoupling of executive and pain-related cortices predicts low pain sensitivity in Zen meditators. *Pain* **2011**, *152*, 150–156. [CrossRef] [PubMed]
71. Grant, J.A.; Rainville, P. Pain sensitivity and analgesic effects of mindful states in Zen meditators: A cross-sectional study. *Psychosom. Med.* **2009**, *71*, 106–114. [CrossRef] [PubMed]
72. Zeidan, F.; Gordon, N.S.; Merchant, J.; Goolkasian, P. The effects of brief mindfulness meditation training on experimentally induced pain. *J. Pain* **2010**, *11*, 199–209. [CrossRef] [PubMed]
73. Zeidan, F.; Grant, J.; Brown, C.; Mchaffie, J.; Coghill, R. Mindfulness meditation-related pain relief: Evidence for unique brain mechanisms in the regulation of pain. *Neurosci. Lett.* **2012**, *520*, 165–173. [CrossRef] [PubMed]
74. Britton, W.B.; Lepp, N.E.; Niles, H.F.; Rocha, T.; Fisher, N.E.; Gold, J.S. A randomized controlled pilot trial of classroom-based mindfulness meditation compared to an active control condition in sixth-grade children. *J. Sch. Psychol.* **2014**, *52*, 263–278. [CrossRef] [PubMed]
75. Sibinga, E.M.; Perry-Parrish, C.; Chung, S.; Johnson, S.B.; Smith, M.; Ellen, J.M. School-based mindfulness instruction for urban male youth: A small randomized controlled trial. *Prev. Med.* **2013**, *57*, 799–801. [CrossRef] [PubMed]

76. Joyce, A.; Etty-Leal, J.; Zazryn, T.; Hamilton, A. Exploring a mindfulness meditation program on the mental health of upper primary children: A pilot study. *Adv. Sch. Ment. Health Prom.* **2010**, *3*, 17–25. [CrossRef]
77. Hooker, K.E.F.; Fodor, I.E. Teaching mindfulness to children. *Gestalt Rev.* **2008**, *12*, 75–91.
78. Montgomery, G.H.; DuHamel, K.N.; Redd, W.H. A meta-analysis of hypnotically induced analgesia: How effective is hypnosis? *Int. J. Clin. Exp. Hypn.* **2000**, *48*, 138–153. [CrossRef] [PubMed]
79. Potié, A.; Roelants, F.; Pospiech, A.; Momeni, M.; Watremez, C. Hypnosis in the Perioperative Management of Breast Cancer Surgery: Clinical Benefits and Potential Implications. *Anesthesiol. Res. Pract.* **2016**, *2016*, 2942416. [CrossRef] [PubMed]
80. Chaves, J.F. Recent advances in the application of hypnosis to pain management. *Am. J. Clin. Hypn.* **1994**, *37*, 117–129. [CrossRef] [PubMed]
81. Kohen, D.P.; Kaiser, P. Clinical hypnosis with children and adolescents—What? Why? How?: Origins, Applications, and Efficacy. *Children* **2014**, *1*, 74–98. [CrossRef] [PubMed]
82. Rogovik, A.L.; Goldman, R.D. Hypnosis for treatment of pain in children. *Can. Fam. Physician* **2007**, *53*, 823–825. [PubMed]
83. Chaves, J.F. Hypnosis in pain management. In *Handbook of Clinical Hypnosis*; Rhue, J.W., Lynn, S.J., Kirsch, I., Eds.; American Psychological Association: Washington, DC, USA, 1993; pp. 511–532.
84. Terhune, D.B.; Cardena, E. Heterogeneity in high hypnotic suggestibility and the neurophysiology of hypnosis. *Neurophysiol. Clin.* **2015**, *45*, 177–178. [CrossRef] [PubMed]
85. Mcgeown, W.J.; Mazzoni, G.; Vannucci, M.; Venneri, A. Structural and functional correlates of hypnotic depth and suggestibility. *Psychiatry Res.* **2015**, *231*, 151–159. [CrossRef] [PubMed]
86. Dillworth, T.; Mendoza, M.E.; Jensen, M.P. Neurophysiology of pain and hypnosis for chronic pain. *Transl. Behav. Med.* **2012**, *2*, 65–72. [CrossRef] [PubMed]
87. Rainville, P.; Hofbauer, R.K.; Paus, T.; Duncan, G.H.; Bushnell, M.C.; Price, D.D. Cerebral mechanisms of hypnotic induction and suggestion. *J. Cogn. Neurosci.* **1999**, *11*, 110–125. [CrossRef] [PubMed]
88. Rainville, P.; Hofbauer, R.K.; Bushnell, M.C.; Duncan, G.H.; Price, D.D. Hypnosis modulates activity in brain structures involved in the regulation of consciousness. *J. Cogn. Neurosci.* **2002**, *14*, 887–901. [CrossRef] [PubMed]
89. Vallath, N. Perspectives on yoga inputs in the management of chronic pain. *Indian J. Palliat. Care* **2010**, *16*, 1–7. [CrossRef] [PubMed]
90. National Center for Complimentary and Integrative Health: Yoga. 2014. Available online: http://nccam.nih.gov/health/yoga (accessed on: 20 June 2017).
91. Nahin, R.L.; Boineau, R.; Khalsa, P.S.; Stussman, B.J.; Weber, W.J. Evidence-based evaluation of complementary health approaches for pain management in the United States. *Mayo Clin. Proc.* **2016**, *91*, 1292–1306. [CrossRef] [PubMed]
92. Kraag, G.; Zeegers, M.P.; Kok, G.; Hosman, C.; Abu-Saad, H.H. School programs targeting stress management in children and adolescents: A meta-analysis. *J. Sch. Psychol.* **2006**, *44*, 449–472. [CrossRef]
93. Woolery, A.; Myers, H.; Sternlieb, B.; Zeltzer, L. A yoga intervention for young adults with elevated symptoms of depression. *Altern. Ther. Health Med.* **2004**, *10*, 60–63. [PubMed]
94. Brands, M.M.; Purperhart, H.; Deckers-Kocken, J.M. A pilot study of yoga treatment in children with functional abdominal pain and irritable bowel syndrome. *Complement. Ther. Med.* **2011**, *19*, 109–114. [CrossRef] [PubMed]
95. Hoffart, C.; Anderson, R.; Wallace, D. A155: Development of an intensive interdisciplinary pediatric pain rehabilitation program: Improving pain, functioning, and psychological outcomes. *Arthritis Rheum.* **2014**, *66*, S201. [CrossRef]
96. Evans, S.; Moieni, M.; Taub, R.; Subramanian, S.K.; Tsao, J.C.; Sternlieb, B.; Zeltzer, L.K. Iyengar yoga for young adults with rheumatoid arthritis: Results from a mixed-methods pilot study. *J. Pain Symptom. Manag.* **2010**, *39*, 904–913. [CrossRef] [PubMed]
97. Lu, D.P.; Lu, G.P. An historical review and perspective on the impact of acupuncture on U.S. medicine and society. *Med. Acupunct.* **2013**, *25*, 311–316. [CrossRef] [PubMed]
98. Niemtzow, R.C. Battlefield Acupuncture. *Med. Acupunct.* **2007**, *19*, 225–228. [CrossRef]
99. Niemtzow, R.C.; Belard, J.L.; Nogier, R. Battlefield Acupuncture in the U.S. Military: A Pain-Reduction Model for NATO. *Med. Acupunct.* **2015**, *27*, 344–348. [CrossRef]

100. Tsai, S.-L.; Misra, S. Auricular Battlefield Acupuncture at the 2016 Pediatric Academic Societies Meeting. *Med. Acupunct.* **2016**, *28*, 173–174. [CrossRef]
101. Tsai, S.; Fox, L.M.; Murakami, M.; Tsung, J.W. Auricular Acupuncture in Emergency Department Treatment of Acute Pain. *Ann. Emerg. Med.* **2016**, *68*, 583–585. [CrossRef] [PubMed]
102. Tsang, P.L. Treatment of chronic pain with acupuncture. *JAMA* **1975**, *232*, 1133–1135. [CrossRef]
103. Golianu, B.; Krane, E.; Seybold, J.; Almgren, C.; Anand, K. Non-pharmacological techniques for pain management in neonates. *Semin. Perinatol.* **2007**, *31*, 318–322. [CrossRef] [PubMed]
104. Lee, M.S.; Ernst, E. Acupuncture for pain: An overview of Cochrane reviews. *Chin. J. Integr. Med.* **2011**, *17*, 187–189. [CrossRef] [PubMed]
105. Manheimer, E.; White, A.; Berman, B.; Forys, K.; Ernst, E. Meta-analysis: Acupuncture for low back pain. *Ann. Intern. Med.* **2005**, *142*, 651–663. [CrossRef] [PubMed]
106. Ezzo, J.; Berman, B.; Hadhazy, V.A.; Jadad, A.R.; Lao, L.; Singh, B.B. Is acupuncture effective for the treatment of chronic pain? A systematic review. *Pain* **2000**, *93*, 198–199. [CrossRef]
107. Andersson, S.; Lundeberg, T. Acupuncture—from empiricism to science: Functional background to acupuncture effects in pain and disease. *Med. Hypotheses* **1995**, *45*, 271–281. [CrossRef]
108. Riet, G.T.; Kleunen, J.; Knipschild, P. Acupuncture and chronic pain: A criteria-based meta-analysis. *J. Clin. Epidemiol.* **1990**, *43*, 1191–1199. [CrossRef]
109. Thomas, M.; Eriksson, S.V.; Lundeberg, T. A comparative study of diazepam and acupuncture in patients with osteoarthritis pain: A placebo controlled study. *Am. J. Chin. Med.* **1991**, *19*, 95–100. [CrossRef] [PubMed]
110. Vickers, A.J.; Linde, K. Acupuncture for chronic pain. *JAMA* **2014**, *311*, 955–956. [CrossRef] [PubMed]
111. Jeanette, C.; Rico, R.C.; Trudnowski, R.J. Acupuncture and pain. *AANA J.* **1976**, *44*, 62–64.
112. Lund, I.; Lundeberg, T. Is acupuncture effective in the treatment of pain in endometriosis? *J. Pain Res.* **2016**, *9*, 157–165. [CrossRef] [PubMed]
113. Dumas, E.O.; Pollack, G.M. Opioid tolerance development: A pharmacokinetic/pharmacodynamic perspective. *AAPS J.* **2008**, *10*, 537. [CrossRef] [PubMed]
114. Han, B.; Compton, W.M.; Jones, C.M.; Cai, R. Nonmedical prescription opioid use and use disorders among adults aged 18 through 64 years in the United States, 2003–2013. *JAMA* **2015**, *314*, 1468–1478. [CrossRef] [PubMed]
115. Freitas, G.R.; Castro, C.G.; Castro, S.M.; Heineck, I. Degree of knowledge of health care professionals about pain management and use of opioids in pediatrics. *Pain Med.* **2014**, *15*, 807–819. [CrossRef] [PubMed]
116. Hui, K.K.; Marina, O.; Liu, J.; Rosen, B.R.; Kwong, K.K. Acupuncture, the limbic system, and the anticorrelated networks of the brain. *Auton. Neurosci.* **2010**, *157*, 81–90. [CrossRef] [PubMed]
117. Han, J.S. Acupuncture and endorphins. *Neurosci. Lett.* **2004**, *361*, 258–261. [CrossRef] [PubMed]
118. Wu, M. Neuronal Specificity of Acupuncture Response: A fMRI Study with Electroacupuncture. *NeuroImage* **2002**, *16*, 1028–1037. [CrossRef] [PubMed]
119. Biella, G.; Sotgiu, M.L.; Pellegata, G.; Paulesu, E.; Castiglioni, I.; Fazio, F. Acupuncture produces central activations in pain regions. *Neuroimage* **2001**, *14*, 60–66. [CrossRef] [PubMed]
120. Napadow, V.; Kettner, N.; Liu, J.; Li, M.; Kwong, K.K.; Vangel, M.; Makris, N.; Audette, J.; Hui, K.K. Hypothalamus and amygdala response to acupuncture stimuli in Carpal Tunnel Syndrome. *Pain* **2007**, *130*, 254–266. [CrossRef] [PubMed]
121. Dhond, R.P.; Yeh, C.; Park, K.; Kettner, N.; & Napadow, V. Acupuncture modulates resting state connectivity in default and sensorimotor brain networks. *Pain* **2008**, *136*, 407–418. [CrossRef] [PubMed]
122. Dhond, R.P.; Kettner, N.; Napadow, V. Do the neural correlates of acupuncture and placebo effects differ? *Pain* **2007**, *128*, 8–12. [CrossRef] [PubMed]
123. Wu, M.T.; Hsieh, J.C.; Xiong, J.; Yang, C.F.; Pan, H.B.; Chen, Y.C.; Tsai, G.; Rosen, B.R.; Kwong, K.K. Central nervous pathway for acupuncture stimulation: Localization of processing with functional MR imaging of the brain–preliminary experience. *Radiology* **1999**, *212*, 133–141. [CrossRef] [PubMed]
124. Carlsson, C. Acupuncture mechanisms for clinically relevant long-term effects—reconsideration and a hypothesis. *Acupunct. Med.* **2002**, *20*, 82–99. [CrossRef] [PubMed]
125. Melzack, R.; Stillwell, D.M.; Fox, E.J. Trigger points and acupuncture points for pain: Correlations and implications. *Pain* **1977**, *3*, 3–23. [CrossRef]

126. Hsieh, J.C.; Tu, C.H.; Chen, F.P.; Chen, M.C.; Yeh, T.C.; Cheng, H.C.; Wu, Y.T.; Liu, R.S.; Ho, L.T. Activation of the hypothalamus characterizes the acupuncture stimulation at the analgesic point in human: A positron emission tomography study. *Neurosci. Lett.* **2001**, *307*, 105–108. [CrossRef]
127. Lundeberg, T.; Stener-Victorin, E. Is there a physiological basis for the use of acupuncture in pain? *Int. Congress Ser.* **2002**, *12*, 3–10. [CrossRef]
128. Zhao, Z.Q. Neural mechanism underlying acupuncture analgesia. *Prog. Neurobiol.* **2008**, *85*, 355–375. [CrossRef] [PubMed]
129. Hui, K.K.; Liu, J.; Makris, N.; Gollub, R.L.; Chen, A.J.; Moore, C.I.; Kennedy, D.N.; Rosen, B.R.; Kwong, K.K. Acupuncture modulates the limbic system and subcortical gray structures of the human brain: Evidence from fMRI studies in normal subjects. *Hum. Brain Mapp.* **2000**, *9*, 13–25. [CrossRef]
130. Adams, D.; Cheng, F.; Jou, H.; Aung, S.; Yasui, Y.; Vohra, S. The safety of pediatric acupuncture: A systematic review. *Pediatrics* **2011**, *128*, e1575–e1587. [CrossRef] [PubMed]
131. Kemper, K.J.; Sarah, R.; Silver-Highfield, E.; Xiarhos, E.; Barnes, L.; Berde, C. On pins and needles? Pediatric pain patients' experience with acupuncture. *Pediatrics* **2000**, *105*, 941–947. [PubMed]
132. Waterhouse, M.W.; Stelling, C.; Powers, M.; Levy, S.; Zeltzer, L.K. Acupuncture and hypnotherapy in the treatment of chronic pain in children. *Clin. Acupunct. Oriental Med.* **2000**, *1*, 139–150. [CrossRef]
133. Zeltzer, L.K.; Tsao, J.C.; Stelling, C.; Powers, M.; Levy, S.; Waterhouse, M. A phase I study on the feasibility and acceptability of an acupuncture/hypnosis intervention for chronic pediatric pain. *J. Pain Symptom. Manag.* **2002**, *24*, 437–446. [CrossRef]
134. Slover, R.; Neuenkirchen, G.L.; Olamikan, S.; Kent, S. Chronic pediatric pain. *Adv. Pediatr.* **2010**, *57*, 141–162. [CrossRef] [PubMed]
135. Wu, S.; Sapru, A.; Stewart, M.A.; Milet, M.J.; Hudes, M.; Livermore, L.F.; Flori, H.R. Using acupuncture for acute pain in hospitalized children. Pediatric critical care medicine. *Pediatr. Crit. Care Med.* **2014**, *10*, 291–296. [CrossRef] [PubMed]
136. Ochi, J.W. Acupuncture instead of codeine for tonsillectomy pain in children. *Int. J. Pediatr. Otorhinolaryngol.* **2013**, *77*, 2058–2062. [CrossRef] [PubMed]
137. Cho, H.K.; Park, I.J.; Jeong, Y.M.; Lee, Y.J.; Hwang, S.H. Can perioperative acupuncture reduce the pain and vomiting experienced after tonsillectomy? A meta-analysis. *Laryngoscope* **2016**, *126*, 608–615. [CrossRef] [PubMed]

5

Multidisciplinary Pain Management for Pediatric Patients with Acute and Chronic Pain: A Foundational Treatment Approach When Prescribing Opioids

Anava A. Wren [1], Alexandra C. Ross [2], Genevieve D'Souza [3], Christina Almgren [3], Amanda Feinstein [3], Amanda Marshall [4] and Brenda Golianu [3,*]

1. Department of Pediatrics, Division of Pediatric Gastroenterology, Hepatology and Nutrition, Stanford University, Palo Alto, CA 94305, USA; awren2@stanford.edu
2. Department of Pediatrics, Child and Adolescent Headache Program, University of California San Francisco, San Francisco, CA 94158, USA; alexandra.ross2@ucsf.edu
3. Department of Anesthesiology Perioperative and Pain Medicine, Stanford University, Palo Alto, CA 94305, USA; gdsouza@stanford.edu (G.D); calmgren@stanfordchildrens.org (C.A.); abfein@stanford.edu (A.F.)
4. Centre for Clinical Brain Sciences, University of Edinburgh, Edinburgh EH16 4SB, UK; a.marshall-15@sms.ed.ac.uk

* Correspondence: bgolianu@stanford.edu

Abstract: Opioid therapy is the cornerstone of treatment for acute procedural and postoperative pain and is regularly prescribed for severe and debilitating chronic pain conditions. Although beneficial for many patients, opioid therapy may have side effects, limited efficacy, and potential negative outcomes. Multidisciplinary pain management treatments incorporating pharmacological and integrative non-pharmacological therapies have been shown to be effective in acute and chronic pain management for pediatric populations. A multidisciplinary approach can also benefit psychological functioning and quality of life, and may have the potential to reduce reliance on opioids. The aims of this paper are to: (1) provide a brief overview of a multidisciplinary pain management approach for pediatric patients with acute and chronic pain, (2) highlight the mechanisms of action and evidence base of commonly utilized integrative non-pharmacological therapies in pediatric multidisciplinary pain management, and (3) explore the opioid sparing effects of multidisciplinary treatment for pediatric pain.

Keywords: multidisciplinary pain management strategies; opioid reduction therapy; non-pharmacological therapy; cognitive behavioral therapy; hypnosis; mindfulness-based stress reduction; acupuncture; pain rehabilitation

---

1. Introduction

Acute and chronic pain are common and often debilitating problems among both pediatric and adult populations according to the Institute of Medicine statement on Relieving Pain in America. The International Association of the Study of Pain (IASP) defines pain as an unpleasant sensory and emotional experience associated with actual or potential tissue damage or described in terms of such damage [1]. Acute pain is the expected physiological response to a noxious chemical, thermal, or mechanical stimulus, and usually accompanies surgery, traumatic injury, tissue damage, or inflammatory processes. It is self-limiting and typically resolves over days to weeks, but it can persist longer as healing occurs [2]. Chronic pain is defined as intractable pain that exists for three or more months despite adequate treatment [1,3].

Opioid therapy is the cornerstone of treatment for acute procedural and postoperative pain in pediatric populations, and is also regularly prescribed for severe and debilitating chronic pain conditions [4]. Despite the benefits of opioids for pain management, opioids have been associated with a range of side effects including respiratory depression, constipation, cognitive dysfunction, and psychiatric comorbidities [5–8]. Persistent opioid use is also associated with physical tolerance, dependence, and addiction [9], as well as heightened pain sensitization [10].

Given the potential for negative outcomes related to opioid use, there have been increased efforts to use multidisciplinary analgesia treatments (i.e., the concurrent use of treatment provided by practitioners from different disciplines) [11]. Combining pharmacological and integrative non-pharmacological therapies, which operate via different modes of action, has been shown to decrease opioid use and related adverse side effects in the perioperative period, as well as improve acute pain symptoms and emotional wellbeing [12]. When acute pain transforms to chronic pain, the consideration of multidisciplinary care may become even more central in facilitating patient comfort, decreasing reliance on opioid therapy, and improving functionality. Of note, in 2016, the CDC published recommended guidelines for prescribing opioids for adults with non-malignant chronic pain in the US stating [13]:

> *"Nonpharmacologic therapy and nonopioid pharmacologic therapy are preferred for chronic pain. Clinicians should consider opioid therapy only if expected benefits for both pain and function are anticipated to outweigh risks to the patient. If opioids are used, they should be combined with nonpharmacologic therapy and nonopioid pharmacologic therapy, as appropriate."*

For patients 18 years and younger, there do not yet exist specific consensus guidelines on prescribing opioids for chronic pain [4,14,15]. Pediatric practitioners are advised to use their best judgment when using opioids after appropriate use of nonopioid alternatives. Opioids are not usually indicated as a first line therapy for primary pain disorders [16]. However, current evidence suggests that opioid prescriptions should not be curtailed for moderately to severely painful conditions [17,18].

Aims

Overall, multidisciplinary treatment is important to consider in the treatment of both acute and chronic pain. The aims of this paper are to: (1) provide a brief overview of a multidisciplinary pain management approach for pediatric patients with acute and chronic pain, (2) highlight the mechanisms of action and evidence base of commonly utilized integrative non-pharmacological therapies in pediatric multidisciplinary pain management, and (3) explore the opioid sparing effects of multidisciplinary treatments for pediatric pain.

This article will discuss the evidence base of several integrative non-pharmacological treatments (cognitive behavioral therapy, mindfulness, medical hypnosis, acupuncture) for the general pediatric practitioner to consider as part of a multidisciplinary treatment plan in the management of complex pain conditions. The therapies discussed were chosen as they are among the most frequently utilized integrative non-pharmacological therapies in pediatric pain clinics [19]. The aim of this review is not to be exhaustive of each integrative non-pharmacological therapy, but rather to provide an overview of the specific therapy, briefly review mechanisms of action as currently understood, and provide relevant research on the topic. While a systematic review of the aforementioned integrative non-pharmacological therapies is outside the scope of this current paper (for several excellent and relevant systematic reviews, please see Fisher et al., 2018 [20] and Kamper et al., 2015 [21]), the overarching goal of this paper is to educate the general pediatric practitioner in evidence-based integrative non-pharmacological therapies included in multidisciplinary pain management to optimize care for youth with acute and chronic pain conditions.

Throughout this paper, we review both pediatric and adult literature. A search was performed using Pubmed, Ovid, Embase, Prospero, Medline, and Cochrane Database on the following topics in both pediatric and adult literature from 2000 to 2018 (see Table 1). Inclusion criteria were: pediatric chronic pain and each of the following: multidisciplinary treatment, cognitive behavioral therapy, mindfulness, hypnosis, acupuncture, and pain rehabilitation. Opioids and opioid reduction therapy were also used as inclusion criteria with each modality. Exclusion criteria were: pediatric procedural pain, acute pediatric pain, pharmacological management of pediatric pain, and regional management of pediatric pain.

Table 1. Search data for pediatric pain articles and selected integrative non-pharmacological therapies (2000–2018).

Modalities	Ovid	Embase	Prospero	Cochrane	Pubmed	Number of Articles Screened	Number of Articles Reviewed
CBT	42	537	2	2	274	48	12
Mindfulness	37	53	2	17	26	45	25
Hypnosis	164	272	1	1	152	28	14
Acupuncture	149	357	2	24	132	32	14
Intensive Rehab	189	164	2	51	87	15	6
Multidisciplinary	324	1232	1	19	546	52	13

CBT = Cognitive Behavioral Therapy.

Regarding article selection criteria, studies were screened and identified by two authors (AW and AR for Cognitive Behavioral Therapy (CBT), mindfulness and hypnosis; CA and GD for multidisciplinary pain management, acupuncture and rehabilitation), and when a consensus could not be reached regarding the inclusion/exclusion of an article in this review BG mediated and made a final decision. The research team prioritized systematic reviews, non-systematic reviews, and randomized controlled studies of these therapies in pediatric pain. Where these were not available, we identified pilot studies in pediatric pain populations to provide the reader with the current state of science and preliminary evidence for a given integrative non-pharmacological therapy. Pediatric pain articles were supplemented with adult articles where systematic reviews were not available, and where studies investigating mechanisms of action were well elucidated in the adult literature and not studied in pediatrics. Of note, adult studies exploring potential mechanisms of action for integrative non-pharmacological therapies are not meant to imply that adult mechanisms are the same as pediatric mechanisms of action, but rather to inform the reader of the current evidence base of this emerging field of research. Due to limitations of space, the use of these interventions to address specific procedural and/or acute pain is not discussed.

2. Multidisciplinary Pain Management Overview

Evidence suggests that multidisciplinary analgesia treatments incorporating nonopioid pharmacological and integrative non-pharmacological therapies can be effective for both acute and chronic pain management, and can improve patients' quality of life and general wellbeing [13,21–24]. Integrative non-pharmacological therapies include modalities such as cognitive behavioral therapy (CBT), mindfulness, medical hypnosis, acupuncture, massage, and music therapy [25]. See Figure 1 for an overview of some elements of multidisciplinary pain management treatment.

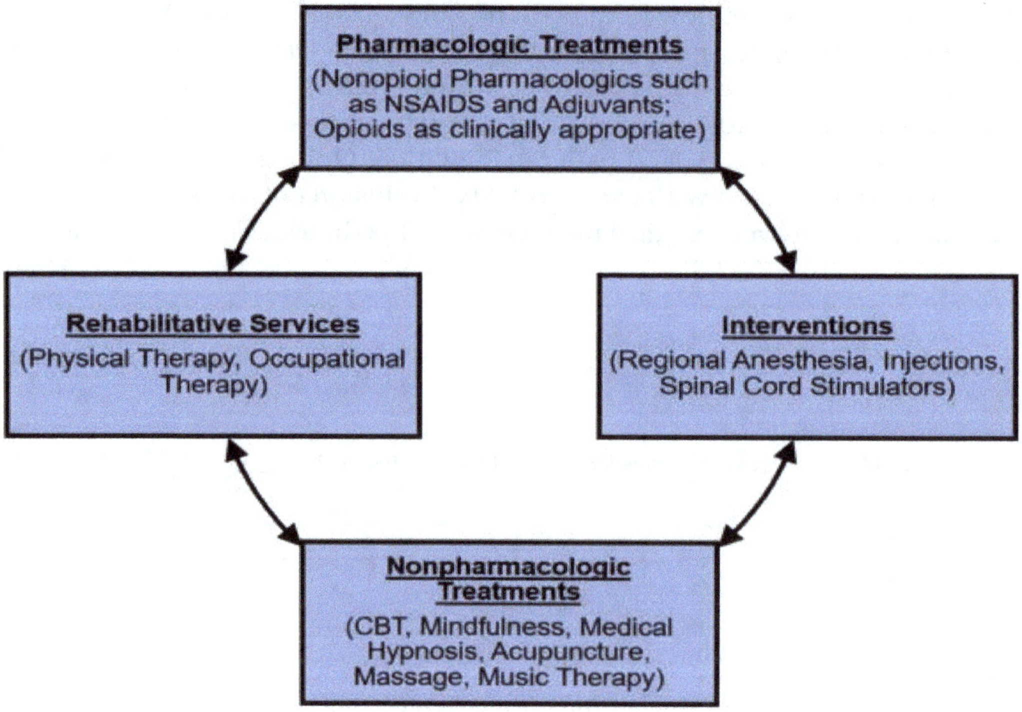

Figure 1. Multidisciplinary pain management treatment: key components in acute and chronic pain management. This figure displays the key treatment components in multidisciplinary treatment for both acute and chronic pain. In the acute setting, in addition to reduction of pain, the efficacy of multidisciplinary treatments is often measured by reduction in needed opioid doses to achieve comfort, while in the setting of chronic pain, the improvements obtained through a multidisciplinary approach are often measured by improvements in function. As is clinically appropriate, in both settings, pharmacologic treatments are combined with regional interventions [26], integrative non-pharmacological techniques, and rehabilitative services as is clinically appropriate to support pain management and improve patients' pain symptoms, functioning and quality of life. Multidisciplinary analgesia treatment aims to ensure patient comfort and wellbeing, while at the same time potentially decreasing the need for opioid use in pediatric populations [25].

2.1. Acute Multidisciplinary Pain Management

Multimodal treatment is defined as "the concurrent use of separate therapeutic interventions with different mechanisms of action within one discipline aimed at different pain mechanisms" [11]. This treatment approach involving multiple medications for pain management is considered optimal in the setting of acute pain (see Figure 2), where the primary goal is immediate analgesia sufficient to allow for the recovery from medical treatments/procedures with minimal side effects.

While acute pain management has historically emphasized the use of opioids, multimodal analgesia treatment incorporates opioid-sparing adjuvants targeting specific aspects of the nociceptive and neuropathic pain physiology. Nociceptive analgesics include acetaminophen, NSAIDS, and glucocorticoids. Neuropathic analgesics commonly include gabapentinoids, lidocaine, ketamine, and alpha 2 agonists. Regional anesthesia and injection of local anesthetics are also regularly utilized to allow targeted analgesia to a specific surgical area. These agents provide safe and effective analgesia and sedation and may help reduce the need for opioid therapies [27–29].

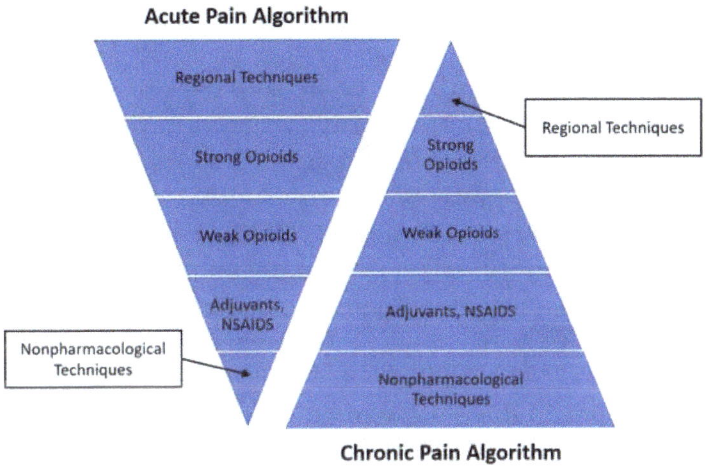

Figure 2. Multidisciplinary pain management: acute and chronic pain algorithms. In acute pain algorithms, the initial treatment begins with regional techniques or intravenous analgesia as a mainstay of therapy. As acute pain improves, therapies are then transitioned as appropriate to varying strengths of PO opioid medications, to adjuvants/NSAIDS, and ultimately integrative non-pharmacological strategies. For situations where severe pain is anticipated, adjuvants and integrative non-pharmacological strategies may be added on at the beginning of treatment, as an opioid sparing strategy, and to increase patient comfort. In chronic pain algorithms, treatment is delivered in the reverse order, beginning with integrative non-pharmacological techniques, then moving to adjuvants, and ultimately progressing to various strengths of opioids and regional techniques and stimulators as clinically appropriate.

Acute pharmacological interventions can be enhanced by the assistance of integrative non-pharmacological interventions (i.e., multidisciplinary treatment). In treatment of pediatric acute pain, the integration of a psychologist or child life specialist into the treatment team can support pain management efforts in the perioperative period by educating the patient in an age appropriate manner about medical procedures, a pain management plan, and implementing behavioral pain management interventions (e.g., distraction, play, active relaxation training) to reduce post-operative pain and anxiety [30]. An acupuncturist or massage therapist can also support acute pediatric pain management following medical procedures and surgeries [31,32]. Incorporating integrative non-pharmacological therapies into multidisciplinary analgesia treatments for acute pediatric pain has been shown to reduce perioperative anxiety and procedural pain [33,34], and thus has the potential to reduce pediatric patients' reliance on pharmacological interventions such as opioids and benzodiazepines. Preliminary evidence supports this notion, demonstrating that even in an acute medical setting such as the management of perioperative pain following a minimally invasive surgery for Pectus Excavatum repair (Nuss procedure) in adolescents, the addition of an integrative non-pharmacological therapy (in this example, self-hypnosis instruction preoperatively) can reduce pain, postoperative opioid use, and even length of hospital stay [35].

2.2. Chronic Multidisciplinary Pain Management

In the management of chronic pain, the emphasis shifts from immediate analgesia to extended pain management services and facilitation of function across domains (e.g., performance of activities of daily living). A multidisciplinary approach to chronic pain management (see Figure 2) has therefore increasingly become the standard of care in pediatric pain management settings. Chronic pain treatment places a central emphasis on integrative non-pharmacological techniques, minimizing side effects, and ideally providing the child skills they can use to more independently manage their symptoms.

Oftentimes, in pain management of complex patients, the utility of integrative non-pharmacological therapies is discussed only when all pharmaceutical therapy options have been exhausted. By then, the patient may begin to feel that medical care is somehow being limited or withdrawn, or that using integrative non-pharmacological therapies indicates that the "pain is in their head". This can lead to patients and families feeling resistant to learning and incorporating these essential integrative non-pharmacological pain management tools. In multidisciplinary chronic pain management, integrative non-pharmacological therapies are incorporated in early phases of treatment, along with appropriate pharmacological interventions to provide optimal care for complex pediatric patients.

Pharmacological interventions in this setting often include analgesics such as acetaminophen and nonsteroidal agents, gabapentinoids, clonidine, tricyclic antidepressants, and where appropriate serotonin-norepinephrine reuptake inhibitors. Another novel adjuvant therapy that deserves mention as a possible opioid sparing agent, cannabidiol (CBD), is gaining popularity in multimodal pain management. CBD is the nonpsychoactive cannabinoid identified in cannabis, while tetrahydrocannabinol or THC is responsible for the hallucinogenic side effects of cannabis [36]. Further research is needed to examine the efficacy and side effect profile of CBD in chronic pain management, and to elucidate side effects and risks.

Opioids are typically minimized in chronic pain management, as the analgesic benefits of opioids are often offset by their long-term negative side effects such as constipation, nausea, vomiting, and sedation, as well as the risk of tolerance, dependence, opioid-induced hyperalgesia, and addiction [5,6]. If opioids are deemed clinically necessary, weak opioids like Tramadol or Hydrocodone can be used in the initial treatment phase but stronger opioids may be needed with recalcitrant pain. Regional anesthesia also may play less of a role, as the duration of the local anesthetic and length of time a catheter can be safely inserted may not provide longer-term analgesic benefit.

3. Integrative Non-Pharmacological Therapies in Pediatric Multidisciplinary Pain Management

Incorporating integrative non-pharmacological interventions into pediatric multidisciplinary chronic pain management has been demonstrated to be feasible and effective and has become the gold standard of care [27,37–39]. These techniques aim to modulate psychological factors, improve coping abilities, and enhance emotional well-being. Specifically, these therapies are thought to target: cognitions (e.g., modifying the child's anxious thoughts related to distressing physical sensations), emotions (e.g., teaching the child emotion regulation strategies and distress tolerance skills to support reductions in negative emotional/somatic symptoms), behaviors (e.g., decreasing pain avoidance behaviors and increasing the use of coping skills), and sensory experiences (e.g., directly targeting pain perceptions through enhanced nervous system inhibitory processes) [37,40]. In contrast to short-term pharmacological management, which provide patients transitory benefit, integrative non-pharmacological techniques can lead to long-term results via changes in neural circuits that regulate habits, affect, and cognitive pain responses [41]. Directly addressing cognitive-affective processes may increase youths' coping repertoire of strategies to manage pain (short-term and long-term), regulate mood, improve psychological well-being and resiliency, and potentially buffer against opioid misuse.

For the purpose of this review, we focus on four frequently utilized interventions in U.S. pain clinics, which include three psychologically based interventions: cognitive behavioral therapy, mindfulness, and medical hypnosis. Acupuncture, an integrative medicine approach widely used in pain management clinics, is additionally reviewed [39,42–45]. Rehabilitative therapies, including physical and occupational therapy (PT, OT), are also an important part of the treatment of chronic pain and are regularly integrated into care to support pain management and increase function [39,46–49]. Of note, rehabilitative therapies are uniquely dependent on the condition being treated (e.g., back pain, ankle sprain, complex regional pain syndrome), and as such, a comprehensive review of PT and OT in pediatric pain was deemed outside the scope of this paper. Overall, there is growing evidence that integrative non-pharmacological techniques can provide lasting pain management benefits, [37] have the potential to decrease reliance on opioids [41], and may minimize side effects [50]. Recent evidence also suggests that interdisciplinary pain management programs can even support effective opioid weaning among youth with chronic pain [14,51]. The importance of integrating non-pharmacologic strategies into the care of youth with acute and chronic pain will be explored below. See Appendix A for a summary of select studies reviewed.

Lastly, it is important to highlight that the integrative non-pharmacological treatments reviewed below often require significant commitment and effort from both children and families, and while frequently effective, improvements typically occur over time. Some barriers to implementation include: patient and family "buy-in" to the proposed treatment; work, family, and scheduling demands; financial challenges; accessibility of local resources (e.g., no accessible providers trained in a particular treatment modality); and the general burden of care. Awareness, sensitivity, and attention to such issues are required on the part of providers to best support patients and families in structuring their multidisciplinary treatment plan.

3.1. *Cognitive Behavioral Therapy*

Cognitive behavioral therapy (CBT) is a form of psychotherapy that has empirical support across a wide range of child, adolescent, and adult populations and is considered an evidence-based intervention in multidisciplinary chronic pain management [52,53]. CBT is based on the premise that thoughts, emotions, and behaviors are closely connected, and how one perceives a situation can significantly influence emotional, behavioral, and physiological responses [54]. When considering CBT for the treatment of chronic pain, protocols often consist of behavioral strategies that encourage engagement in normal daily activities (e.g., activity pacing to increase functioning across domains), cognitive techniques that support challenging and reframing negative "self-talk" statements (e.g., acknowledging catastrophic pain-related thoughts—"This pain is ruining my life"—and using evidence to determine more helpful responses—"This pain is bothersome, but I can handle it and go forward"), and self-regulation skills that help decrease physiological arousal and increase relaxation and wellbeing (e.g., diaphragmatic breathing, progressive muscle relaxation). Acceptance and Commitment Therapy (ACT), an extension of CBT, aims to improve functioning by increasing the ability to act effectively in the presence of pain and distress (i.e., psychological flexibility) [55]. CBT strategies are effective with a wide age range when adapted to the specific developmental level of the child or adolescent [56].

Of note, in the adult literature, neuroimaging data suggest that cognitive reappraisal of pain, a central CBT strategy for patients with chronic pain, may impact pain experiences through top-down processes resulting in increased prefrontal cortex gray matter [57]. CBT has also been linked to increased activation in the ventrolateral prefrontal and lateral orbitofrontal cortices, providing additional support for the role of a cortical control mechanism in CBT [58]. Additionally, CBT for chronic pain has led to changes in somatosensory cortices, potentially reflecting alterations in the perception of noxious signals (i.e., adaptive responses to pain signals) [57].

3.1.1. Evidence for CBT and Pain Management

There is a strong evidence base for the effectiveness of CBT among adults with chronic pain. A meta-analysis of 25 randomized controlled trials of CBT for adults with chronic pain noted significant changes in patients' reported pain experiences, cognitive coping, and behavioral expressions of pain as compared to wait list controls [59].

CBT is also the most well-established psychological intervention among youth with chronic pain [20,60]. A growing evidence base of systematic reviews and meta-analyses have documented that behavioral and cognitive behavioral interventions can produce a medium to large effect on pain outcomes and small effect on disability in chronic pain populations (e.g., headache, abdominal pain). [37,61,62]. In one strong meta-analytic review of randomized controlled trials of psychological therapies for the management of chronic pain in children and adolescents, Palermo and colleagues noted positive effects of CBT on clinically significant pain reduction, with an odds ratio of 4.13 across 9 studies with 406 participants [61]. Recent research is also beginning to explore various models of treatment delivery for CBT for chronic pain including online modules [63] and group-based formats [64,65]. As compared to other evidence-based psychological therapies, CBT is currently the dominant therapeutic model implemented in both medical and non-medical settings and is viewed as well accepted by patients and providers alike [60].

3.1.2. CBT Summary

In sum, while additional research is needed (e.g., larger RCTs with varying treatment delivery modes and monitoring of longer-term follow-up), a growing body of literature demonstrates the efficacy of CBT protocols for children, teenagers, and adults with chronic pain. This evidence-based treatment is well accepted by patients and providers and is increasingly available to pediatric patients. Although youth in more remote areas may have limited access to cognitive behavioral interventions for chronic pain, the advent of web-based treatments holds promise for reaching a wider pediatric audience [63].

3.2. *Mindfulness*

Mindfulness has been described as the ability to be aware of the present moment and one's experiences (e.g., thoughts, emotions, body sensations) in a purposeful, non-judgmental manner [66]. Research demonstrates associations between mindfulness, psychological and physical well-being, and improved health outcomes [67–69]. Interventions and training programs targeting the cultivation of mindfulness (i.e., mindfulness-based interventions; MBIs) have received increasing attention in pain management in recent years. The primary goal of MBIs is to teach individuals mindfulness via a series of breathing, meditation, and movement exercises, all of which cultivate present-moment, compassionate awareness [66,70]. Bringing attention to the present in this manner aims to serve as a buffer from ruminating on bothersome physical symptoms such as pain, negative cognitions, and perceived stress that can contribute to the experience of pain [71–73].

Neuroimaging studies in adults have provided further support for the mechanisms by which mindfulness meditation practice can lead to change. Specifically, regions of the brain associated with sensory processing and the cognitive modulation of pain (e.g., thalamus, insula, anterior cingulate cortex, orbitofrontal cortex) [74,75] have high concentrations of opioid receptors, [75,76] prompting hypotheses that mindfulness practice may modulate the endogenous opioid system [77]. Other neuroimaging research proposes that mindfulness-induced analgesia is due to a more complex process engaging multiple brain networks and neurochemical mechanisms [78].

3.2.1. Evidence for MBIs and Pain Management

An increasing body of literature has demonstrated that mindfulness interventions are feasible and efficacious in adult pain populations. Systematic reviews and meta-analyses have documented that mindfulness-based protocols can significantly improve pain outcomes (e.g., pain severity, interference, and sensitivity), psychological distress (e.g., depression), and quality of life among adults [79–81].

In pediatric populations, pilot studies have demonstrated initial feasibility and acceptability of mindfulness-based interventions for children and adolescents experiencing a range of chronic pain conditions (e.g., musculoskeletal, neuropathic, headache, abdominal pain) [82–84]. These mindfulness protocols have also garnered preliminary empirical support for their efficacy in improving pain-related outcomes such as fibromyalgia symptoms, functional disability, cortisol levels, pain acceptance, and emotional distress among youth with pain symptoms [82–86]. The existing research is promising. For example, in one pilot randomized trial of a mindfulness-based intervention for female adolescents with chronic pain, patients reported improvements in coping with pain, and reductions in pre- and post-mindfulness session salivary cortisol levels ($p < 0.001$) [83]. The quality of this research; however, has varied from randomized controlled trials to pilot studies and is limited in generalizability by small sample sizes, lack of a control groups, and lack of random assignment [83,86–88].

Given the more robust body of literature supporting the use of mindfulness interventions with youth to address symptoms of anxiety and depression [89], MBIs have become increasingly popular and available in recent years. Many schools are beginning to implement skills-based learning for stress management, including mindfulness, bringing developmentally appropriate adaptations (e.g., teaching is varied and interactive) of the intervention directly to groups of children with little cost [90]. A recent well controlled sizable RCT compared the application of mindfulness-based stress reduction (MBSR) to a health education control group in 300 5th- to 8th-grade students in an urban public school setting and found significantly lower levels of somatization, depression, negative affect, negative coping, rumination, self-hostility, and post-traumatic symptom severity (all $p < 0.05$) as compared to control [91]. Attention to cultural and developmental aspects of the child and family are important in the successful implementation of these therapies as well. There is also increasing availability of mindfulness-based self-administered electronic resources that may help bring this intervention to the most underserved areas. While free or low cost and easily accessible, there is unfortunately little evidence yet available on the efficacy of these electronic resources [92].

3.2.2. Mindfulness Summary

Substantive findings support the use of mindfulness interventions among adults with chronic pain. While preliminary research among pediatric pain populations demonstrates feasibility and acceptability of MBI's among youth, further research to investigate adaptations of mindfulness protocols for children and adolescents with chronic pain is needed. Clinical judgment is recommended until published research can better guide the use of MBIs among youth with pain. That being said, mindfulness interventions may be low cost or free adjunctive treatments that have fewer side effects as compared to pharmacologic interventions.

3.3. Hypnosis

Hypnosis is another integrative non-pharmacological treatment increasingly used in multidisciplinary pain management. Hypnosis has been defined as a state of attentive and receptive concentration generating changes in individuals' experiences of themselves and their environment [93,94]. While hypnosis usually (but not always) involves relaxation, [95] this treatment modality differs from mindfulness meditation in the thoughtful and deliberate use of therapeutic suggestions to facilitate change in a targeted domain (in the case of hypnotic analgesia, the patient's sensory experience) [40].

Similar to the impact of opioids on the brain, hypnotic analgesia is hypothesized to enhance nervous system inhibitory processes that attenuate pain experiences [96] through a variety of brain areas involved in pain processing (for a detailed review, see Jensen and Patterson, 2015) [97]. Neuroimaging studies in adults conducted during hypnotic experiences have noted significant signal changes associated with sensation and perception (e.g., primary somatosensory cortex, thalamus, insula), as well as in sensorimotor integration pain systems (e.g., supplementary motor cortex) [97–99].

3.3.1. Evidence for Hypnosis and Pain Management

There is a growing evidence base supporting the efficacy of hypnotically induced analgesia, identifying medical hypnosis as a "well established treatment" for pain in adult populations [100,101]. A meta-analysis investigating hypnosis for acute and chronic pain management found that for 75% of patients across studies (18 studies; $n = 933$) hypnosis provided substantial pain relief and was shown to be superior to non-hypnotic psychological interventions [52].

While there is a significantly smaller pediatric research base, extant controlled studies indicate positive results for pain reduction using this treatment modality among pediatric populations.

Supportive findings for pain reduction have been noted in youth undergoing surgery, cancer patients, and young people diagnosed with irritable bowel syndrome (IBS) [102–105]. In one noteworthy randomized controlled trial of hypnosis for children with functional abdominal pain or IBS, hypnosis was demonstrated as highly superior to standard medical therapy in reducing both pain frequency and pain intensity ($p < 0.001$) [104]. Additionally, one recent randomized controlled trial examined self-hypnosis training for 22 self-selected adolescents hospitalized for the Nuss procedure [35]. The results of this study indicated that in addition to better pain control, self-hypnosis training was associated with use of fewer milligrams per hour of morphine equivalents throughout a patient's five-day hospitalization ($p = 0.005$). A smaller and earlier study exploring this same procedure (five treatment patients and five control patients) noted no significant difference between opioid use in these two groups, but did document a shorter hospital stay for adolescents in the self-hypnosis group [95]. Numerous uncontrolled trials report results that trend in a positive direction including additional trials of hypnosis for abdominal pain, cancer, headaches, and juvenile classic migraine [106–109].

National training for pediatric hypnosis exists to teach providers across disciplines (e.g., physicians, psychologists, nurses, child life specialists) to use hypnosis tools and integrate them into clinical practice. In-person provider training with a child and adolescent focus is recommended before implementing this modality. Notably, in many geographic locations, patients may not have access to a provider trained in pediatric hypnosis.

3.3.2. Hypnosis Summary

Like mindfulness-based interventions, hypnosis is a well-established integrative non-pharmacological intervention for chronic pain management among adults [100], and there is a smaller but growing research base for pediatric pain management and hypnosis [103,104]. While preliminary evidence is promising, more research will be necessary before providers can confidently assert that hypnosis aides in pain management in pediatric populations.

3.4. Acupuncture

Acupuncture is an ancient medical procedure that has been practiced in China and other East Asian countries for over 2000 years. The technique involves the placement of small needles at various locations in the body. Traditional explanations suggest that acupuncture works by activating and engaging movement in the body's own energy resources, termed "Qi" [110]. Traditionally, acupuncture has been employed for the prevention of disease, as well as an early intervention in emerging illness. As an adjunct to current medical practice, acupuncture is often employed late in the course of illness (e.g., to assist with pain, loss of function), as well as to support withdrawal from opioid therapy. Related therapies include electroacupuncture, acupressure, moxibustion (i.e., burning of an herb near an acupoint to create local warming), laser stimulation of acupoints, and non-invasive stimulation of acupoints utilizing a transcutaneous electrical nerve stimulator (TENS, referred to as TEAS).

Studies exploring the mechanisms of action involved in acupuncture to better understand how acupuncture can lead to improvements in symptoms such as pain and withdrawal have focused on several areas. First, fMRI studies have demonstrated that acupuncture can lead to changes in brain blood flow, including the activity of the default mode network (DMN), and normalization of activity in areas of the limbic system often referred to as the "pain matrix" (e.g., insula, anterior cingulate gyrus, prefrontal cortex) [47,111,112]. Other work has shown that acupuncture can stimulate endorphin release in the central nervous system [113]. Research has not elucidated exactly how the needling procedures lead to these changes in brain activity; however, one possible explanation suggests activation of the cholinergic anti-inflammatory pathway—a neural pathway that modulates the body's immune response to injury [114,115].

3.4.1. Evidence for Acupuncture and Pain Management

In 1997, the NIH conducted a Consensus Meeting, where studies of acupuncture were reviewed by an expert panel. It was determined that sufficient evidence was present to recommend acupuncture for the treatment of adult postoperative pain, postoperative dental pain, and nausea and vomiting [116]. Other promising indications included the treatment of addiction. Since that time, multiple clinical studies have demonstrated that acupuncture was efficacious in the treatment of chronic back pain, headaches, and osteoarthritis among adults [117–119].

Pediatric applications have centered on the use of acupuncture for both acute and chronic pain [120]. Of particular relevance, research has demonstrated that acupuncture can decrease acute postoperative pain among pediatric populations. In a prospective randomized controlled study, Lin and colleagues found that acupuncture led to a statistically significant reduction in pain and agitation ($p < 0.001$) among 60 children undergoing bilateral myringotomy and tympanostomy compared to a control condition [121]. Additionally, fewer youth required additional analgesia in the acupuncture versus control condition. In another randomized controlled trial, acupuncture led to significantly less pain ($p < 0.001$) following tonsillectomy compared to a sham acupuncture condition [122].

Acupuncture treatment may also be useful in reducing opioid-related withdrawal symptoms among pediatric populations. In a randomized controlled trial to treat Neonatal Abstinence Syndrome, acupuncture led to a shorter duration of morphine treatment (28 days vs. 39 days in the control group; $p = 0.019$) and hospital stay (35 vs. 50 days in the control group; $p = 0.048$) [123]. Another study demonstrated that a course of acupuncture was helpful in supporting infants wean off a high dose opioid infusion in the intensive care unit [43].

Several randomized studies have explored in more detail the effect of acupuncture on pediatric chronic pain. Gottschling and colleagues performed a randomized trial using laser acupuncture, a non-invasive type of acupuncture, with 43 children who suffered from either migraine or tension type headache. The mean number of headaches per month decreased by 6.4 days in the group which received acupuncture treatment, and by 1 day in the placebo group ($p < 0.001$). Secondary outcomes of headache severity likewise decreased and were statistically significant at all time points [124].

In a small randomized controlled trial comparing acupuncture with sham acupuncture, 14 adolescents with pelvic pain due to endometriosis experienced a 4.8 (SD 2.4) point reduction in pain (on an 11-point numeric rating scale) after 4 weeks, which differed significantly from the control group who experienced an average reduction of 1.4 (SD 2.1) ($p = 0.004$). Reduction in pain was found to persist six months post-intervention; however, after four weeks the differences were not clinically significant, suggesting continued acupuncture may be necessary for a more prolonged therapeutic effect [125].

3.4.2. Acupuncture Summary

Acupuncture appears to be an effective integrative non-pharmacological therapy in the management of acute postoperative pain and neonatal abstinence syndrome, and there is some preliminary evidence for chronic pediatric pain. Additional basic and clinical research is needed to adequately characterize the mechanisms of acupuncture and clinical effects on pain and withdrawal symptoms in pediatric populations. Given that acupuncture has been shown to be a well-tolerated and acceptable intervention among youth, feasible to implement in clinics, and has a low side effect profile, it should be considered for incorporation into multidisciplinary analgesia for youth with acute and chronic pain.

4. Intensive Interdisciplinary Pediatric Pain Rehabilitative Programs

As described above, the primary goal of pediatric pain management is functional restoration in concert with the management of discomfort. When multimodal analgesia and multidisciplinary outpatient care have not successfully met these goals, some youth are referred to comprehensive interdisciplinary pain programs. Interdisciplinary care involves "multimodal treatment provided by a multidisciplinary team collaborating in assessment and treatment using a shared biopsychosocial model and goals" [11]. This interdisciplinary approach involves escalation of intensity and quantity of standard therapies to better meet the need for this vulnerable population.

Intensive interdisciplinary pain treatment (IIPT) programs are becoming a popular treatment choice for children with chronic pain who exhibit significant functional disability and are unable to progress in an outpatient setting or for those who lack the proper resources in their local environment. IIPT involves patient and family participation in either an inpatient or outpatient day hospital setting with coordinated interventions among at least three disciplines including pain or rehabilitation physicians, psychologists, and physical and occupational therapists [38]. Logan et al. performed a longitudinal case series of 56 patients ages 8 to 18 suffering from Complex Regional Pain Syndrome (CRPS) and showed that an IIPT program led to improvements in functional disability, pain symptoms, medication use, and emotional functioning (all $p < 0.01$) [126]. Simons et al. showed that IIPT was superior to outpatient treatment with significantly larger improvements in functional disability, pain-related fear, and readiness to change among children with chronic pain [127]. Of note, Bruce et al. demonstrated that patients in a three-week IIPT program who were receiving opioids were able to be weaned off these medications and remained opioid-free at the 3-month follow-up [51]. While these results are promising, these studies require further investigation and corroboration. In the United States, 11 pediatric pain centers exist that offer this high level of coordinated treatment, varying in treatment duration (2–12 weeks) and daily treatment components [128].

5. Discussion

This article provides an overview of a multidisciplinary pain management approach for pediatric patients with acute and chronic pain, and highlights the evidence base of commonly utilized integrative non-pharmacological therapies for the treating pediatrician, primary health care pediatric provider, or non-pain pediatric specialist. The review explores a topic that is often overlooked in the medical literature, resulting in a noteworthy gap of knowledge among many providers caring for pediatric patients with complex medical and pain conditions. As such, this review aims to further inform providers about multidisciplinary pain management and highlight the role of integrative non-pharmacological therapies in medically complex situations by summarizing and synthesizing relevant literature. Currently, many patients often receive a medical cocktail including opioids, benzodiazepines, gabapentinoids, and other medications for pain management. The early incorporation of the integrative non-pharmacological therapies reviewed in this paper may help in lowering the doses of medications needed to attain comfort for this young and vulnerable population. Of note, there is preliminary evidence that some of the integrative non-pharmacological therapies reviewed, specifically hypnosis and acupuncture, may decrease the need for opioid therapy in inpatient populations (e.g., Nuss procedure, neonatal abstinence syndrome). While additional research is needed to explore the efficacy and generalizability of these results, these studies are encouraging and suggest that practitioners should specifically consider incorporating multidisciplinary pain management strategies where possible and feasible for patients for whom prolonged opioid therapy is being considered or prescribed for acute or chronic pain.

Additionally, many of the integrative non-pharmacological therapies reviewed consist of teaching skills that are applicable beyond an individual pain episode. The patient is taught to implement pain management skills themselves, which may increase the patient's personal efficacy, coping resources, and overall resilience. These integrative non-pharmacological therapies can provide effective pain relief and give patients the feeling that they are able to have some "control" over a difficult pain management problem. Through increased knowledge and familiarity with these therapies and multidisciplinary pain management, the general pediatric practitioner is better equipped to help pediatric patients feel empowered to explore evidence-based integrative non-pharmacological options, creating an integrative process of care that is holistic, safe, and effective.

Limitations

Although this paper is not a formal systematic review, it provides a thorough review of the literature that may be most pertinent to our intended audience—the general pediatric practitioner. The data base for the therapies described above in pediatric pain is still in its infancy, and therefore, few RCT's exist within several the integrative non-pharmacological topic areas described (see Table A1). In addition, the heterogeneity of study population and design precludes a systematic comparison that would be of value to the general reader. In some instances, there was no pediatric data available on a particular topic. While mechanisms of action may differ between adult and pediatric populations due to developmental effects, adult data was reviewed where it was available and felt to contribute to an understanding of a mechanism of action of the therapy.

6. Conclusions

Multidisciplinary pain management, including pharmacological and integrative non-pharmacological therapies, has been demonstrated to be efficacious in the treatment of both acute and chronic pain. Pharmacological interventions include opioids and opioid-sparing agents that target specific aspects of the nociceptive and neuropathic pain physiology. Simultaneously, integrative non-pharmacological interventions such as CBT, MBIs, hypnosis, and acupuncture target the cognitive-affective and physiologic components of the pain experience, and support the cultivation of coping tools that can lead to long-term improvements in pain, psychological functioning, and quality of life. Given extant research, the incorporation of multidisciplinary pain management treatment including both multimodal pharmacological and integrative non-pharmacological therapies is recommended early in the process of caring for youth experiencing acute and chronic pain.

Suggested future directions include performance of larger pediatric trials across integrative non-pharmacological pain interventions, assessing the potential synergistic nature of combined integrative non-pharmacological therapies, and conducting further research on the transition from acute to chronic pain management. It is also recommended that studies more directly explore the associations and effects of multidisciplinary treatment on the necessity for and use of opioid therapies in pediatric pain, especially in chronic pain management, and on the possible utility of these therapies in weaning from opioids and other therapies. Overall, additional societal resources are urgently needed to increase availability of multidisciplinary pain management services to all youth impacted by acute and chronic pain.

Author Contributions: Conceptualization, A.W., A.R. and B.G., Methodology, A.W., A.R., B.G., G.D.; Diagrams, G.D.; Writing—Original Draft Preparation, all; Writing—Review & Editing, all.; Visualization, B.G.; Supervision, B.G.

Appendix A

Table A1. Selection of important studies in pediatric integrative non-pharmacological therapies reviewed for this paper. From all the articles screened, the articles with the highest level of evidence are summarized below.

Therapy Type	Authors (Reference Number)	Study Type (Grade of Evidence)	Study Population	Outcome	Key Results
CBT	Eccleston et al. [37]	Cochrane systematic review (1)	Cochrane systematic review of psychological therapies (37 RCTs; 2111 participants, mean age 12.45, SD 2.2)	Pain intensity; Disability	Reduced headache pain (RR 2.47, CI 1.97–3.09, $p < 0.01$; Reduced disability in headache pain (SMD −0.49, CI −0.74 to −0.24, $p < 0.01$); Reduced nonheadache pain (SMD −0.57, CI −0.86 to −0.27, $p < 0.01$); Reduced disability in nonheadache pain (SMD −0.45, CI −0.71 to −0.19, $p < 0.01$
	Palermo et al. [61]	Meta-analysis (1)	Meta-analysis (25 RCTs; 1247 participants, 9–17 yo)	Pain intensity	Decreased headache (OR 6.1, CI 4.06 to 9.15, $p < 0.0001$); Decreased abdominal pain (OR 7.5, CI 3.29 to 17.16, $p < 0.001$)
	Fisher et al. [62]	Systematic review and meta-analysis (1)	Meta-analysis (37 RCTs; 1005 participants, mean age 9.4, SD 1.14)	Pain intensity; Disability	Decreased non-headache pain (SMD −0.60, CI −0.91to −0.29, $p < 0.001$); Decreased nonheadache pain disability (SMD −0.27, CI −0.46 to −0.08, $p < 0.01$); Decreased headache (RR 2.9, CI 2.25 to 3.73, $p < 0.001$); Decreased headache at follow-up (RR 3.34, CI 2.02 to 5.53, $p < 0.001$
Mindfulness	Ruskin et al. [82]	Prospective pre-post interventional study (2)	21 adolescents, 12–18 yo with chronic pain	Feasibility; Acceptability	90.5% treatment completion rate; No dropouts; Compliance with home practice (M = 60 min/week); Would recommend group to a friend
	Chadi et al. [83]	RCT (2)	19 adolescents, 13.9–17.8 yo with chronic pain	Quality of life; Depression; Anxiety; Pain perception; Psychological distress; Salivary cortisol	No significant changes in quality of life, depression, anxiety, pain perception, or psychological distress; Cortisol levels decreased from an average of 3.37 (±1.72) pre-intervention nmol/L to 1.95 (±1.13) nmol/L post-intervention; Cohen's d = 0.77, $p < 0.001$).
	Ali et al. [84]	Pilot (3)	15 adolescents, 10–18 yo with fibromyalgia, chronic fatigue, musculoskeletal pain, headache, or abdominal pain	Functional disability; Fibromyalgia symptoms; Quality of life; Mindfulness	Decreased functional disability (33% improvement, $p = 0.026$); improved fibromyalgia symptoms (26% improvement, $p = 0.03$), and improved mindfulness (child: 12% improvement, $p = 0.02$; parent: 17% improvement, $p = 0.03$).
	Waelde et al. [85]	Pilot (3)	20 adolescents, 13–17 yo with chronic pain	Feasibility and Acceptability Parental assessment	Feasible and acceptable; Decreased parental worry about child ($p < 0.01$)
	Hesse et al. [86]	Pilot (3)	20 adolescent females, 11–16 yo, with recurrent headaches	Quality of life; Pain acceptance; Depression	Improved quality of life, Parent assess PedsQL, $p = 0.049$; Improved child acceptance of pain, CPAQ-A $p = -0.005$; Improved child depression, CES-DC $p = 0.009$
Hypnosis	Manworren et al. [35]	RCT (2)	24 adolescents, 10–18 yo undergoing Nuss procedure	Pain intensity; Morphine equivalent/hour; Length of stay (LOS)	Lower mean pain intensity (−1.72, 95% CI 2.89–0.55, $p = 0.0047$); Lower maximum pain intensity (−2.27, 95% CI 3.73–0.82, $p = 0.0028$); Less morphine equivalents/hour (−0.13, 95% CI −0.25–0.00, $p = 0.046$); Shorter LOS ($p = 0.0013$)
Acupuncture	Tsao et al. [122]	RCT (2)	59 children, 3–12 yo undergoing tonsillectomy	Pain, Oral food intake	Improvement in pain control and oral intake ($p = 0.0065$ and 0.001, respectively)
	Raith et al. [123]	RCT (2)	28 newborns with neonatal abstinence syndrome	Duration of morphine treatment; Length of stay	Shorter duration of morphine treatment (28 days vs. 39 days; $p = 0.019$) and hospital stay (35 vs. 50 days; $p = 0.048$)

Table A1. *Cont.*

Therapy Type	Authors (Reference Number)	Study Type (Grade of Evidence)	Study Population	Outcome	Key Results
Rehabilitation	Hechler, et al. [38]	Systematic review (1)	10 studies (1020 adolescents, mean age 13.9, SD 1.5)	Pain intensity; Pain-related disability	Decreased pain intensity (d = −1.33, CI −2.28 to −0.38, $p = 0.01$); Decreased pain related disability (d = −1.09, CI −1.71 to −0.48, $p < 0.001$)
	Logan et al. [126]	Longitudinal case series (3)	56 children and adolescents, 8–18 yo with CRPS	Pain intensity; Functional disability; Subjective report of limb function, timed running, occupational performance, medication use, use of assistive devices, emotional functioning, anxiety and depression	Statistically significant improvements from admission to discharge in pain intensity, functional disability, subjective report of limb function, timed running, occupational performance, medication use, use of assistive devices, emotional functioning, anxiety, and depression. (all $p < 0.01$). (multiple outcomes)
	Simons et al. [127]	Comparative study (case-controlled) (3)	100 children and adolescents, mean age 13.9 (SD 2.17)	Functional disability; Fear of pain; Readiness to change	Improved functional disability ($p = 0.00$); Improved fear of pain ($p = 0.00$); Increased readiness to change (precontemplation $p = 0.01$, action/maintenance $p = 0.00$) (multiple outcomes)
	Bruce et al. [51]	Prospective longitudinal case series (3)	171 adolescents 12–18, mean age 15.3 (SD 1.73)	Functional disability; depressive symptoms; catastrophizing; Changes in opioid medication	Improved functional disability ($p < 0.001$) Improved depressive symptoms ($p < 0.0001$) Improved catastrophizing ($p < 0.0001$) Reduced pain severity ($p = 0.0001$) Decreased opioid medication (Out of 30 patients on opioids, 21 were weaned off medication, 1 did not finish program)

Notes: RCT, randomized controlled trials; SD, standard deviation; RR, risk ratio; CI, confidence interval; SMD, standardized mean difference; yo, years old; OR, odds ratios; M, mean; PedsQL, Pediatric Quality of Life Inventory; CPAQ-A, Chronic Pain Acceptance Questionnaire-Activity Engagement; CES-DC, Center for Epidemiological Studies of Depression Scale for Children; LOS, length of stay; d, effect sizes; CRPS, complex regional pain syndrome.

References

1. Pain terms: A list with definitions and notes on usage. Recommended by the IASP Subcommittee on Taxonomy. *Pain* **1979**, *6*, 249.
2. Anwar, K. Pathophysiology of pain. *Dis. Mon.* **2016**, *62*, 324–329. [CrossRef] [PubMed]
3. IASP Pain Terminology. International Association for the Study of Pain Committee on Taxonomy. Available online: http://www.iasp-pain.org/Taxonomy#Pain (accessed on 1 December 2018).
4. Slater, M.E.; De Lima, J.; Campbell, K.; Lane, L.; Collins, J. Opioids for the management of severe chronic nonmalignant pain in children: A retrospective 1-year practice survey in a children's hospital. *Pain Med.* **2010**, *11*, 207–214. [CrossRef] [PubMed]
5. Berde, C.; Nurko, S. Opioid side effects—Mechanism-based therapy. *N. Engl. J. Med.* **2008**, *358*, 2400–2402. [CrossRef] [PubMed]
6. Moore, R.A.; McQuay, H.J. Prevalence of opioid adverse events in chronic non-malignant pain: Systematic review of randomised trials of oral opioids. *Arthritis Res. Ther.* **2005**, *7*, R1046–R1051. [CrossRef] [PubMed]
7. Gomes, T.; Mamdani, M.M.; Dhalla, I.A.; Paterson, J.M.; Juurlink, D.N. Opioid dose and drug-related mortality in patients with nonmalignant pain. *Arch. Intern. Med.* **2011**, *171*, 686–691. [CrossRef] [PubMed]
8. Grunkemeier, D.M.; Cassara, J.E.; Dalton, C.B.; Drossman, D.A. The narcotic bowel syndrome: Clinical features, pathophysiology, and management. *Clin. Gastroenterol. Hepatol.* **2007**, *5*, 1126–1139. [CrossRef]
9. Fudin, J.; Raouf, M.; Wegrzyn, E.L. *Opioid Dosing Policy: Pharmacological Considerations Regarding Equianalgesic Dosing*; American Academy of Integrative Pain Management: Lenexa, KS, USA, 2017.
10. Lee, M.; Silverman, S.M.; Hansen, H.; Patel, V.B.; Manchikanti, L. A comprehensive review of opioid-induced hyperalgesia. *Pain Physician* **2011**, *14*, 145–161.
11. Task Force on Multimodal Pain Treatment Defines Terms for Chronic Pain Care. Available online: http://www.iasp-pain.org/PublicationsNews/NewsDetail.aspx?ItemNumber=6981 (accessed on 1 December 2018).
12. Friedrichsdorf, S.J. Contemporary pediatric palliative care: Myths and barriers to integration into clinical care. *Curr. Pediatr. Rev.* **2016**, *13*, 8–12. [CrossRef]
13. Dowell, D.; Haegerich, T.M.; Chou, R. CDC guideline for prescribing opioids for chronic pain—United States, 2016. *MMWR Recomm. Rep.* **2016**, *65*, 1–49. [CrossRef]
14. Dash, G.F.; Wilson, A.C.; Morasco, B.J.; Feldstein Ewing, S.W. A Model of the Intersection of Pain and Opioid Misuse in Children and Adolescents. *Clin. Psychol. Sci.* **2018**, *6*, 629–646. [CrossRef] [PubMed]
15. Schechter, N.L.; Walco, G.A. The Potential Impact on Children of the CDC Guideline for Prescribing Opioids for Chronic Pain: Above All, Do No Harm. *JAMA Pediatr.* **2016**, *170*, 425–426. [CrossRef] [PubMed]
16. Friedrichsdorf, S.J.; Giordano, J.; Desai Dakoji, K.; Warmuth, A.; Daughtry, C.; Schulz, C.A. Chronic Pain in Children and Adolescents: Diagnosis and Treatment of Primary Pain Disorders in Head, Abdomen, Muscles and Joints. *Children (Basel)* **2016**, *3*, 42. [CrossRef] [PubMed]
17. Chung, C.P.; Callahan, S.T.; Cooper, W.O.; Dupont, W.D.; Murray, K.T.; Franklin, A.D.; Hall, K.; Dudley, J.A.; Stein, C.M.; Ray, W.A. Outpatient Opioid Prescriptions for Children and Opioid-Related Adverse Events. *Pediatrics* **2018**, *142*. [CrossRef] [PubMed]
18. Krane, E.J.; Weisman, S.J.; Walco, G.A. The National Opioid Epidemic and the Risk of Outpatient Opioids in Children. *Pediatrics* **2018**, *142*. [CrossRef] [PubMed]
19. Lin, Y.C.; Lee, A.C.; Kemper, K.J.; Berde, C.B. Use of complementary and alternative medicine in pediatric pain management service: A survey. *Pain Med.* **2005**, *6*, 452–458. [CrossRef] [PubMed]
20. Fisher, E.; Law, E.; Dudeney, J.; Palermo, T.M.; Stewart, G.; Eccleston, C. Psychological therapies for the management of chronic and recurrent pain in children and adolescents. *Cochrane Database Syst. Rev.* **2018**, *9*. [CrossRef]
21. Kamper, S.J.; Apeldoorn, A.T.; Chiarotto, A.; Smeets, R.J.; Ostelo, R.W.; Guzman, J.; van Tulder, M.W. Multidisciplinary biopsychosocial rehabilitation for chronic low back pain: Cochrane systematic review and meta-analysis. *BMJ* **2015**, *350*, h444. [CrossRef]
22. Lee, C.; Crawford, C.; Swann, S. Active Self-Care Therapies for Pain (PACT) Working Group. Multimodal, integrative therapies for the self-management of chronic pain symptoms. *Pain Med.* **2014**, *15* Suppl. 1, S76–S85. [CrossRef]

23. Nicol, A.L.; Hurley, R.W.; Benzon, H.T. Alternatives to opioids in the pharmacologic management of chronic pain syndromes: A narrative review of randomized, controlled, and blinded clinical trials. *Anesth. Analg.* **2017**, *125*, 1682–1703. [CrossRef]
24. Gardiner, P.; Lestoquoy, A.S.; Gergen-Barnett, K.; Penti, B.; White, L.F.; Saper, R.; Fredman, L.; Stillman, S.; Lily Negash, N.; Adelstein, P.; et al. Design of the integrative medical group visits randomized control trial for underserved patients with chronic pain and depression. *Contemp. Clin. Trials* **2017**, *54*, 25–35. [CrossRef] [PubMed]
25. Tick, H.; Nielsen, A.; Pelletier, K.R.; Bonakdar, R.; Simmons, S.; Glick, R.; Ratner, E.; Lemmon, R.L.; Wayne, P.; Zador, V.; et al. Evidence-Based Nonpharmacologic Strategies for Comprehensive Pain Care: The Consortium Pain Task Force White Paper. *Explore (NY)* **2018**, *14*, 177–211. [CrossRef] [PubMed]
26. Waldman, S. *Pain Management*, 2nd ed.; Elsevier: Philadelphia, PA, USA, 2011; ISBN 9781437736038.
27. Odell, S.; Logan, D.E. Pediatric pain management: The multidisciplinary approach. *J. Pain Res.* **2013**, *6*, 785–790. [CrossRef] [PubMed]
28. Gritsenko, K.; Khelemsky, Y.; Kaye, A.D.; Vadivelu, N.; Urman, R.D. Multimodal therapy in perioperative analgesia. *Best Pract. Res. Clin. Anaesthesiol.* **2014**, *28*, 59–79. [CrossRef] [PubMed]
29. Brooks, M.R.; Golianu, B. Perioperative management in children with chronic pain. *Paediatr. Anaesth.* **2016**, *26*, 794–806. [CrossRef] [PubMed]
30. Panella, J.J. Preoperative care of children: Strategies from a child life perspective. *AORN J.* **2016**, *104*, 11–22. [CrossRef] [PubMed]
31. Suresh, S.; Wang, S.; Porfyris, S.; Kamasinski-Sol, R.; Steinhorn, D.M. Massage therapy in outpatient pediatric chronic pain patients: Do they facilitate significant reductions in levels of distress, pain, tension, discomfort, and mood alterations? *Paediatr. Anaesth.* **2008**, *18*, 884–887. [CrossRef]
32. Wang, S.M.; Escalera, S.; Lin, E.C.; Maranets, I.; Kain, Z.N. Extra-1 acupressure for children undergoing anesthesia. *Anesth. Analg.* **2008**, *107*, 811–816. [CrossRef]
33. Brewer, S.; Gleditsch, S.L.; Syblik, D.; Tietjens, M.E.; Vacik, H.W. Pediatric anxiety: Child life intervention in day surgery. *J. Pediatr. Nurs.* **2006**, *21*, 13–22. [CrossRef]
34. Yip, P.; Middleton, P.; Cyna, A.M.; Carlyle, A.V. Non-pharmacological interventions for assisting the induction of anaesthesia in children. *Cochrane Database Syst. Rev.* **2009**, CD006447. [CrossRef]
35. Manworren, R.C.B.; Girard, E.; Verissimo, A.M.; Ruscher, K.A.; Santanelli, J.P.; Weiss, R.; Hight, D. Hypnosis for postoperative pain management of thoracoscopic approach to repair pectus excavatum: Retrospective analysis. *J. Pediatr. Surg. Nurs.* **2015**, *4*, 60–69. [CrossRef]
36. Jensen, B.; Chen, J.; Furnish, T.; Wallace, M. Medical marijuana and chronic pain: A review of basic science and clinical evidence. *Curr. Pain Headache Rep.* **2015**, *19*, 50. [CrossRef] [PubMed]
37. Eccleston, C.; Palermo, T.M.; Williams, A.C.; Lewandowski, H.A.; Morley, S.; Fisher, E.; Law, E. Psychological therapies for the management of chronic and recurrent pain in children and adolescents. *Cochrane Database Syst. Rev.* **2014**, CD003968. [CrossRef] [PubMed]
38. Hechler, T.; Kanstrup, M.; Holley, A.L.; Simons, L.E.; Wicksell, R.; Hirschfeld, G.; Zernikow, B. Systematic review on intensive interdisciplinary pain treatment of children with chronic pain. *Pediatrics* **2015**, *136*, 115–127. [CrossRef] [PubMed]
39. Lee, B.H.; Scharff, L.; Sethna, N.F.; McCarthy, C.F.; Scott-Sutherland, J.; Shea, A.M.; Sullivan, P.; Meier, P.; Zurakowski, D.; Masek, B.J.; et al. Physical therapy and cognitive-behavioral treatment for complex regional pain syndromes. *J. Pediatr.* **2002**, *141*, 135–140. [CrossRef] [PubMed]
40. Kuttner, L. Pediatric hypnosis: Pre-, peri-, and post-anesthesia. *Paediatr. Anaesth.* **2012**, *22*, 573–577. [CrossRef] [PubMed]
41. Garland, E.L. Disrupting the downward spiral of chronic pain and opioid addiction with mindfulness-oriented recovery enhancement: A review of clinical outcomes and neurocognitive targets. *J. Pain Palliat. Care Pharmacother.* **2014**, *28*, 122–129. [CrossRef]
42. Agoston, A.M.; Sieberg, C.B. Nonpharmacologic treatment of pain. *Semin. Pediatr. Neurol.* **2016**, *23*, 220–223. [CrossRef]
43. Golianu, B.; Seybold, J.; Almgren, C. Acupucture helps reduce need for sedative medications in neonates and infants undergoing treatment in the intensive care unit. *Med. Acupunct.* **2014**, *26*, 279–285. [CrossRef]

44. Schmitt, Y.S.; Hoffman, H.G.; Blough, D.K.; Patterson, D.R.; Jensen, M.P.; Soltani, M.; Carrougher, G.J.; Nakamura, D.; Sharar, S.R. A randomized, controlled trial of immersive virtual reality analgesia, during physical therapy for pediatric burns. *Burns* **2011**, *37*, 61–68. [CrossRef]
45. Brown, M.L.; Rojas, E.; Gouda, S. A Mind-body approach to pediatric pain management. *Children (Basel)* **2017**, *4*, 50. [CrossRef] [PubMed]
46. Rabin, J.; Brown, M.; Alexander, S. Update in the treatment of chronic pain within pediatric patients. *Curr. Probl. Pediatr. Adolesc. Health Care* **2017**, *47*, 167–172. [CrossRef] [PubMed]
47. Dhond, R.P.; Yeh, C.; Park, K.; Kettner, N.; Napadow, V. Acupuncture modulates resting state connectivity in default and sensorimotor brain networks. *Pain* **2008**, *136*, 407–418. [CrossRef] [PubMed]
48. Jiang, H.; White, M.P.; Greicius, M.D.; Waelde, L.C.; Spiegel, D. Brain activity and functional connectivity associated with hypnosis. *Cereb. Cortex* **2017**, *27*, 4083–4093. [CrossRef] [PubMed]
49. Kucyi, A.; Salomons, T.V.; Davis, K.D. Cognitive behavioral training reverses the effect of pain exposure on brain network activity. *Pain* **2016**, *157*, 1895–1904. [CrossRef] [PubMed]
50. Becker, W.C.; Dorflinger, L.; Edmond, S.N.; Islam, L.; Heapy, A.A.; Fraenkel, L. Barriers and facilitators to use of non-pharmacological treatments in chronic pain. *BMC Fam. Pract.* **2017**, *18*, 41. [CrossRef] [PubMed]
51. Bruce, B.K.; Ale, C.M.; Harrison, T.E.; Bee, S.; Luedtke, C.; Geske, J.; Weiss, K.E. Getting back to living: Further evidence for the efficacy of an interdisciplinary pediatric pain treatment program. *Clin. J. Pain* **2017**, *33*, 535–542. [CrossRef]
52. Chambless, D.L.; Hollon, S.D. Defining empirically supported therapies. *J. Consult. Clin. Psychol.* **1998**, *66*, 7–18. [CrossRef]
53. Butler, A.C.; Chapman, J.E.; Forman, E.M.; Beck, A.T. The empirical status of cognitive-behavioral therapy: A review of meta-analyses. *Clin. Psychol. Rev.* **2006**, *26*, 17–31. [CrossRef]
54. Beck, J.S. *Cognitive Behavior Therapy: Basics and Beyond*; Guilford Press: New York, NY, USA, 2011.
55. Wicksell, R.K.; Greco, L.A. Acceptance and commitment therapy for pediatric chronic pain. In *Acceptance and Mindfulness Treatments for Children and Adolescents: A Practitioner's Guide*; New Harbinger Publications: Oakland, CA, USA, 2008; pp. 89–113. ISBN 978-1-57224-541-9.
56. Grave, J.; Blissett, J. Is cognitive behavior therapy developmentally appropriate for young children? A critical review of the evidence. *Clin. Psychol. Rev.* **2004**, *24*, 399–420. [CrossRef]
57. Seminowicz, D.A.; Shpaner, M.; Keaser, M.L.; Krauthamer, G.M.; Mantegna, J.; Dumas, J.A.; Newhouse, P.A.; Filippi, C.G.; Keefe, F.J.; Naylor, M.R. Cognitive-behavioral therapy increases prefrontal cortex gray matter in patients with chronic pain. *J. Pain* **2013**, *14*, 1573–1584. [CrossRef] [PubMed]
58. Jensen, K.B.; Kosek, E.; Wicksell, R.; Kemani, M.; Olsson, G.; Merle, J.V.; Kadetoff, D.; Ingvar, M. Cognitive Behavioral Therapy increases pain-evoked activation of the prefrontal cortex in patients with fibromyalgia. *Pain* **2012**, *153*, 1495–1503. [CrossRef] [PubMed]
59. Williams, A.C.; Eccleston, C.; Morley, S. Psychological therapies for the management of chronic pain (excluding headache) in adults. *Cochrane Database Syst. Rev.* **2012**, *11*, CD007407. [CrossRef] [PubMed]
60. Coakley, R.; Wihak, T. Evidence-based psychological interventions for the management of pediatric chronic pain: New directions in research and clinical practice. *Children (Basel)* **2017**, *4*, 9. [CrossRef] [PubMed]
61. Palermo, T.M.; Eccleston, C.; Lewandowski, A.S.; Williams, A.C.; Morley, S. Randomized controlled trials of psychological therapies for management of chronic pain in children and adolescents: An updated meta-analytic review. *Pain* **2010**, *148*, 387–397. [CrossRef] [PubMed]
62. Fisher, E.; Heathcote, L.; Palermo, T.M.; de C Williams, A.C.; Lau, J.; Eccleston, C. Systematic review and meta-analysis of psychological therapies for children with chronic pain. *J. Pediatr. Psychol.* **2014**, *39*, 763–782. [CrossRef] [PubMed]
63. Palermo, T.M.; Wilson, A.C.; Peters, M.; Lewandowski, A.; Somhegyi, H. Randomized controlled trial of an Internet-delivered family cognitive-behavioral therapy intervention for children and adolescents with chronic pain. *Pain* **2009**, *146*, 205–213. [CrossRef]
64. Huestis, S.E.; Kao, G.; Dunn, A.; Hilliard, A.T.; Yoon, I.A.; Golianu, B.; Bhandari, R.P. Multi-Family Pediatric Pain Group Therapy: Capturing Acceptance and Cultivating Change. *Children (Basel)* **2017**, *4*, 106. [CrossRef]
65. Coakley, R.; Wihak, T.; Kossowsky, J.; Iversen, C.; Donado, C. The Comfort Ability Pain Management Workshop: A Preliminary, Nonrandomized Investigation of a Brief, Cognitive, Biobehavioral, and Parent Training Intervention for Pediatric Chronic Pain. *J. Pediatr. Psychol.* **2018**, *43*, 252–265. [CrossRef]
66. Kabat-Zinn, J. *Wherever You Go, There You Are*; Hyperion: New York, NY, USA, 1994.

67. Black, D.S.; Slavich, G.M. Mindfulness meditation and the immune system: A systematic review of randomized controlled trials. *Ann. N. Y. Acad. Sci.* **2016**, *1373*, 13–24. [CrossRef]
68. Grossman, P.; Niemann, L.; Schmidt, S.; Walach, H. Mindfulness-based stress reduction and health benefits. A meta-analysis. *J. Psychosom. Res.* **2004**, *57*, 35–43. [CrossRef]
69. Ahola Kohut, S.; Stinson, J.; Davies-Chalmers, C.; Ruskin, D.; van Wyk, M. Mindfulness-based interventions in clinical samples of adolescents with chronic illness: A systematic review. *J. Altern. Complement. Med.* **2017**, *23*, 581–589. [CrossRef] [PubMed]
70. Baer, R.A. Mindfulness training as a clinical intervention: A conceptual and empirical review. *Clin. Psychol. Sci. Pract.* **2003**, *10*, 125–143. [CrossRef]
71. Garland, E.L.; Froeliger, B.; Zeidan, F.; Partin, K.; Howard, M.O. The downward spiral of chronic pain, prescription opioid misuse, and addiction: Cognitive, affective, and neuropsychopharmacologic pathways. *Neurosci. Biobehav. Rev.* **2013**, *37*, 2597–2607. [CrossRef] [PubMed]
72. Garland, E.L.; Gaylord, S.A.; Palsson, O.; Faurot, K.; Douglas Mann, J.; Whitehead, W.E. Therapeutic mechanisms of a mindfulness-based treatment for IBS: Effects on visceral sensitivity, catastrophizing, and affective processing of pain sensations. *J. Behav. Med.* **2012**, *35*, 591–602. [CrossRef] [PubMed]
73. Holzel, B.K.; Lazar, S.W.; Gard, T.; Schuman-Olivier, Z.; Vago, D.R.; Ott, U. How does mindfulness meditation work? Proposing mechanisms of action from a conceptual and neural perspective. *Perspect. Psychol. Sci.* **2011**, *6*, 537–559. [CrossRef] [PubMed]
74. Zeidan, F.; Martucci, K.T.; Kraft, R.A.; Gordon, N.S.; McHaffie, J.G.; Coghill, R.C. Brain mechanisms supporting the modulation of pain by mindfulness meditation. *J. Neurosci.* **2011**, *31*, 5540–5548. [CrossRef] [PubMed]
75. Zeidan, F.; Vago, D.R. Mindfulness meditation-based pain relief: A mechanistic account. *Ann. N. Y. Acad. Sci.* **2016**, *1373*, 114–127. [CrossRef]
76. Wager, T.D.; Scott, D.J.; Zubieta, J.K. Placebo effects on human mu-opioid activity during pain. *Proc. Natl. Acad. Sci. USA* **2007**, *104*, 11056–11061. [CrossRef]
77. Sharon, H.; Maron-Katz, A.; Ben Simon, E.; Flusser, Y.; Hendler, T.; Tarrasch, R.; Brill, S. Mindfulness meditation modulates pain through endogenous opioids. *Am. J. Med.* **2016**, *129*, 755–758. [CrossRef]
78. Zeidan, F.; Adler-Neal, A.L.; Wells, R.E.; Stagnaro, E.; May, L.M.; Eisenach, J.C.; McHaffie, J.G.; Coghill, R.C. Mindfulness-meditation-based pain relief is not mediated by endogenous opioids. *J. Neurosci.* **2016**, *36*, 3391–3397. [CrossRef] [PubMed]
79. Veehof, M.M.; Trompetter, H.R.; Bohlmeijer, E.T.; Schreurs, K.M. Acceptance- and mindfulness-based interventions for the treatment of chronic pain: A meta-analytic review. *Cogn. Behav. Ther.* **2016**, *45*, 5–31. [CrossRef] [PubMed]
80. Hilton, L.; Hempel, S.; Ewing, B.A.; Apaydin, E.; Xenakis, L.; Newberry, S.; Colaiaco, B.; Maher, A.R.; Shanman, R.M.; Sorbero, M.E.; et al. Mindfulness meditation for chronic pain: Systematic review and meta-analysis. *Ann. Behav. Med.* **2017**, *51*, 199–213. [CrossRef] [PubMed]
81. Anheyer, D.; Haller, H.; Barth, J.; Lauche, R.; Dobos, G.; Cramer, H. Mindfulness-based stress reduction for treating low back pain: A systematic review and meta-analysis. *Ann. Intern. Med.* **2017**, *166*, 799–807. [CrossRef] [PubMed]
82. Ruskin, D.A.; Gagnon, M.M.; Kohut, S.A.; Stinson, J.N.; Walker, K.S. A mindfulness program adapted for adolescents with chronic pain: Feasibility, acceptability, and initial outcomes. *Clin. J. Pain* **2017**. [CrossRef] [PubMed]
83. Chadi, N.; McMahon, A.; Vadnais, M.; Malboeuf-Hurtubise, C.; Djemli, A.; Dobkin, P.L.; Lacroix, J.; Luu, T.M.; Haley, N. Mindfulness-based intervention for female adolescents with chronic pain: A pilot randomized trial. *J. Can. Acad. Child Adolesc. Psychiatry* **2016**, *25*, 159–168. [PubMed]
84. Ali, A.; Weiss, T.R.; Dutton, A.; McKee, D.; Jones, K.D.; Kashikar-Zuck, S.; Silverman, W.K.; Shapiro, E.D. Mindfulness-based stress reduction for adolescents with functional somatic syndromes: A pilot cohort study. *J. Pediatr.* **2017**, *183*, 184–190. [CrossRef] [PubMed]
85. Waelde, L.C.; Feinstein, A.B.; Bhandari, R.; Griffin, A.; Yoon, I.A.; Golianu, B. A pilot study of mindfulness meditation for pediatric chronic pain. *Children (Basel)* **2017**, *4*, 32. [CrossRef]

86. Hesse, T.; Holmes, L.G.; Kennedy-Overfelt, V.; Kerr, L.M.; Giles, L.L. Mindfulness-based intervention for adolescents with recurrent headaches: A pilot feasibility study. *Evid. Based Complement. Alternat. Med.* **2015**, *2015*, 508958. [CrossRef]
87. Jastrowski Mano, K.E.; Salamon, K.S.; Hainsworth, K.R.; Anderson Khan, K.J.; Ladwig, R.J.; Davies, W.H.; Weisman, S.J. A randomized, controlled pilot study of mindfulness-based stress reduction for pediatric chronic pain. *Altern. Ther. Health Med.* **2013**, *19*, 8–14.
88. Ruskin, D.; Lalloo, C.; Amaria, K.; Stinson, J.N.; Kewley, E.; Campbell, F.; Brown, S.C.; Jeavons, M.; McGrath, P.A. Assessing pain intensity in children with chronic pain: Convergent and discriminant validity of the 0 to 10 numerical rating scale in clinical practice. *Pain Res. Manag.* **2014**, *19*, 141–148. [CrossRef] [PubMed]
89. Zoogman, S.; Goldberg, S.B.; Hoyt, W.T.; Miller, L. Mindfulness interventions with youth: A meta-analysis. *Mindfulness* **2015**, *6*, 290–302. [CrossRef]
90. Zenner, C.; Herrnleben-Kurz, S.; Walach, H. Mindfulness-based interventions in schools-a systematic review and meta-analysis. *Front. Psychol.* **2014**, *5*, 603. [CrossRef] [PubMed]
91. Sibinga, E.M.; Webb, L.; Ghazarian, S.R.; Ellen, J.M. School-Based Mindfulness Instruction: An RCT. *Pediatrics* **2016**, *137*. [CrossRef] [PubMed]
92. Mani, M.; Kavanagh, D.J.; Hides, L.; Stoyanov, S.R. Review and Evaluation of Mindfulness-Based iPhone Apps. *JMIR Mhealth Uhealth* **2015**, *3*, e82. [CrossRef] [PubMed]
93. Hilgard, E.R. *Hypnotic Susceptibility*; Harcourt, Brace & World Inc.: New York, NY, USA, 1965.
94. Spiegel, H.; Spiegel, D. *Trance and Treatment: Clinical Uses of Hypnosis*; American Psychistric Publishing: Washington, DC, USA, 1987; ISBN 978-1585621903.
95. Lobe, T.E. Perioperative hypnosis reduces hospitalization in patients undergoing the Nuss procedure for pectus excavatum. *J. Laparoendosc. Adv. Surg. Tech. A* **2006**, *16*, 639–642. [CrossRef] [PubMed]
96. Gruzelier, J.H. A working model of the neurophysiology of hypnosis: A review of the evidence. *Contemp. Hypn.* **1998**, *15*, 3–21. [CrossRef]
97. Jensen, M.P.; Patterson, D.R. Hypnotic approaches for chronic pain management: Clinical implications of recent research findings. *Am. Psychol.* **2014**, *69*, 167–177. [CrossRef]
98. Crawford, H.J.; Horton, J.E.; Harrington, G.C.; Vendemia, J.M.C.; Plantec, M.B.; Jung, S.; Shamro, C.; Downs, J.H., III. Hypnotic analgesia (Disattending pain) impacts neuronal network activation: An fMRI study of noxious somatosensory TENS stimuli. *Neuroimage* **1998**, *7*, S436. [CrossRef]
99. Rainville, P.; Duncan, G.H.; Price, D.D.; Carrier, B.; Bushnell, M.C. Pain affect encoded in human anterior cingulate but not somatosensory cortex. *Science* **1997**, *277*, 968–971. [CrossRef]
100. Montgomery, G.H.; DuHamel, K.N.; Redd, W.H. A meta-analysis of hypnotically induced analgesia: How effective is hypnosis? *Int. J. Clin. Exp. Hypn.* **2000**, *48*, 138–153. [CrossRef] [PubMed]
101. Adachi, T.; Fujino, H.; Nakae, A.; Mashimo, T.; Sasaki, J. A meta-analysis of hypnosis for chronic pain problems: A comparison between hypnosis, standard care, and other psychological interventions. *Int. J. Clin. Exp. Hypn.* **2014**, *62*, 1–28. [CrossRef] [PubMed]
102. Lambert, S.A. The effects of hypnosis/guided imagery on the postoperative course of children. *J. Dev. Behav. Pediatr.* **1996**, *17*, 307–310. [CrossRef] [PubMed]
103. Liossi, C.; Hatira, P. Clinical hypnosis versus cognitive behavioral training for pain management with pediatric cancer patients undergoing bone marrow aspirations. *Int. J. Clin. Exp. Hypn.* **1999**, *47*, 104–116. [CrossRef] [PubMed]
104. Vlieger, A.M.; Menko-Frankenhuis, C.; Wolfkamp, S.C.; Tromp, E.; Benninga, M.A. Hypnotherapy for children with functional abdominal pain or irritable bowel syndrome: A randomized controlled trial. *Gastroenterology* **2007**, *133*, 1430–1436. [CrossRef] [PubMed]
105. Vlieger, A.M.; Rutten, J.M.; Govers, A.M.; Frankenhuis, C.; Benninga, M.A. Long-term follow-up of gut-directed hypnotherapy vs. standard care in children with functional abdominal pain or irritable bowel syndrome. *Am. J. Gastroenterol.* **2012**, *107*, 627–631. [CrossRef]
106. Anbar, R.D. Self-hypnosis for the treatment of functional abdominal pain in childhood. *Clin. Pediatr. (Phila)* **2001**, *40*, 447–451. [CrossRef]
107. Olness, K. Imagery (self-hypnosis) as adjunct therapy in childhood cancer: Clinical experience with 25 patients. *Am. J. Pediatr. Hematol. Oncol.* **1981**, *3*, 313–321.

108. Kohen, D.P.; Zajac, R. Self-hypnosis training for headaches in children and adolescents. *J. Pediatr.* **2007**, *150*, 635–639. [CrossRef]
109. Olness, K.; MacDonald, J.T.; Uden, D.L. Comparison of self-hypnosis and propranolol in the treatment of juvenile classic migraine. *Pediatrics* **1987**, *79*, 593–597.
110. Lin, Y.C.; Wan, L.; Jamison, R.N. Using integrative medicine in pain management: An evaluation of current evidence. *Anesth. Analg.* **2017**, *125*, 2081–2093. [CrossRef]
111. Hui, K.K.; Liu, J.; Marina, O.; Napadow, V.; Haselgrove, C.; Kwong, K.K.; Kennedy, D.N.; Makris, N. The integrated response of the human cerebro-cerebellar and limbic systems to acupuncture stimulation at ST 36 as evidenced by fMRI. *Neuroimage* **2005**, *27*, 479–496. [CrossRef]
112. Napadow, V.; Kettner, N.; Liu, J.; Li, M.; Kwong, K.K.; Vangel, M.; Makris, N.; Audette, J.; Hui, K.K. Hypothalamus and amygdala response to acupuncture stimuli in Carpal Tunnel Syndrome. *Pain* **2007**, *130*, 254–266. [CrossRef] [PubMed]
113. Wang, S.M.; Kain, Z.N.; White, P. Acupuncture analgesia: I. The scientific basis. *Anesth. Analg.* **2008**, *106*, 602–610. [CrossRef] [PubMed]
114. Oke, S.L.; Tracey, K.J. The inflammatory reflex and the role of complementary and alternative medical therapies. *Ann. N. Y. Acad. Sci.* **2009**, *1172*, 172–180. [CrossRef] [PubMed]
115. Chavan, S.S.; Tracey, K.J. Regulating innate immunity with dopamine and electroacupuncture. *Nat. Med.* **2014**, *20*, 239–241. [CrossRef] [PubMed]
116. NIH consensus conference: Acupuncture. *JAMA* **1998**, *280*, 1518–1524. [CrossRef]
117. Haake, M.; Muller, H.H.; Schade-Brittinger, C.; Basler, H.D.; Schafer, H.; Maier, C.; Endres, H.G.; Trampisch, H.J.; Molsberger, A. German Acupuncture Trials (GERAC) for chronic low back pain: Randomized, multicenter, blinded, parallel-group trial with 3 groups. *Arch. Intern. Med.* **2007**, *167*, 1892–1898. [CrossRef]
118. Zhao, L.; Chen, J.; Li, Y.; Sun, X.; Chang, X.; Zheng, H.; Gong, B.; Huang, Y.; Yang, M.; Wu, X.; et al. The long-term effect of acupuncture for migraine prophylaxis: A randomized clinical trial. *JAMA Intern. Med.* **2017**, *177*, 508–515. [CrossRef]
119. Berman, B.M.; Lao, L.; Langenberg, P.; Lee, W.L.; Gilpin, A.M.; Hochberg, M.C. Effectiveness of acupuncture as adjunctive therapy in osteoarthritis of the knee: A randomized, controlled trial. *Ann. Intern. Med* **2004**, *141*, 901–910. [CrossRef]
120. Golianu, B.; Yeh, A.M.; Brooks, M. Acupuncture for pediatric pain. *Children (Basel)* **2014**, *1*, 134–148. [CrossRef] [PubMed]
121. Lin, Y.C.; Tassone, R.F.; Jahng, S.; Rahbar, R.; Holzman, R.S.; Zurakowski, D.; Sethna, N.F. Acupuncture management of pain and emergence agitation in children after bilateral myringotomy and tympanostomy tube insertion. *Paediatr. Anaesth.* **2009**, *19*, 1096–1101. [CrossRef] [PubMed]
122. Tsao, G.J.; Messner, A.H.; Seybold, J.; Sayyid, Z.N.; Cheng, A.G.; Golianu, B. Intraoperative acupuncture for posttonsillectomy pain: A randomized, double-blind, placebo-controlled trial. *Laryngoscope* **2015**, *125*, 1972–1978. [CrossRef] [PubMed]
123. Raith, W.; Schmolzer, G.M.; Resch, B.; Reiterer, F.; Avian, A.; Koestenberger, M.; Urlesberger, B. Laser acupuncture for neonatal abstinence syndrome: A randomized controlled trial. *Pediatrics* **2015**, *136*, 876–884. [CrossRef] [PubMed]
124. Gottschling, S.; Meyer, S.; Gribova, I.; Distler, L.; Berrang, J.; Gortner, L.; Graf, N.; Shamdeen, M.G. Laser acupuncture in children with headache: A double blind, randomized, bicenter, placebo-controlled trial *Pain* **2008**, *137*, 405–412. [CrossRef] [PubMed]
125. Wayne, P.M.; Kerr, C.E.; Schnyer, R.N.; Legedza, A.T.; Savetsky-German, J.; Shields, M.H.; Buring, J.E.; Davis, R.B.; Conboy, L.A.; Highfield, E.; et al. Japanese-style acupuncture for endometriosis-related pelvic pain in adolescents and young women: Results of a randomized sham-controlled trial. *J. Pediatr. Adolesc. Gynecol.* **2008**, *21*, 247–257. [CrossRef] [PubMed]
126. Logan, D.E.; Carpino, E.A.; Chiang, G.; Condon, M.; Firn, E.; Gaughan, V.J.; Hogan, M.; Leslie, D.S.; Olson, K.; Sager, S.; et al. A day-hospital approach to treatment of pediatric complex regional pain syndrome: Initial functional outcomes. *Clin. J. Pain* **2012**, *28*, 766–774. [CrossRef]

127. Simons, L.E.; Sieberg, C.B.; Pielech, M.; Conroy, C.; Logan, D.E. What does it take? Comparing intensive rehabilitation to outpatient treatment for children with significant pain-related disability. *J. Pediatr. Psychol.* **2013**, *38*, 213–223. [CrossRef]

128. American Pain Society. Pain in Infants, Children, and Adolescents SIG. Available online: http://americanpainsociety.org/get-involved/shared-interest-groups/pediatric-adolescent-pain (accessed on 1 December 2018).

6

Pediatric Integrative Medicine: Vision for the Future

Anna Esparham [1,*], Sanghamitra M. Misra [2], Erica Sibinga [3], Timothy Culbert [4], Kathi Kemper [5], Hilary McClafferty [6], Sunita Vohra [7] and Lawrence Rosen [8]

1 Division of Child Neurology-Headache Section, Children's Mercy Hospital, University of Missouri School of Medicine-Kansas City, Kansas City, MO 64108, USA
2 Mobile Clinic Program, Texas Children's Hospital, Baylor College of Medicine, Houston, TX 77054, USA; smisra@bcm.edu
3 Department of Pediatrics, Johns Hopkins School of Medicine, Baltimore, MD 21205, USA; esibinga@jhmi.edu
4 Integrative Medicine, Prairie Care, University of Minnesota Medical School, Chaska, MN 55318, USA; tculbert@prairie-care.com
5 Department of Pediatrics, College of Medicine, Ohio State University, Columbus, OH 43210, USA; kathi.kemper@osumc.edu
6 Department of Medicine, Arizona Center for Integrative Medicine, University of Arizona, Tucson, AZ 85724, USA; hmcclafferty@email.arizona.edu
7 Integrative Health Institute, CARE Program, PedCAM Network, Department of Pediatrics, Medicine, and Psychiatry, Faculty of Medicine and Dentistry, University of Alberta, Edmonton, AB T6G 2C8, Canada; svohra@ualberta.ca
8 Whole Child Center, Oradell, NJ 07649, USA; ldrdoc@alum.mit.edu
* Correspondence: aeesparham@cmh.edu

Abstract: Pediatric integrative medicine (PIM) is of significant interest to patients, with 12% of the general pediatric population and up to 80% of children with chronic conditions using PIM approaches. The field of PIM has evolved over the past 25 years, approaching child health with a number of guiding principles: preventive, context-centered, relationship-based, personalized, participatory, and ecologically sustainable. This manuscript reviews important time points for the field of PIM and reports on a series of meetings of PIM leaders, aimed at assessing the state of the field and planning for its future. Efforts in the first decade of the 2000s led to increased visibility in academic and professional pediatric organizations and through international listservs, designed to link those interested in and practicing PIM, all of which continue to flourish. The PIM leadership summits in recent years resulted in specific goals to advance PIM further in the following key areas: research, clinical practice, professional education, patient and family education, and advocacy and partnerships. Additionally, goals were developed for greater expansion of PIM professional education, broader support for pediatric PIM research, and an expanded role for PIM approaches in the provision of pediatric care.

Keywords: pediatric integrative medicine; vision; clinical practice; education; advocacy; complementary therapies

1. Introduction

Integrative medicine is defined as relationship-centered care that focuses on the whole person, is informed by evidence, and makes use of all appropriate therapeutic approaches, healthcare professionals and disciplines to achieve optimal health and healing, including evidence-based complementary and alternative medicine. Pediatric integrative medicine (PIM) develops and promotes this approach within the field of pediatrics [1,2].

The field of pediatrics is at a crossroads. The health of our children—our future—is at stake. The prevalence rates of myriad chronic pediatric health conditions continue to rise at an unprecedented pace [3,4]. Chronic health conditions contribute to the global burden of disability [5]. Historically, the conventional solution has favored a 'disease-treatment system' that often incentivizes more invasive care at higher cost, an approach poorly aligned with the needs of today's children. Health care transformation is no longer optional; it is an absolute imperative. Advocates and stakeholders in search of better health care require new approaches to meet the complex health challenges faced by children. We are searching for safer and more cost-effective paradigms to optimize the health and well-being of children everywhere. Multidisciplinary healthcare models that implement integrative and complementary therapies for patients with chronic illness have shown improved clinical outcomes and quality of life [6,7]. In addition, health outcomes are improved through patient empowerment [8,9]. Integrative medicine promotes relationship-centered care and empowers individuals to incorporate wellness strategies such as improving nutrition, physical activity, and sleep hygiene.

Pediatric integrative medicine (PIM) represents an evolution in pediatric care, a paradigm that embodies a philosophy consistent with long-standing holistic principles of quality medical care. As Dr. Kathi Kemper noted in her Presidential Address to the Ambulatory Pediatric Association nearly 20 years ago, "Holistic medicine is really just good medicine. It means caring for the whole child in the context of that child's values, their family's beliefs, their family system, and their culture in the larger community, and considering a range of therapies based on the evidence of their benefits and cost" [10] (p. 214).

PIM is defined by several core guiding principles [2,11]:

- Preventive: True primary care pediatrics is proactive rather than reactive. Prescribing lifestyle solutions to prevent disease is generally preferable to costly and potentially risky treatments. Lifestyle prescriptions may include food, activity, nature, creativity, rest, mindfulness, and connection with others.
- Context-centered: Children must be nurtured within the context of healthy families, communities, and schools. Health in mind, body, and spirit depends on how suitable the environment is for the child.
- Relationship-based: Only through open communication and building trust are we best able to work together to ensure each child's optimal health. The connection between health professionals and families has its own healing potential.
- Personalized: Health is not a one-size-fits-all proposition. Each child carries a unique potential based on a complex interplay of genetic and environmental factors. There is no medical treatment that can be guaranteed as safe for 100% of any population. Each family has the inherent right to make health care decisions for their children, keeping in mind the best interests of the child as well as legitimate public health concerns that ethically inform these decisions.
- Participatory: Creating health should be a collaborative process, actively encouraging participation and putting children and families back in control of their own health. Patient-centered care creates hope and empowers families to make sustainable changes, inspiring children to create the future they deserve.
- Ecologically sustainable: How we practice healthcare affects the environment, which has a measurable and cyclical impact on our health. The health and well-being of all the Earth's inhabitants are intimately tied to the health of our planet.
- Evidence-informed: Therapies that are evidence-informed while using the safety-effectiveness rubric (Figure 1) are considered as part of the treatment plan.

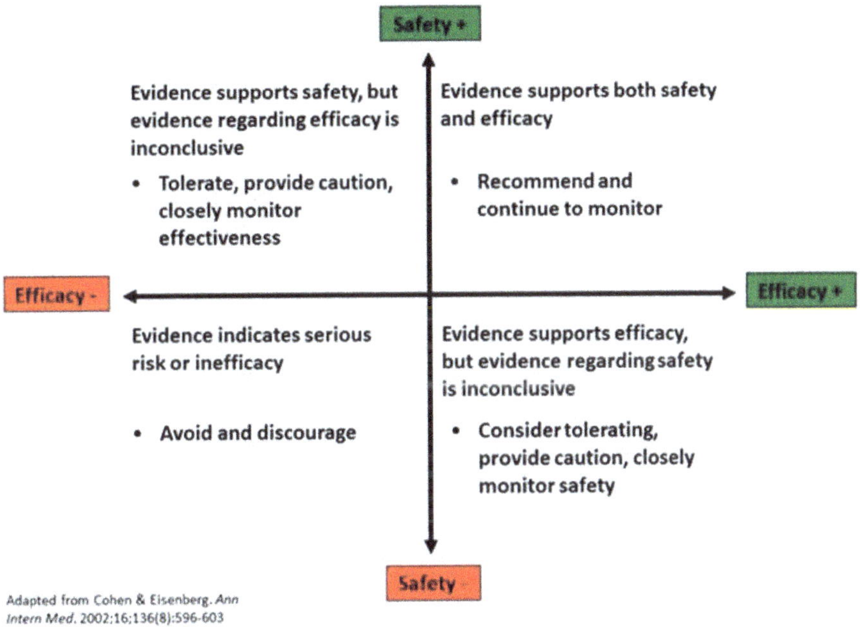

Figure 1. Safety–effectiveness therapy evaluation rubric.

2. Background

The field of PIM has developed organically over the last 25 years owing to pressing need and interest from pediatric health professionals, parents, and children. We have clear and compelling data that complementary therapies are of great interest to parents [12]. Use of these therapies in pediatrics is significant, as the 2012 National Health Interview Survey revealed that 12% of children use complementary therapies [13]. Studies in specific chronically ill populations have reported complementary therapy use in up to 80% of study participants [14,15]. We use the term "complementary" specifically to delineate these therapies from those offered within conventional Western medical care systems. PIM, by definition, embodies the integration of complementary therapies with conventional pediatric health care in a way that is informed by best available evidence and centered on the individual patient and family. Truly effective and safe patient-centered care demands that we talk with our patients about therapies of interest to them and know where to find evidence to inform these conversations.

Critics maintain that integrative therapies do not have sufficient evidence to support their use in pediatric populations. We recognize that all health interventions would benefit from more high quality pediatric research to assess both effectiveness and safety. We do not agree that, by definition, all conventional care is evidence-based and that complementary therapies, by definition, lack evidence, or else they would be incorporated as part of conventional care. Research published in reputable journals has shown over the last 30 years that myriad complementary therapies are safe and effective for a variety of pediatric conditions and symptoms. Pediatric health professionals are encouraged to ask their patients and families about complementary therapy use [12]. In a national survey sent to members of the American Academy of Pediatrics (AAP), most pediatric healthcare professionals (87%) had been asked about complementary and alternative (CAM) therapies by a patient/parent within three months of the survey [16]. In addition, over 80% of the pediatric healthcare professionals desired additional information on CAM, with fewer than 5% reporting being knowledgeable about individual CAM therapies [16]. Of the whether or not professionals 'believe' in these therapies is immaterial;

patient-centered care and patient safety demand that professionals know what health approaches are being used and considered. Health professionals must remember that evidence-informed medicine is a triad: best available evidence, clinical experience, and patient preference [17]. Dr. Kathi Kemper and Mr. Cohen, JD, MBA, MFA published a now well-established rubric to evaluate the use of therapies [18], see Figure 1.

As demonstrated in the graphic, use of therapies should be recommended if the intervention is known to be safe and effective based on best available evidence. If the therapy is known to be safe but efficacy has not yet been conclusively established, it is reasonable to tolerate use while monitoring response. If a therapy is known to be effective but its safety is questionable, after a careful informed consent discussion, use may be considered if monitored closely. Finally, a therapy is to be avoided and discouraged if it has no proven efficacy and known adverse effects. Relative risks and benefits should always be considered in light of best available evidence, and professionals can use the graphic to help guide decision-making in collaboration with patients and families. It is important to note that this rubric applies to all therapies—not just those deemed complementary—as complementary therapies may not apply to all pediatric conditions.

We recognize there are pediatric health professionals who would like to know how to discuss and apply these therapies in clinical practice, where to seek further training, and when to refer patients for these therapies. In addition, several barriers may exist for both professionals and families, such as adequate coverage of therapies and availability of PIM resources for the underserved or for those living in resource-poor locations [19,20]. The PIM Leadership Initiative (PIMLI) has developed this position statement to provide a unified vision for PIM to meet the needs of professionals in the service of pediatric patients and families. As PIM is still growing, although 20 years old, providing structure and vision is imperative for the continued, sustainable development of the field.

3. Evolution of Pediatric Integrative Medicine

The field of PIM has evolved tremendously over the past two decades. The sentinel events that have shaped the current PIM landscape are noted below.

Pediatric integrative medicine timeline, 1995–2017:

- 1995 Ambulatory Pediatric Association establishes Holistic Pediatrics Special Interest Group
- 1996 "The Holistic Pediatrician" published (Kemper)
- 1998 Boston Children's Hospital establishes Center for Holistic Pediatric Education and Research
- 1999 First PIM Conference hosted by University of Arizona; Dr. Kemper's APA Presidential Address (*Holistic Pediatrics = Good Medicine*)
- 2000 Second PIM Conference hosted by Children's Hospitals and Clinics (Minneapolis) and University of Minnesota, AAP Task Force on CAM established and AAP NCE CAM sessions start
- 2004 First PIMLI Summit in St. Paul, MN; Pediatric Complementary and Alternative Medicine Research & Education (PedCAM) Network (Vohra) and International Pediatric Integrative Medicine (IPIM) Network (Rosen) started
- 2005 AAP Provisional Section on Complementary, Holistic, and Integrative Medicine (CHIM) and Integrative Pediatrics Council (IPC) established
- 2005–2008 International PIM/Pangea conferences hosted by IPC
- 2006 *Pediatrics in Review* series on PIM debuts (Vohra, editor)
- 2007 *Pediatric Clinics of North America* volume on PIM published (Rosen, Riley ed.)
- 2008 AAP Section on CHIM official (name later changed to Section on Complementary and Integrative Medicine, or SOCIM); *The Use of Complementary and Alternative Medicine in Pediatrics* AAP Clinical Report published in *Pediatrics*, IPC dissolves
- 2009 "Textbook on Integrative Pediatrics" published (Culbert, Olness ed.)
- 2012 PIM program survey published (*Pediatric integrative medicine: pediatrics' newest subspecialty?* Vohra S, et al.); University of Arizona Center for Integrative Medicine launches Pediatric

Integrative Medicine in Residency (PIMR) curriculum; AAP SOCIM name changed to Section on Integrative Medicine (SOIM)
- 2014 *Physician Health and Wellness* AAP Clinical Report published in *Pediatrics*; inaugural AAP SOIM Pioneer Award given to Dr. Kemper; "A Guide to Integrative Pediatrics" textbook published (Misra, Verissimo)
- 2015 PIMLI Summit II in Boston, MA
- 2016 PIMLI Summit III in Hackensack, NJ; "The Holistic Pediatrician, 20th Anniversary Edition" published (Kemper); *Mind-Body Therapies in Children and Youth* AAP Clinical Report published in *Pediatrics*
- 2017 "Integrative Pediatrics: Art, Science, and Clinical Application" textbook published (McClafferty)

All events are listed to the best of the PIMLI's Summit collective knowledge and may not include all international PIM events.

As noted, the first official meeting of PIM leaders in the United States was held in 2004 and termed the Pediatric Integrative Medicine Leadership Initiative (PIMLI) Summit. The first PIMLI Summit spawned several major initiatives: A Section on Integrative Medicine within the AAP, an interprofessional PIM nonprofit (the IPC), and two international online resources (the IPIM-Network and PedCAM). These entities spearheaded numerous educational programs, including (1) PIM content at the AAP's National Conferences and Pangea PIM Conferences; (2) publication of key PIM books and scholarly articles; and (3) the establishment of the PIM in Residency (PIMR) training program. The decade of significant progress following this first PIMLI Summit coupled with the desire to nurture sustainable growth in the field prompted PIM leaders to systemically revisit the vision for the future of PIM [2,21,22].

4. 2015 PIMLI Summit

Supported by a generous grant from the Marino Health Foundation, Drs. Kathi Kemper and Lawrence Rosen—in partnership with the AAP—developed the second PIMLI Summit held in Boston, MA in June 2015 to accomplish the following objectives: (1) develop a long-term vision for PIM addressing gaps and future needs for clinical, educational, research, and advocacy domains; and (2) develop future PIM leaders who can achieve the vision through practical strategies and partnerships.

A group of fifteen PIM leaders from the United States and Canada were invited to attend the Summit. These physicians had a varying range of expertise in PIM with different stages of career development, and practiced in a variety of settings. They also represented the AAP Section on Integrative Medicine, Academy of Integrative Health and Medicine, University of Arizona Pediatric Integrative Medicine in Residency program, various North American pediatric academic programs, and the PedCAM and IPIM Networks. An intentional effort was made to incorporate a balance of early career and established leaders. Representatives from many other professions and partner organizations were consulted during meeting preparation to optimize long-term sustainability and success and to embody the interprofessional philosophy inherent in integrative care. Specifically, with organizational support by John Weeks, a pioneer in collaborative interprofessional IM efforts over several decades, representatives from the Academic Collaborative for Integrative Health (ACIH) participated in a comprehensive pre-Summit survey.

4.1. Professional Pre-Summit Survey Summary

In May 2015, more than 30 integrative health professionals provided feedback on the definition of integrative medicine, the state of child health, and a vision for PIM through a pre-Summit survey developed by Drs. Kemper and Rosen (unpublished data). In addition to pediatricians, these professionals represented expertise in Ayurvedic Medicine, botanical medicine, chiropractic, education, energy medicine, family medicine, health policy, massage therapy, mental health, naturopathy, Traditional Chinese Medicine, and yoga. Drs. Kemper and Rosen coordinated a conference call with John Weeks and a specially-designed 15-member interprofessional task force to discuss the survey and provide guidance for the Summit. A wordcloud (Figure 2) was created from stakeholder comments about what integrative medicine meant to them (unpublished data).

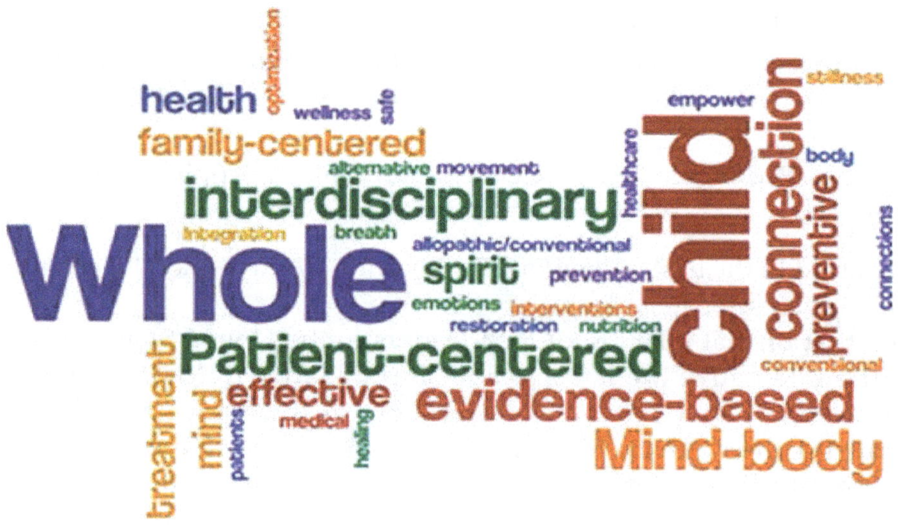

Figure 2. What does integrative medicine mean to you?

Regarding the current state of children's health, respondents noted that while pediatric acute care is 'good', both the quality and quantity of medical care for children and youth with chronic conditions often is not optimal. Survey participants felt the current conventional health care system is failing to adequately address the rising prevalence of chronic illnesses in children. They believed there is a need for a larger workforce of PIM health professionals to meet the challenges of complex childhood conditions while also promoting wellness. They also highlighted the importance of educating families about lifestyle approaches including healthy nutrition, physical activity, sleep, and stress coping skills. A need for more effective advocacy for improving children's health globally was mentioned, including a push for healthier modes of transportation, sustainable agriculture and food sources, and addressing health related environmental factors.

When asked how pediatricians can more effectively work with other stakeholders to best serve children's needs, survey participants responded that collaboration with other health professionals, parent groups, third-party payers, and community organizations is key. PIM stakeholders' vision for what pediatric integrative medicine would look like in 10 years included the wish that "decisions regarding a child's healthcare would be made from an integrative perspective, taking all possible healthcare options into account". Pediatric clinics would provide integrative care as part of the medical home with respect for all members of the patient's health care team. In addition, schools that train health professionals will incorporate integrative medicine training and provide interprofessional learning environments to build trust and facilitate patient-centered collaborative care. Finally, increased public and private funding would be available to support the investigation of all evidence-informed approaches that are personalized to the individual, given their health, preferences, and goals.

4.2. Parent Survey Summary

Parents are key PIM stakeholders and, therefore, a national parent online survey was conducted just prior to the PIMLI Summit to guide the meeting, with the logistical support of Kiwi Magazine, a publication focused on healthy lifestyle approaches for families. A sample of 1500 parents solicited through Kiwi's Moms Meet network (https://momsmeet.com, unpublished data) answered questions regarding their knowledge of PIM, PIM therapies they'd like to see offered in pediatric practices, and their willingness to advocate for insurance coverage of PIM therapies. Of note, even in this sample of natural health oriented parents, nearly one in four respondents were not familiar with IM. Fewer than one in seven definitively consider their pediatrician integrative while approximately 60% of parents believe having an integrative pediatrician for their children is important. Information about therapies is most commonly found online, and the two most desired in-office therapies are nutritional counseling and behavioral/mental health services. Key survey findings are shown in Figure 3a–d below.

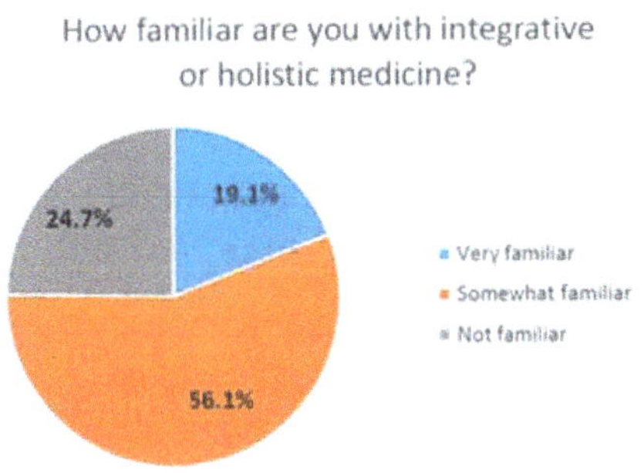

(a)

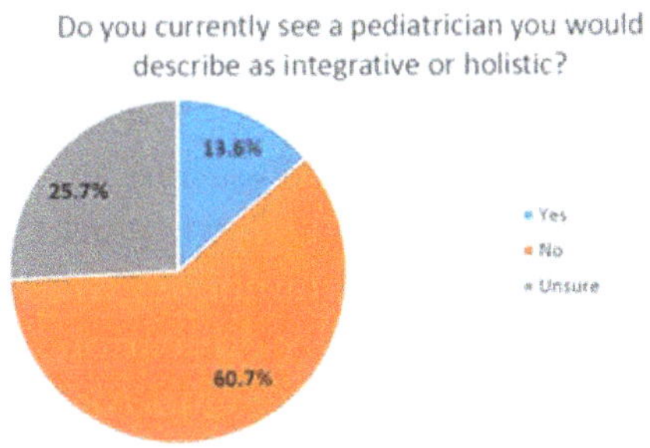

(b)

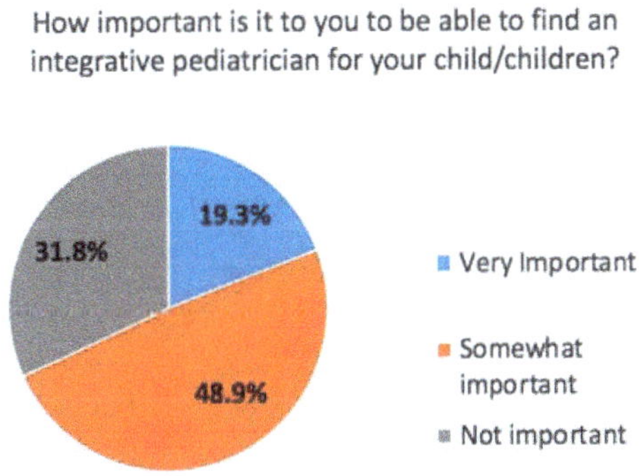

(c)

Figure 3. *Cont.*

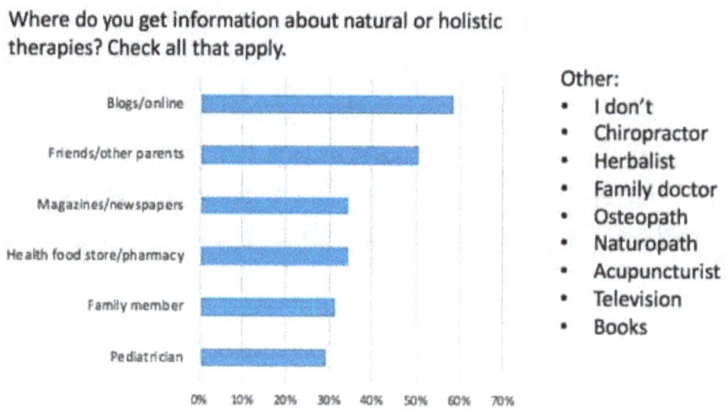

(d)

Figure 3. (**a**) Parent response to question "how familiar are you with integrative or holistic medicine?" Answer options included: very familiar, somewhat familiar, and not familiar; (**b**) Parent response to question "do you currently see a pediatrician you would describe as integrative or holistic?" Answer options included: yes, no, and unsure; (**c**) Parent response to question "how important is it to you to be able to find an integrative pediatrician for your child/children?" Answer options included: very important, somewhat important, and not important; (**d**) Parent response to question "where do you get information about natural or holistic therapies?" Answer options included all options that applied to parents: blogs/websites, friends/other parents, magazines/newspapers, health food store/pharmacy, family member, pediatrician, and other (as outlined above).

4.3. 2015 PIMLI Summit Summary

At the opening of the 2015 Summit, the 15 PIM leaders in attendance reviewed the professional survey as well as the evolution of the field to date. Using a World Café meeting paradigm, participants explored five strategic domains critical to the sustainable growth of the PIM field: research, clinical practice, professional education, patient and family education, and advocacy and partnerships [23]. Small groups were tasked with describing the existing gaps for each domain with specific strategies to address those gaps. The whole group then worked to clarify gaps and strategies to identify realistic and specific action steps to address each domain.

The following strategies were ultimately identified within each domain:

Research

- Expand the AAP Section on Integrative Medicine research and education grant program.
- Explore the development of a multi-center PIM research network.
- Publish PIM research articles in mainstream academic journals.

Clinical practice

- Promote use of existing quality clinical resources such as *Pediatrics in Review* articles, special issues in professional journals, well-designed research trials on complementary therapies, and integrative pediatrics textbooks.
- Compile and distribute sample encounter forms, handouts, and smart phrases for electronic health records to support PIM clinical care.
- Develop an interprofessional online clinical resource repository.

Professional education

- Maximize distribution and utilization of PIM residency curriculum and fellowship programs.

- Facilitate a regularly occurring interprofessional conference to advance PIM education, leadership development, and to embrace and grow the PIM community.
- Present PIM content at pediatric subspecialty meetings and other health professional conferences, including those targeting the underserved.
- Participate in initiatives to address policy development for modern health problems such as chronic pain and opioid addiction that significantly impact children.

Patient and Family Education

- Develop multilingual descriptions of PIM therapies in child-friendly language.
- Increase PIM content on the AAP's parent information website (healthychildren.org) by adapting existing *Pediatrics in Review* articles.
- Develop an online video series featuring children and families discussing integrative care success stories.
- Develop a robust library of PIM patient handouts for widespread use in the clinical setting.

Advocacy and Partnerships

- Establish an online presence to serve as a strong independent voice advocating for PIM as mainstream pediatric healthcare, including a repository for research, clinical, and educational resources.
- Partner with disease-specific organizations to spread knowledge of PIM therapies that may improve quality of life for their stakeholders.
- Cultivate strong relationships with specialties also serving children, such as family medicine, medicine/pediatrics, and obstetrics/gynecology.
- Work with federal and state organizations to develop and promote preventive lifestyle policies for children and families.
- Contribute to resource development and advocacy efforts that support payment for PIM services and models of care.
- Explore sustainable resources for philanthropy to support ongoing growth of the field.

The group noted that these are considerable tasks and that an organization does not currently exist to oversee and coordinate all of these strategies. Meeting participants unanimously expressed a strong desire to explore the creation of an ongoing, sustainable PIMLI leadership group to coordinate this work. Immediate next steps were debated, leading to the development of specific action plans related to the above strategies and the delegation to participants. Finally, meeting participants prioritized the following activities most needing financial support:

- Sustainable support for the AAP SOIM research and education grant program.
- Re-printing and redistribution of the "Talk with Your Doctor" PIM poster (http://www.cpsp.cps.ca/uploads/publications/Posters-CAM.pdf) to pediatricians.
- Establishment of a new organization as the independent voice advocating for PIM as mainstream pediatric health care, engaging and nurturing current and future leaders of the PIM movement.

The first two activities were delegated to the AAP SOIM Executive Committee. A PIMLI steering committee was formed to pursue the third priority.

5. 2016 PIMLI Summit

With additional generous funding by the Marino Health Foundation, members of the PIMLI steering committee met in July 2016 at the Hackensack University Medical Center in New Jersey to further discuss the establishment of a new organization to coordinate PIM initiatives. In preparation for this meeting, key PIM stakeholders were consulted via an online survey to assess current community needs (unpublished data). Survey participants were recruited from two professional listservs: the IPIM Network and the AAP Section on Integrative Medicine listserv.

2016 Professional Survey Highlights

- A total 93 health professionals completed the survey.
- Approximately 75% identified as pediatricians (MD/DO) with a total of 17 professional disciplines represented.
- Approximately 50% had been in practice more than 20 years, and more than 80% had been in practice more than 10 years.
- Over 75% stated that currently available PIM resources online are not sufficient to support their pediatric practice.
- The top two most valuable current online PIM resources were the two listservs noted above; no current website was rated as valuable by more than 25% of respondents.

Conversations with key stakeholders and advisors confirmed the need and desire for an independent organization focused specifically on PIM education and advocacy, directed at the broad 'middle' of the professional and consumer populations. Challenges identified included: (1) prioritizing PIM both within a larger pediatric organization and within a larger integrative organization; (2) securing funding for administrative support given the significant ongoing clinical, research, and educational commitments of PIM leadership—creating a balanced interprofessional leadership group; and (3) nurturing leadership development to ensure sustainability of the organization. Understanding these obstacles, the PIMLI steering committee evaluated and debated potential partners to host this initiative, concluding that no existing group ideally met our needs. They proposed exploration of hosting an independent nonprofit organization as the first option. Paramount to the success of this organization would be the design and launch of a robust multimedia website that serves as a hub for all PIM activities, including:

- Membership for pediatric healthcare professionals providing specialized access to educational and community-building resources, including integrating existing interprofessional and international PIM networks (IPIM Network, PedCAM network).
- Consumer and policymaker engagement via media tools and the development of short promotional videos profiling PIM "success stories".
- Educational and Research Resource Repository, including professional presentations and a searchable PIM publication bibliography.
- Continuing education online conferences and webinars.
- Professional consultative service assisting the development of academic PIM centers and clinical practices.
- Coordination of PIM efforts with the AAP SOIM and other reputable national/international organizations.

Organizational structure and funding needs were discussed including potential funding partners and self-sustainable sources of support and leadership. Given the huge scope of the proposed activities above and the clearly expressed needs in the 2016 professional survey, the scope was initially narrowed to online PIM professional education, because opportunities to fill the gap of online educational resources currently exist. At this time, PIM education exists through the University of Arizona Center for Integrative Medicine: Pediatric Integrative Medicine in Residency (PIMR) curriculum for pediatric resident physicians, various continuing education conferences, and online resources [24]. The PIMR program consists of a 100-h online educational curriculum initially piloted in five diverse pediatric residency training programs in the United States. In 2016, the PIMR program had grown to include more than 500 residents nationally and internationally in nine residency programs. Of note, the PIMR program is specifically limited to pediatric resident physicians. The AAP SOIM sponsors PIM educational sessions each year at the AAP National Conference to a broader group of pediatricians, though these sessions are not accessible to many other PIM professional groups nor to nonmembers of the AAP. Ultimately, collaborative efforts to reinforce interactive and online curricula at various steps during training and practice may help to meet the demand for therapeutic options that are safe, effective, and aligned with patients' values. A comprehensive, accessible online professional PIM education hub would be optimally situated to meet the needs of the larger PIM community.

6. Vision for the Future

Based on work at the 2015 and 2016 Summits, long-range visions for PIM's next decade are outlined:

- PIM exemplifies a mainstream model of comprehensive care that emphasizes a personalized, participatory, and evidence-informed approach to the whole child.
- PIM emphasizes preventive health, understanding of the etiology of underlying illness, and exploration of all appropriate treatment options to optimize health and well-being.
- PIM promotes a cohesive, respectful, and interprofessional team approach focused on the well-being of the child as a growing, developing individual in the context of the family.
- Professionals collaborate across disciplines and geographic boundaries in advocating for the needs of patients and families from all socioeconomic and cultural backgrounds.
- Integrative professionals embrace self-care as a cornerstone of health.
- Integrative professionals support identification of and access to reliable PIM educational, clinical, and research resources for all those interested in maximizing patient health and wellness.

To achieve this vision, proposed tangible outcomes include:

- Establishment of an international and interprofessional pediatric group to coordinate and advance the work of PIM in collaboration with the AAP SOIM. This two-pronged approach ultimately represents the optimal strategy to ensure the sustainable growth, evolution, and impact of PIM within the field of Pediatrics.
- Medical schools, residencies, and other professional training programs teach PIM routinely and widely.
- Hospitals, clinics, and academic centers promote co-located PIM services (e.g., credentialing nurses and/or other providers and staff in biofeedback, aromatherapy, clinical hypnosis, etc.).
- Pediatric training programs implementing the PIMR curriculum and PIM fellowship programs experience high enrollment and active participation of alumni.
- A yearly interprofessional symposium is established and brings together PIM professionals for collaborative learning.
- PIM materials (e.g., description of therapies, licensing/credentialing information, clinical guidance, patient educational materials, research summaries, and updates) are compiled and hosted on an independent website for ready access by professionals, patients, and institutions.
- PIM research is adequately funded to develop the science of utilization, safety, efficacy, and cost-effectiveness of PIM therapies, and a multi-center research network is established to facilitate the acquisition of this knowledge.
- Safe, effective, and cost-effective PIM therapies and health care systems receive endorsement from national organizations, hospital leadership, and other decision makers to judiciously expand PIM as appropriate.

Author Contributions: A.E., S.M.M., and L.R. were the authors responsible for the conceptualization and writing of this manuscript; E.S., T.C., K.K., H.M., and S.V. contributed to the writing and editing of this manuscript.

Acknowledgments: The Pediatric Integrative Medicine Leadership Initiative would like foremost to thank the Marino Health Foundation for its generous support of the 2015 and 2016 Summits and related work. The PIMLI would also like to acknowledge the American Academy of Pediatrics, in particular Teri Salus and Anne Gramiak, for their logistical support coordinating and facilitating the 2015 PIMLI Summit. PIMLI leaders are extremely grateful to John Weeks and the ACIH committee who helped in preparation for the 2015 Summit, and to *Kiwi Magazine* and the Moms Meet Network for assistance with the 2015 Parent Survey. Finally, the PIMLI group thanks the members of the PIM community who participated in the 2015 and 2016 professional surveys. Thank you to all the PIMLI leaders involved, in addition to the authors: Michelle Bailey, David Becker, Anu French, Scott Shannon, David M. Steinhorn, Minal Vazirani, and Ana Maria Verissimo.

References

1. Academic Consortium for Integrative Medicine and Health. Available online: https://imconsortium.org/about/introduction/ (accessed on 27 August 2018).
2. Vohra, S.; Surette, S.; Mittra, D.; Rossen, L.D.; Gardiner, P.; Kemper, J.K. Pediatric integrative medicine: Pediatrics' newest subspecialty? *BMC Pediatr.* **2012**, *15*, 12–123. [CrossRef] [PubMed]
3. National Center for Health Statistics. *Health United States with Chartbook on Trends in the Health of Americans*; Table 58. Md; National Center for Health Statistics: Hyattsville, MA, USA, 2006.
4. Perrin, J.M.; Bloom, S.R.; Gortmaker, S.L. The increase of childhood chronic conditions in the United States. *JAMA* **2007**, *27*, 2755–2759. [CrossRef] [PubMed]
5. GBD 2015 DALYs and HALE Collaborators. Global, regional, and National disability-adjusted life-years (DALYs) for 315 diseases and injuries and healthy life expectancy (HALE), 1990–2015: A systematic analysis for the Global Burden of Disease Study 2015. *Lancet* **2016**, *8*, 1603–1658. [CrossRef]
6. Rabin, J.; Brown, M.; Alexander, S. Update in the treatment of chronic pain with pediatric patients. *Curr. Probl. Pediatr. Adolesc. Health Care* **2017**, *47*, 167–172. [CrossRef] [PubMed]
7. Jacobs, H.; Gladstein, J. Pediatric headache: A clinical review. *Headache* **2012**, *52*, 333–339. [CrossRef] [PubMed]
8. Powers, T.L.; Bendall, D. Improving health outcomes through patient empowerment. *J. Hosp. Mark. Public Relat.* **2003**, *15*, 45–59. [CrossRef]
9. Maizes, V.; Rakel, D.; Niemiec, C. Integrative medicine and patient-centered care. *Explore* **2009**, *5*, 277–289. [CrossRef] [PubMed]
10. Kemper, K.J. Holistic pediatrics = good medicine. *Pediatrics* **2001**, *105*, 214–218.
11. Becker, D.K. Pediatric Integrative Medicine. *Prim. Care* **2017**, *44*, 337–350. [CrossRef] [PubMed]
12. Kemper, K.J.; Vohra, S.; Walls, R.; Task Force on Complementary and Alternative Medicine; Provisional Section on Complementary, Holistic, and Integrative Medicine. American Academy of Pediatrics. The use of complementary and alternative medicine in pediatrics. *Pediatrics* **2008**, *122*, 1374–1386. [CrossRef] [PubMed]
13. NCCIH Children and the Use of Complementary Health Approaches. Available online: https://nccih.nih.gov/health/children#hed1 (accessed on 31 March 2017).
14. Slader, C.A.; Reddel, H.K.; Jenkins, C.R.; Armour, C.L.; Bosnic-Anticevich, S.Z. Complementary and alternative medicine use in asthma: Who is using what? *Respirology* **2006**, *11*, 373–387. [CrossRef] [PubMed]
15. Post-White, J.; Fitzgerald, M.; Hageness, S.; Sencer, S.F. Complementary and alternative medicine use in children with cancer and general and specialty pediatrics. *J. Pediatr. Oncol. Nurs.* **2009**, *26*, 7–15. [CrossRef] [PubMed]
16. Kemper, K.J.; O'Connor, K.G. Pediatricians' recommendations for complementary and alternative medical (CAM) therapies. *Ambul Pediatr.* **2004**, *4*, 482–487. [CrossRef] [PubMed]
17. Sackett, D.L.; Rosenberg, W.M.; Gray, J.A.; Haynes, R.B.; Richardson, W.S. Evidence-based medicine: What it is and what it isn't. *BMJ* **1996**, *13*, 71–72. [CrossRef]
18. Kemper, K.J.; Cohen, M. Ethics meet complementary and alternative medicine: New light on old principles. *Contem. Pediatr.* **2004**, 482–487.
19. Cost. Use of Complementary Health Approaches in U.S. Available online: https://nccih.nih.gov/research/statistics/NHIS/2012/cost (accessed on 13 August 2018).
20. Birdee, G.S.; Phillips, R.S.; Davis, R.B.; Gardiner, P. Factors associated with pediatric use of complementary and alternative medicine. *Pediatrics* **2010**, *125*, 249–256. [CrossRef] [PubMed]

21. Highfield, E.S.; McLellan, M.C.; Kemper, K.J.; Risko, W.; Woolf, A.D. Integration of complementary and alternative medicine in a major pediatric teaching hospital: An initial overview. *J Altern. Complement Med.* **2005**, *11*, 373–380. [CrossRef] [PubMed]
22. Lin, Y.C.; Lee, A.C.; Kemper, K.J.; Berde, C.B. Use of complementary and alternative medicine in pediatric pain management service: A survey. *Pain Med.* **2005**, *6*, 452–458. [CrossRef] [PubMed]
23. World Café Method. Available online: http://www.theworldcafe.com/key-concepts-resources/world-cafe-method (accessed on 31 March 2017).
24. McClafferty, H.; Dodds, S.; Brooks, A.J.; Brenner, M.G.; Brown, M.L.; Fraizer, P.; Mark, J.D.; Weydert, J.A.; Wilcox, G.M.G.; Lebensohn, P.; et al. Pediatric Integrative Medicine in Residency (PIMR): Description of a New Online Educational Curriculum. *Children* **2015**, *17*, 98–107. [CrossRef] [PubMed]

7

Medical Yoga Therapy

Ina Stephens

Department of Pediatrics, University of Virginia Medical Center, Charlottesville, VA 22903, USA; is8n@virginia.edu

Abstract: Medical yoga is defined as the use of yoga practices for the prevention and treatment of medical conditions. Beyond the physical elements of yoga, which are important and effective for strengthening the body, medical yoga also incorporates appropriate breathing techniques, mindfulness, and meditation in order to achieve the maximum benefits. Multiple studies have shown that yoga can positively impact the body in many ways, including helping to regulate blood glucose levels, improve musculoskeletal ailments and keeping the cardiovascular system in tune. It also has been shown to have important psychological benefits, as the practice of yoga can help to increase mental energy and positive feelings, and decrease negative feelings of aggressiveness, depression and anxiety.

Keywords: yoga; yogic practice; anxiety; depression; mindfulness; meditation; arthritis; ADHD; cardiovascular disease; inflammation

---

1. Introduction

Within the past decade, yoga has infiltrated not only Western culture, but also Western medicine. The more we learn about this ancient practice, the more we realize that its benefits go far beyond increased flexibility and muscle tone. A common misunderstanding is that yoga predominantly focuses on increasing flexibility; however, although Hatha Yoga, or the physical practice of yoga, does emphasize appropriate postural alignment, musculoskeletal strength and endurance as well as balance, the study and practice of yoga incorporates mindfulness-based practices such as mindful breathing techniques, focused concentration, meditation and self-reflection.

Modern medicine has made enormous progress in controlling communicable diseases over the past century, such that it is now the non-communicable diseases (NCDs) that have reached epidemic proportions and cause the majority of deaths worldwide. The World Health Organization (WHO) estimates that 80% of NCD deaths are due to four main disease types: cardiovascular disease, cancer, diabetes, and respiratory diseases [1]. Unfortunately, lifestyle is the major causative factor in NCDs, including tobacco use, sedentary lifestyle, lack of regular exercise, unhealthy diets and chronic psychosocial stress [1,2]. Chronic inflammation and stress is a common factor of many of the NCDs, and an area where yoga has been found to be extremely beneficial.

Recent research has shown that yogic and mindfulness-based practices can positively impact the body in many ways, including helping to regulate blood glucose levels and keeping the cardiovascular system healthy. It also has been shown to have important psychological benefits, as the practice of yoga can help to increase alertness and positive feelings, and decrease negative feelings of aggressiveness, depression and anxiety [3–8]. Some healthcare providers are responding to these positive findings—as well as the growing patient demand for an alternative approach to wellness that is natural, low-tech, relatively inexpensive and generally very safe—by incorporating medical yoga into their practices [1].

2. Prescription: Yoga

Medical yoga is defined as the use of yoga practices for the prevention and potential treatment of medical conditions. Beyond the physical elements of yoga, which are important and effective for strengthening the body, medical yoga also incorporates appropriate breathing techniques, mindfulness, meditation and self-reflection/study in order to achieve the maximum benefits. Medical Yoga Therapy or "Yoga Chikitsa" is the dynamic state of physical and mental ease, coupled with spiritual well-being. Yoga helps one to develop a positive state of health by not only treating illness, but also helping one to understand the underlying causes of disease. Medical yoga therapy, ideally, is an individualized, personalized and holistic approach that takes into account not only the patient's mind, body and spirit, but also their family, support network, work situation, and culture, as part of the patient's individualized treatment plan. As an example, if one is diagnosed with anxiety, a physician trained in medical yoga may prescribe specific breathing techniques (pranayamas), calming postures (asanas), mindfulness-based practices and/or meditation, as well as other lifestyle guidance. This type of therapy does not incur the potentially adverse effects of medications, and can produce benefits to the patient, long after their relationship with the health provider ends.

The mindfulness and meditation aspects of yoga are ways of training the mind so that one is not distracted and caught up in its endless churning thought stream. These practices build resilience, help the patient cope with stress and manage potential triggers for anxiety. They can also promote self-reflection that may uncover the source(s) of one's anxiety. If necessary, anti-anxiety medications and/or psychotherapy may be used in tandem; medical yoga in such cases is strongly adjunctive and complementary.

Yoga is most powerful when it changes the patient's general health outlook, changing the emphasis from reactive to proactive health management. The yogic definition of health or "svastha" is when the functions of the body and mind are in harmony so that they can turn inward to reach the goal of Self-realization. In yogic terms, when you are really your "Self", you are truly at "ease". It is the loss of the Self that creates "dis-ease". This is a bit different than the Western concept of health, which is often defined as "the absence of disease." In contrast, the yogic concept is that "disease is the absence of vibrant health". Accordingly, this way of thinking reaffirms the understanding that the nature of yoga is to find one's eternal Self of health, peace and well-being [1].

This review article will focus on: (1) The science behind medical yoga; (2) The relationship of stress to health and healing; (3) The yogic approach to health care; and (4) The research behind medical yoga therapy.

3. What Is Yoga

Yoga is not a particular denomination or religion, but an age-old practice based on a harmonizing system for the body, mind, and spirit to attain inner peace and liberation [9,10]. Yoga is a tool that can deepen and benefit anyone, of any religion. It does not conflict with personal beliefs; it is simply a vehicle to help one transform oneself by promoting conscious connection with oneself, the world, and the highest truth. There are many traditional paths of yoga, including tantra, mantra, kundalini, bhakti, jnana, karma, raja yoga, and others, all of which have their own techniques to awaken these connections. According to the classic text of the *Yoga Sutras of Patanjali*, "yoga" is the complete "inhibition of the modifications of the mind" [9] or quieting of the constant chatter in one's mind so that our True Selves can manifest, rest in our own true nature and be free of suffering. Disease, as described in the sutras, is said to be an impediment to spiritual practice, growth and freedom from suffering [9]. Traditional yogic practices include breath control and techniques (pranayama), meditation (including mindfulness), the adoption of specific bodily postures (asanas) and self-reflection (scriptural or self-study) [9,10].

As a mindfulness practice, yoga requires one to be fully aware in the present moment. This practice helps to diffuse anxiety (which largely concerns the future), and sadness (which largely concerns the past). All the yogic practices use present moment, non-judgmental awareness as the foundation.

Of course, such presence benefits the healthcare provider as much as the patient: if one can learn to pay attention to oneself, one can really pay attention to one's patients. One can then teach the patient to pay attention to him or herself as well.

4. Medical Yoga Prescription

Medical yoga as considered here comprises the use of traditional yogic practices to prevent, cure, and/or ameliorate disease. The ideal medical yoga prescription includes the yogic practices of breathing techniques, bodily postures, meditation techniques and self-reflection; a healthy, nourishing diet; reducing substances such as caffeine, tobacco, drugs and alcohol; healthy sleep hygiene and appropriate support, which may include family, spouse, children, friends and/or support groups, with or without psychotherapy. It is important that medical yoga therapy should start gently and with self-compassion.

For providers considering adding yoga to their therapeutic armamentarium, the best place to start is to consider yoga therapy as a complement to their patient's current medical treatment. Yoga alone should not be considered a substitute for appropriate medication or psychotherapy. However, in situations where a patient is at risk of an illness but does not currently need more intensive therapy, introduction of yogic practices may forestall or prevent progression to the point where medical therapy is needed. Patients whose daily activities produce back strain or who have inherently stressful lives may benefit from yoga as a prophylactic strategy, thereby potentially avoiding more intensive interventions. It is also important to remember that not all yoga is appropriate for all patients and that yoga therapy is different than simply taking a group yoga class where the yoga instructor may not be aware of an individual student's health concerns or problems. Most certified yoga teachers, or instructors, have received some training in anatomy and physiology; however, this training can be quite varied and is not equivalent to the training required by the yoga therapist or healthcare practitioner. As noted previously, yoga therapy, different from a yoga class, starts with a detailed history and physical examination and assessment from the health practitioner.

Yoga brings the autonomic nervous system into healthy balance by stimulating the parasympathetic nervous system [11,12]. The sympathetic nervous system, or our "emergency response system," is activated when our body or mind feels threatened or perceives being stressed, whether that be a "positive" or a "negative" stress. This "flight or fight" response results in vasoconstriction, causing decreased blood flow to the extremities and the digestive system in order to prepare one for survival [11]. One's heart rate and blood pressure increase, the liver converts glycogen to glucose and releases glucose into the bloodstream, the bronchioles dilate, and the blood flow pattern changes, leading to decreased digestive system activity and reduced urine output. In contrast, the parasympathetic system is stimulated when one relaxes; it is often called the "rest and digest" mechanism of our nervous system. The parasympathetic system stimulates blood flow to the digestive system, brain, extremities and sexual organs [11]. As many of us go through our day, what is happening on the "outside"—i.e., what we may think or what we may encounter—causes a constant interaction between the two facets of the nervous system. Yogic practices work by decreasing physiologic arousal and quieting down this continual play of the autonomic system. They can reduce one's heart rate and blood pressure, ease one's respirations and increase heart rate variability—all signs of improved parasympathetic tone [13].

5. Stress

Many in today's society live in "sympathetic overdrive." This occurs when the body perceives a continuous stressor, and the short-term sympathetic stress response persists all day long [11]. Unfortunately, our bodies were not really set up in a way to handle these continual stressors [12]. Due to the continued excitation, one of the major neuroendocrine systems of the body, the hypothalamic-pituitary-adrenal (HPA) axis is set in motion. The HPA axis regulates and helps to control many different bodily processes including one's reaction to stress, immune function, digestion and energy expenditure and storage. The axis is set in motion with release of corticotropin-releasing factor (CRF) from the hypothalamus. CRF then stimulates the anterior pituitary gland to release adrenocorticotropic hormone (ACTH), which subsequently stimulates the adrenal cortex to produce and release cortisol [14]. In response to the stress, cortisol functions by aiding in the metabolism of fat, protein, and carbohydrates by converting them to glucose through gluconeogenesis. This longer-term stress response subsequently raises blood glucose levels, suppresses the immune system, and causes retention of sodium and water by the kidneys, with subsequent increased blood volume and blood pressure. At a certain blood concentration, cortisol will exert a negative feedback to the hypothalamus and the pituitary gland with decreased discharging of both CRF and ACTH. At this point, homeostasis returns to the body and entire system. If, however, the body continues to be in a state of stress, real or perceived, this cycle perpetuates with subsequent sustained HPA axis activation [14,15].

Not all stress has unfavorable effects, of course. When the body is able to tolerate the stress, and can use it to boost one's performance, the positive effects are numerous and impressive. There are over >1400 biochemical reactions that the body has in response to stress, with subsequent effects on one's body, mind, emotions and behavior [12]. However, stress becomes negative when it exceeds one's ability to cope. At this point, the body systems can become fatigued, causing multiple problems, both physically and emotionally [15,16].

Chronic stress is experienced when there is a mismatch between a perceived demand and one's ability to cope with that demand; it includes one's emotional and mental response to the outside situation. When one is continually stressed, whether that stress is real or perceived, his or her nervous system can be shifted towards the state of sympathetic overdrive [11,12]. At this point, the actual activity of the sympathetic nervous system decreases with a decline in the release of epinephrine, but corticosteroid release continues to be activated at above-normal levels. In such a case, the individual may no longer even recognize that they are in a stressful state. Moreover, chronic stress can be precipitated by any number of factors and conditions, some regular and unavoidable: constant worry, daily life hassles, frustrations over one's job or family, traffic jams, finances, poor sleep or eating habits, demands on time, and challenging life situations all create stress [12]. Stress can even also be triggered by one's memory of difficult or scary past situations that have previously occurred. This state of high stress causing continuous sympathetic stimulation is epidemic in our society, from the corporate executive down to the young child on a busy school and activity schedule.

So stress is part of our lives—does it matter? In fact, the burden due to stress-related illness is quite concerning. The Centers for Disease Control and Prevention estimates that stress accounts for about 75% of all physician visits [12,16,17], and up to 80% of all visits to primary care providers are for stress-related complaints [12,17]. These involve a wide spectrum of complaints, including headache, back pain, hypertension, arrhythmias, irritable bowel syndrome, insomnia, depression, anxiety, skin problems, fatigue, obesity, migraines, hyperlipidemia and accidents.

Research has shown that continued and chronic stress can result in a generalized immunosuppressive effect that prevents the body to initiate a timely and appropriate immune reaction [16,18–20]. During acute stress, norepinephrine, epinephrine and ACTH are released, signaling certain kinds of cells to become mobilized into the bloodstream, potentially preparing the body for the "fight or flight" response [1]. Acute stress increases levels of pro-inflammatory cytokines in the bloodstream [21]. Whereas inflammation is a necessary short-term response for eliminating pathogens and initiating healing, chronic systemic inflammation causes dysregulation of the immune system and increases one's risk for chronic diseases [20–22]. Chronic stress, like acute stress, is associated with high levels of pro-inflammatory cytokines, but with potentially different health consequences [22]. Type 1 cytokine protective immune responses have been shown to be suppressed during times when the body is undergoing challenges of chronic stress, while pro-inflammatory and type-2 cytokine responses are activated [23,24]. Chronic or long-term stress can also suppress immunity by decreasing the number of immune cells as well as their function. These phenomenon may exacerbate pro-inflammatory diseases and thus potentially increase one's susceptibility to infections and possibly different types of cancer [24].

Chronically high levels of cortisol can also be neurotoxic [14]. These high levels have been associated with accelerated aging, cognitive inhibition, impaired memory and the ability to learn, increased anxiety and fear, as well as depression and anhedonia [25–27]. Areas of the brain, including the hippocampus and the prefrontal cortex (PFC), both with high cortisol receptors, can become impaired with high cortisol levels. Prolonged stress, both physiological and psychological, with continued high levels of blood cortisol can induce lowered metabolic rates and decreased synaptic densities in the hippocampus and the PFC [25,28–30]. Even perceived stress has been shown to negatively correlate with overall PFC volume, specifically in white matter volume of the PFC, specifically in the ventrolateral and dorsolateral PFC [31].

Cortisol activates the amygdala, the body's "threat center." The amygdala is an almond-shaped brain structure that is crucial in the stress response. An enlarged and hyperactive amygdala is often observed during stressful conditions placed on the body [14,32–35]. Of interest, studies performed on decreasing stress revealed that following stress-reduction interventions, where patients reported significantly reduced perceived stress, decreases basolateral amygdala gray matter density, as seen on Magnetic Resonance Imaging (MRI) scans [32,36].

Stress, of all kinds, is thought to play a significant role in the development of depression by depleting the body's "positive" neurotransmitters, such as gamma-aminobutyric acid (GABA), serotonin and dehydroepiandrosterone (DHEA) [37–42]. Dysregulation of the HPA axis is often seen and reported in those with depressive disorders. In addition, both the dopaminergic and serotonergic systems are thought to be involved in the development of depression if they become dysfunctional or dysregulated [43]. Studies done in rats have shown that chronic stress can induce a depressive state, along with notable dysregulation of both their HPA axes and their dopaminergic and serotonergic systems in the PFC. Release of GABA has also shown to be impaired in these rats as well [40,43]. Other mood disorders, including anxiety, are also thought to be aggravated by stress-induced modifications of the PFC. Of note, stress may impact the prefrontal GABA pathways. This can impair the function of the limbic structures, which are known to control one's emotions and behavior [44,45].

6. How Do Yogic Practices Work?

Yoga-based practices of postures (asanas) and movement sequences are usually taught in conjunction with some type of breathing and/or meditation technique [1]. This type of mindful movement with slow, rhythmic breathing is more likely to promote parasympathetic and vagal tone compared to other forms of exercise [1,11,46,47]. Improved vagal tone is reflected by increased heart rate variability (HRV), which is the variation in the time interval between heartbeats. This physiologic phenomenon can be predictive of how readily the heart rate returns to normal, or quiets down, after increasing in response to a stressor. Decreased HRV is associated with poorer myocardial function, often seen after a myocardial infarction, and is seen with increased sympathetic activity. Increased HRV with high frequency activity is associated with increased parasympathetic activity. Yogic breathing techniques—in particular, alternate nostril breathing, which involves breathing through the left and right nostril alternately—has been associated with increased parasympathetic activity, increased HRV and decreased systolic blood pressure [48]. Slow and rhythmic breathing has also been shown to promote the release of prolactin and the hormone oxytocin, which can foster feelings of friendship, calmness and bonding to others (released during childbirth which may help the mother relax and bond with her newborn during a very painful process) [1,49]. These yoga practices also reduce circulating levels of cortisol and have been demonstrated to reduce the manifestations of stress. With practice, there is decreased firing from the locus coeruleus, which is the principal site in the brain for synthesis of norepinephrine in response to stress and panic. This decreased norepinephrine output helps the body to relax and quiet down with reduced respiratory rates and heart rates. The decreased sympathetic output decreases the release of corticotropin releasing factor, with resultant decrease in cortisol output [50–52].

An open-label study from 2013 performed on a cohort of 54 outpatients with clinical depression at a tertiary care psychiatric hospital revealed that, as a group, this cohort had higher levels of serum cortisol compared to healthy controls [50]. These 54 subjects were offered yoga classes as adjunctive therapy for their depressive symptoms. The yoga module was taught to the group over a month's time and subjects were advised to practice daily at home. Antidepressant medication was prescribed in addition if advised by the subject's psychiatrist. The cohort was broken down into three groups: Group (G) 1 received conventional drug therapy (DT) alone (N-16), G2 received yoga therapy (YT) alone (N-19), and G3 received DT along with YT (N-19). A G4 group was used as healthy controls (N-18). The Hamilton Depression Rating Scale (HDRS) was used to rate subject's depressive symptoms, along with measurements of serum cortisol, obtained both at baseline and after three months of intervention. In the total sample, with good adherence, and irrespective of treatment method, the cortisol levels were found to be decreased significantly at the end of treatment in all subjects. Of interest, however, is that more subjects in the yoga groups (both YT and YT plus DT) had significantly greater drops in their cortisol levels as compared to the drug-only (DT) group ($p < 0.008$). In the YT-only group, there was also a high correlation between decreased cortisol levels and lower scores on the HDRS surveys, indicating a positive antidepressant effect as well ($p < 0.001$) [50].

7. Meditation

It appears that formal meditation practice can change both brain structure and function [53]. It has been found that people who do more meditation practice develop more robust brain structures in certain areas. Multiple studies have shown that yogic practices such as mindful meditation can increase both cortical thickness and gray matter, particularly in areas controlling emotional regulation and executive functioning. These regions notably include the insula, the ventromedial pre-frontal cortex and anterior cingulate cortex (ACC) [53,54]. The insula is involved with proprioception, self-awareness and emotional regulation. The ventromedial PFC is the brain's center for executive functioning, including planning, problem solving and emotional regulation. The ACC is the self-regulatory process center, giving one the ability to monitor attention conflicts and allow for more cognitive flexibility [55–58].

Meditation has been shown to increase the thickness of the left hippocampus, the region of the brain that functions in the formation of long-term memory, emotional regulation and cognition, as well as being a critical area of the brain that plays a vital role in the resiliency to chronic stress and depressive states, possibly due to expression of hippocampal neurotrophic protein (brain-derived neurotropic factor or BDNF) [59]. Resiliency to stress, stress-related depression and post-traumatic stress are housed in the hippocampus—multiple studies have shown that increased hippocampal activation correlated negatively with post-traumatic stress disorder (PTSD) and depression symptoms, and positively with resilience [25,55,60–62]. PTSD patients show considerable reduction in volume of the hippocampus, decreased ventromedial PFC activity and insufficient inhibition of the amygdala, all resulting in increased fear, persistent negative emotions, impulsivity, anxiety and depressive rumination.

Mindfulness meditation, particularly in long-term expert meditators, has been shown to diminish activity and size in anxiety-related areas of the brain such as the amygdala, as well as to increase the size of the PFC and insular cortex, both controlling emotional regulation. These meditators have also been shown to have diminished functional connections between the amygdala and the PFC, allowing for less reactivity to stressors [55,63,64]. Meditation also appears to be effective for PTSD and depression symptoms, although more high-quality studies are needed [65,66].

A recent study suggested that hatha yoga postures (asanas) alone can also improve stress and increase relaxation dispositions. This randomized controlled trial performed in 2015 among college students with high psychological stress assessed the effects of sun salutations or suryanamaskar (defined as a series of 12 physical postures) on relaxation dispositions (R-dispositions). Suryanamaskar is a traditional asana sequence that is a well-known yogic exercise; however, there are few studies on the physiologic effects of regular suryanamaskar practice [67,68]. In this study, the intervention group was to practice a daily suryanamaskar session for 14 days, which was composed of a short warm up, 13 rounds of suryanamaskar with mantras and breathing, followed by a cool down in a sitting position. The set of exercises took approximately 20 min to complete daily. No specific activity was given for the control arm to perform. After 14 days, the experimental group scored higher on multiple aspects on the surveys with increased points compared to the control group for: physical relaxation, mental calmness, feeling at ease and peace, being more well-rested and refreshed, improved strength, awareness and joy. In addition, the intervention group scored lower on fatigue, somatic stress, worry, and negative emotional feelings when compared with the control group [69].

8. Yoga and Neurotransmitters

Yoga practices can increase multiple neurotransmitters and hormones such as GABA, serotonin, and dopamine—all natural anti-depressants [11]. They have been shown to increase levels of melatonin, helping to initiate sleep, improving sleep quality and sleep regulation, as well as increasing levels of oxytocin, the "bonding hormone", thus helping with feelings of connectedness and "being seen and heard" [70–74].

GABA is one of the body's chief inhibitory neurotransmitters, working to reduce neuronal excitability and activity throughout the central nervous system (CNS). GABA acts as an important player in the body's response to stress, fear, depression, anxiety and sleep regulation. Lower-than-normal levels of GABA in the brain have been associated with schizophrenia, depression, anxiety, post-traumatic stress disorder, epilepsy and sleep disorders [73].

Multiple kinds of both anxiolytic and anti-depressant medications work by increasing GABA levels in the central nervous system. As mentioned earlier, yoga practices seem to be effective by bringing the parasympathetic and sympathetic systems into balance (often by increasing parasympathetic tone and decreasing sympathetic firing), and does this in large part by increasing GABA activity [75]. Meditation increases activity in the PFC as well as stimulates the thalamus (in particular, the reticular nucleus), which increases production and delivery of GABA throughout the CNS. Studies have shown that GABAergic inhibitory interneurons result in cortical inhibition which has been implicated in improved cognitive performance and enhanced emotional regulation capabilities [76]. Multiple studies have shown that the practice of yoga and meditation may work as well as other therapies in increasing GABA levels in the brain [77–79].

9. Yoga and Telomeres

As meditation, mindfulness practices and yoga have been moving more and more into the mainstream, it is becoming more apparent that these practices may work to keep our minds and bodies from withering with age by potentially stabilizing, and even lengthening telomeres. Telomeres are small, repetitive, chromosomal sequences found at the end of chromosomes which protect the chromosome from deterioration and cell death. They keep the chromosome stable. Telomere shortening, or unraveling, affects how quickly cells age. As they shorten, the chromosome's structural integrity weakens. Telomere length has been found to be a prognostic marker of aging, disease and premature morbidity in humans. Shorter telomeres are associated with cell aging, cell death, premature aging and a broad range of aging-related diseases, including cardiovascular disease, cancer, stroke, dementia, obesity, osteoporosis, Alzheimer's, macular degeneration, acquired immunodeficiency syndrome (AIDS), and osteoarthritis. They have also been associated with pediatric syndromes such as Progeria, Cri-du-chat, Down's syndrome, tuberous sclerosis, dyskeratosis congenita and Fanconi anemia. Telomere shortening is prevented by the enzyme telomerase. Of note, chronic stress may potentially speed up the aging process through decreased telomerase activity and telomere shortening [80].

In 2008, Dean Ornish found a significant association between comprehensive lifestyle changes (including yoga, meditation, breathing, stress management and a healthy whole-food, plant-based diet), and increased telomerase activity in human peripheral blood mononuclear cells. Of interest, the participants of this study also showed significant reductions in psychological distress and low-density lipoprotein cholesterol [81]. In 2013, a five-year follow-up study was completed on the same participants and controls. The participants were found to have persistently increased telomere length and telomerase activity over their age-matched controls. The study also compared blood samples from 2008 and 2013, evaluating both relative telomere length (RTL) and telomerase enzymatic activity per cell. Of interest, after five years, RTL was found to have increased in the lifestyle intervention group and to have decreased in the control group with the difference between the two groups as statistically significant [82]. This was the first controlled trial to show that any lifestyle intervention might lengthen telomeres over time.

Meditation has also been shown to be potentially protective regarding RTL. An intriguing study from 2013 evaluated a group of 15 subjects practicing Loving-Kindness Meditation (LKM) compared to a control group of non-meditators (n-22). LKM, or *Metta bhavana* from the Buddhist tradition, is a method of developing compassion by directing well-wishes towards others. It can be practiced by anyone, regardless of religious affiliation. It is a meditation of care, concern, friendship and compassion for oneself and others. Peripheral blood leukocytes were then measured for RTL in both groups. The LKM practitioners were found to have significantly longer RTLs than the control group, particularly for the women ($p = 0.007$). Although this study was limited by its small sample size, these results are exciting as they suggest that meditation—in particular, LKM practice—might increase RTL, a biomarker associated with aging and longevity [83].

10. Yoga and Inflammation

As noted above, inflammation is the body's natural immune response to infection, injury, and stress. However, inflammation can have serious health implications when it becomes prolonged and chronic. Chronic systemic inflammation may not be as apparent as acute inflammation, and can persist undetected at low levels for years. This can slowly damage the body, lead to the development of chronic diseases and increase one's risk for type II diabetes, atherosclerosis, cardiovascular disease, autoimmune disease and age-related diseases.

As previously discussed, yoga is beneficial for decreasing both acute and chronic stress levels. In multiple studies, yoga has been found to decrease inflammatory markers such as C-reactive protein and other inflammatory cytokines in the blood, while increasing levels of multiple immunoglobulins and natural killer cells [11,84–86]. Recent research has also shown that those who practice yoga regularly have higher levels of leptin and adiponectin in their bodies, both natural chemicals that work to alleviate inflammation in the body. Adiponectin has been found to be a key component of endothelial function and is cardioprotective [1,87,88].

A very interesting recent discovery is that even a small amount of practice may make a significant difference. A notable study by Yadav et al. in 2012 looked at how even a very brief (10-day) yoga-based lifestyle intervention can reduce the inflammatory markers of stress in patients with chronic diseases. In this trial, 86 patients (44 female/42 male) with chronic inflammatory diseases, including those who were overweight/obese received a ten-day yoga-based intervention program, including yoga asanas, pranayama and both individual and group stress management sessions. Statistically significant changes ($p < 0.05$) were seen after this short ten-day intervention with decreased cortisol, tumor necrosis factor-alpha (TNF-α) and interleukin-6 (IL-6) levels, and elevated levels of β-endorphins [89].

Another randomized, controlled clinical trial from 2014 also showed that practicing yoga for as little as three months can not only lower markers of inflammation, but can also make big differences in symptoms of fatigue in breast cancer survivors [90]. In this trial, 200 women were recruited and randomly assigned to either 12 weeks of 90-min hatha yoga classes twice per week, or a wait-list control. Breast cancer treatments were fully completed before the onset of the study.

Multiple inflammatory markers were evaluated as part of the outcome of this trial as well as multiple different surveys assessing both fatigue and depression. At three months post-treatment, comparing the yoga group to the control group, fatigue was found to be lower as well as a number of inflammatory markers such as IL-6, TNF-α and IL-1 β and scores for vitality were found to be higher (all statistically significant with $p < 0.05$) [90].

Of particular interest, this study also showed that the more yogic practices that the women did, the better their outcomes. Also significant was that the results were sustained: after six months post-intervention, both fatigue and inflammation were still lower in the intervention group as compared to controls (decreased by 57% and 20%, respectively) [90]. This suggests that yogic practices can continue to make significant sustained differences in signs and symptoms of inflammation even months later.

11. Yoga and Back Pain/Arthritis

The American College of Rheumatology states that exercise and physical activity is a necessary part of an effective treatment program for patients with both osteoarthritis and rheumatoid arthritis [91,92]. In these patients, exercise has been shown to have a vital role in promoting joint health without worsening disease. Patients suffering from arthritis who exercise regularly have less joint pain, more vitality, better sleep, reduced morning joint stiffness and improved daily living function. In particular, yoga incorporates important elements of body awareness such as proprioception, coordination, balance and postural alignment, all of which are particularly important in individuals with joint disease [93].

A comprehensive review of randomized controlled trials that evaluated yoga as an intervention for chronic low back pain (CLBP) supported the practices and found them to be efficacious on short-term improvements in functional disability [94]. In fact, yoga therapy has been shown to improve pain, back function, spinal mobility, depression and anxiety in patients with CLBP to a greater degree than physical therapy [95,96].

The largest, most rigorously conducted randomized controlled trial (RCT) of yoga and arthritis to date was published in 2015 by Moonaz et al. at Johns Hopkins University. Most importantly, this trial examined the safety, efficacy and feasibility of yoga for sedentary patients with both rheumatoid and osteoarthritis, with significant outcomes revealing important physical and mental health benefits in these individuals with regular yoga practice. After eight weeks of intervention, improvements were seen in physical pain, general health, vitality, ability to carry out Activities of Daily Living (ADLs), balance, upper body strength and mental health scales ($p < 0.05$). Of great interest, almost all benefits that were seen were still observable nine months after study completion [97].

12. Yoga and Cardiac Disease

Cardiovascular disease (CVD) encompasses a broad spectrum of syndromes, including atherosclerosis, stroke, arrhythmia, hypertension, hyperlipidemia, heart disease and peripheral vascular disease, and is the leading cause of mortality, morbidity and disability worldwide [1]. Although there have been tremendous advancements in medications, treatment plans and programs for both the prevention and treatment of CVD, there are still a number of challenges in implementation of these programs, and limitations of the treatments. Multiple risk factors are known to cause oxidative stress, leading to endothelial disruption and dysfunction. These include dyslipidemia, diabetes, hypertension, obesity, smoking and psychological stress, which can in turn start a cascade of events involving inflammatory and vasoactive mediators, in particular, interleukin-6, fibrinogen, C-reactive protein and tumor necrosis factor-alpha, that lead to the development of CVD [1]. Yoga therapy may be a significant and cost-effective therapy for CVD by interrupting a number of these different events along this cascade [1,11,88,98–100].

Of interest is a study done by Sarvottam et al. suggesting that even a short-term yoga-based program may reduce the risk for CVD. In this trial, a ten-day yoga intervention program was found to significantly reduce the body mass indices and systolic blood pressures in 51 overweight and obese men. These men were also found to have significant changes in certain inflammatory markers with decreases in IL-6 and elevation of adiponectin [88].

According to the American Heart Association, yoga practices can help to lower blood pressure, increase lung capacity, improve respiratory function and heart rate, improve circulation and boost muscle tone [101]. As previously discussed, yoga can reduce stress both by balancing the autonomic nervous system with increased parasympathetic and reduced sympathetic activities, respectively, thus optimizing and restoring the body's homeostasis (decreasing allostatic load), as well as decreasing the reactivity of the HPA axis. By decreasing both of these pathways, yoga can interrupt multiple different inflammatory events on the cascade toward CVD and enhance cardiovagal function [102].

An intriguing study by Krishna et al. in 2014 evaluated the effects of yoga therapy in patients with heart failure. Parameters including heart rate, blood pressure, heart rate variability (HRV) and rate pressure product (RPP) were measured before and after yoga intervention. As mentioned above, increased HRV is predictive of how readily the heart rate returns to normal, or quiets down, after increasing in response to a stressor—a sign of parasympathetic tone—and RRP is an index of myocardial O_2 consumption and load on the heart. Both of these are measures of cardiac autonomic function. In this trial of 130 heart failure patients, randomly assigned to receive either a yoga intervention program or standard medical therapy alone, heart rate (HR), blood pressure (BP), and measures of cardiac autonomic function were assessed before and after the 12-week intervention. The results were quite significant with p values all <0.05 regarding decreases in HR, BP and RPP in the yoga group compared to the controls. Sympathetic nervous system modulation (measured by Lfnu—low-frequency normalized unit) decreased significantly and parasympathetic nervous system modulation (measured by Hfnu—high frequency normalized unit) increased significantly as well in the intervention compared to the controls—both signs indicating improved HRV [103].

This study suggests that there could be a great benefit of yoga therapy as an adjunct to medical treatment in patients with heart failure. In addition, because it is important to consider that in patients with severe and/or decompensated heart failure physical exercise may not be well tolerated, yoga, particularly gentle asanas, breathing exercises and meditation, may be easily tolerated by these individuals [1].

As a complementary and integrative therapy, yoga for the management of hypertension has been studied in numerous randomized controlled trials. On average, the overall effect of yoga therapy results in a reduction of systolic BP of approximately 10 mmHg and approximately an 8 mmHg reduction in diastolic BP [75,104]. Of note, yoga seems to be efficacious only for hypertension, not for pre-hypertension. It is also important to recognize that at this time yoga therapy can only be recommended as an adjunct to antihypertensive pharmacological treatment, not as an alternative therapy alone. Breathing and meditation seem to be the important components of the yoga interventions as well rather than physical yoga asanas for hypertensive patients. These are the components of the yogic practice that can increase parasympathetic activity and decrease sympathetic tone, which counteracts the surplus of sympathetic activity associated with hypertension. In addition, the specific components of yoga practice may help one to self-regulate, so that the mind and body can work to bring one's physical, emotional, autonomic and psychological systems into balance, which is most critical when the body is under stress [105]. An interesting study conducted in 2013 on the effects of Iyengar yoga supports this theory. After an eight-week yoga program intervention, outcomes from surveys strongly suggested that the yoga practice helped to benefit self-regulation in terms of physical function, enriched sleep quality, dietary improvements with improved lifestyle choices, reduction of stress and anxiety and enhanced calm mental/emotional states in the study participants [106]. Despite the increasing evidence that yogic practices may reduce blood pressure, it is important to recognize that many of the studies done have also included diet modifications, exercise and/or supportive guidance and counseling—all part of the "yogic lifestyle". The exact mechanisms as to the potential benefits of yoga in controlling blood pressure remain unknown at this time. Additional rigorously controlled trials are needed to further investigate the potential benefits of yoga for improving blood pressure in those individuals with both pre-hypertension and hypertension to help determine optimal yogic practices, yoga program design and treatment plan [1,75,105,107].

Yoga therapy may also be quite useful as a complementary therapy for atrial fibrillation (AF). It is well known that the autonomic nervous system plays a pivotal role in the pathophysiology of AF, and it has been proposed that an imbalance in both the sympathetic and parasympathetic nervous systems contribute to the disease entity [108,109]. In a trial performed in 2013 by Lakkireddy et al. the impact of a three-month yoga intervention program was evaluated in 49 patients with paroxysmal AF. Both symptomatic and asymptomatic AF episodes were assessed for a three-month control period prior to the intervention, and during the intervention. Statistically significant decreases in both symptomatic and asymptomatic AF episodes were observed with p values < 0.001. Of interest, feelings of both depression and anxiety were also found to be reduced significantly in study subjects as well as improvements on several measures of quality of life including general health, physical functioning, vitality, social functioning and mental health [108]. The benefits of yoga therapy in these patients with AF are thought to be due to restoration of sympathetic and parasympathetic balance at the level of HPA axis as well as decreasing both inflammation and oxidative stress, resulting in the suppression of atrial remodeling, micro-reentry circuits and triggers for AF; however, the exact mechanism remains unknown [1,108].

13. Yoga for Pediatrics

A growing amount of evidence is showing that yoga and other mindfulness-based practices are paramount for today's children. Due to various new demands and standards in today's society, children and adolescents experience stress and mental health challenges that have not been seen in generations past. In a society exploding with technology, children now are confronted with many daily distractions and temptations, with resultant overstimulation and pressures from their peers. There are more stresses on families with reduced downtime and quiet time caused by the overscheduling of activities, overvaluing productive time and greater pressure to succeed academically. Recent research shows that the current generation of young adults is the most "stressed-out" generation, compared with their predecessors [110]. There is constant stimulation through technology, internet and social media, as well as extensive media usage by children and adolescents in today's world. Not only are children and young adults under more stress, but they also have fewer coping skills to manage these stressors. As with adults, when children internalize stress, it is often manifested physically, resulting in health issues such as insomnia, chronic abdominal pain, headaches, depression, anxiety and mood swings [103,111]. For the past number of years, schools have been cutting programs such as life skills courses and physical education classes. When these stress management skills are not learned at an early age, it only becomes harder to learn them as the children get older. Yoga may help children, adolescents and young adults cope with stress by teaching them self-regulation skills to control emotions and stress at a young age. These practices would, in turn, help their well-being and mental health, improve overall resiliency and help to positively keep their lives in balance. Yogic practices help the body to connect to the mind by helping one to focus on the present moment and clearing the mind of overwhelming thoughts. Even very young children can learn to benefit from yogic breathing techniques, which can help to calm and distract toddlers from a temper tantrum or help them to sleep. According to the National Institutes of Health, children who practice yoga have an increased sense of self-awareness and self-confidence. Concentration skills are enhanced [104,112]. These learned mind-body skills can also help a child reexamine a difficult, or even painful, experience into one that bolsters their sense of resiliency [105,113]. This, in turn, may contribute to improved attention, self-esteem, empowerment and good mental health [114–116].

According to the 2007 National Health Interview Survey (NHIS), mind-body therapies, including yoga, were the most favored complementary and alternative medicine (CAM) practices among children with behavioral, emotional or mental health problems. Per the 2012 NHIS, the use of yoga and yoga therapy in children had increased since 2007 from 2.5% to 3.2% (more than 400,000 children) [113]. Of note, older children between the ages of 13 and 17 were noted to use these mind-body therapies more often, and were more commonly used by female patients versus male patients (5.7% vs. 1.7%) [117].

Of interest, a survey taken in 2007 showed that in children and adolescents with chronic pain, over 60% of the subjects tried at least one CAM approach for pain. Of these practices, yogic practices and therapies were used by 32% as their first choice of CAM therapy [118].

Compared to research performed in adults, there is unfortunately a lack of good RCTs on the safety and efficacy of yoga among the pediatric population. In 2008, Galantino et al. performed a systematic review and found 24 studies of yoga for children which included case-control studies, pilot studies, cohort studies and RCTs. Although this review concluded that there was certainly positive evidence regarding the use of yoga in the pediatric population, more research is imperative [119,120]. Since then, there have been no recent systematic reviews of pediatric therapeutic yoga [114]; however, a growing number of RCTs are being performed. In a recent bibliometric analysis of yoga studies published between 1975 and 2014, there were 366 studies found with 31 of the studies (9.9%) including children [121]. In 2010, Kaley-Isley et al. performed a comprehensive review, and subsequently summarized applicable studies with children and adolescents treated with yoga therapy practices as an intervention. The majority of these studies showed benefit as well as very few adverse effects. Among these studies, the areas for which yoga was used for therapy in children include physical fitness, cardiac and respiratory symptoms, mental and behavioral health, developmental syndromes, irritable bowel syndrome, eating disorders including obesity, anorexia and bulimia, cancer and prenatal effects on birth outcomes [1]. In 2016, 14 individual controlled studies were evaluated, showing that yoga, as a CAM treatment and approach, appears to be an encouraging therapy and stress management intervention for children and adolescents, again with a very low rate of reported adverse effects. Yoga therapy can have significantly favorable effects on psychological and cognitive functioning, particularly in patients with emotional, mental and behavioral disorders [117]. Of note, many of the studies reviewed had methodological limitations, small sample sizes, lack of randomization and much variability between yoga practice intervention methods so that clear conclusions were not possible, and it was suggested that to obtain the most benefits from therapeutic yoga in children, more regulated research efforts are warranted [117,122].

There has been increasing interest in the use of mind-body techniques and therapies for children and adolescents with focusing, concentration and attention disorders. If yoga and mindfulness helps one to focus inward and pay attention, it would be only natural to assume that these types of therapies would be of great benefit to those who have difficulty with inattentiveness. Ideally, this increased focus would potentially increase attention naturally, even in children with challenging attention disorders.

In 2012, a systematic review of 124 trials examining the evidence for efficacy of yoga in the treatment of a number of different pediatric psychiatric disorders, of which 16 met appropriate criteria for the final review, showed emerging evidence (Grade B) to support a role for yoga in treating children with Attention Deficit and Hyperactivity Disorder (ADHD) in two RCTs [123]. Among these two RCTs was an intriguing randomized trial from 2004, published in the *Journal of Attention Disorders*, which showed that boys diagnosed with ADHD, on appropriate medication, reduced their symptoms in inattentiveness and behavior when practicing yoga regularly. In this trial, 16 boys with ADHD were randomized to receive either yoga therapy (YG) or cooperative activities (CG) in addition to their previously prescribed medications for a total of 20 weeks. The YG received one hour of hatha yoga per week along with breathing and relaxation techniques. Assessments were performed both pre- and post-intervention using the Conners' Parent and Teacher Rating Scales (CPRS and CTRS). Although there was improvement in both groups, the YG group showed significant improvement on five subscales of the CPRS. Positive changes on the CTRS were also seen in those who attended more yoga sessions and who engaged in more home practice. Although this was a small study, the trial did suggest that yoga may be a useful CAM therapy for adjunctive management, along with medical management, in children with ADHD. Larger and more collaborative studies on yoga's potential benefits for these children are needed [124].

Another trial from 2006 by Haffner et al. evaluated 19 children with ADHD and randomized them to receive either YG or conventional motor training (CG), along with their current medication regimens. The YG received 2 h of hatha yoga weekly for a period of 34 weeks. Outcome measures here included test scores on a task requiring focused attention, as well as both parent and teacher ratings of ADHD symptoms. Results from this trial revealed that the yoga training was superior to the conventional motor training. This pilot study also demonstrated that yoga can be an impressive adjunctive treatment for ADHD, though again limited by its small sample size. These researchers advocate for further research into the impact of yoga on children with ADHD [125].

What about the possibilities of yoga entering the school curriculum? It has become increasingly commonplace for large companies and offices to incorporate yoga and meditation facilities for their employees as a means to help improve concentration, refresh focus, improve motivation and counteract prolonged sitting at a desk orworkbench all work-day long. Schoolchildren, who also spend hours working and sitting all day, may benefit to the same degree.

There have been a few RCTs have evaluated the effects yoga within a school curriculum particularly in the prevention of mental health problems and enhancement of psychosocial well-being. One RCT from 2012 by Khalsa et al. studied 109 students randomly assigned to receive either an 11-week yoga education program versus regular physical education. In this trial, students were asked to self-report measures of mental health parameters including mood, anxiety, stress, and resilience both at baseline and post-intervention. Results were remarkable for statistically significant differences in measures of the students' feelings of anger control, fatigue and inertia [126]. Of note, this is one of a few trials that compares the effects of yoga to that of another form of exercise (in this case, physical education as an exercise control group). More studies comparing the yoga with standard exercise are warranted as benefits can certainly be seen for both.

Another interesting study from 2010 examined a school-based mindfulness and yoga intervention program in four inner city public schools in Baltimore, MD. Each of the schools was randomly assigned to undergo either a 12-week yoga/mindfulness intervention program or a wait-list control. Mental health parameters were also assessed in the trial including stress responses, feelings of depression, emotional arousal, control of thoughts and student social interactions. Positive outcomes were again seen in the intervention group compared to the controls in a number of these different psychological variables. Both of these studies are significant in that they suggest that mindfulness-based programs may be of great benefit for youths, especially in helping them to cope with daily stressors. In addition, both studies illustrate that a school-based mindfulness/yoga program is easily accessible, acceptable to students/staff and feasible to incorporate into schools that serve underprivileged and stressed youth [127].

A landmark study was recently performed in 2016, again in two inner-city public schools in Baltimore, MD. This large RCT examined in 300 students, randomized to receive either the Mindfulness Based Stress Reduction (MBSR) program, developed by Jon Kabat-Zinn, or a healthy education program (Healthy Topics (HT)) for an intervention period of 12 weeks. The two groups were comparable at baseline: average age was 12 years, 50.7% female, 99.7% African American, and 99% eligible for free lunch. After the 12-week intervention program, the results were quite significant with the MBSR students reporting lower levels of depression, self-hostility and other negative affective complaints than the group who received HT education ($p < 0.05$) [128]. These outcomes suggested that underprivileged, vulnerable and disadvantaged youths could significantly benefit from mindfulness-based programs in school, particularly with negative psychological symptoms and developing improved coping mechanisms for stress.

Of great significance is the impact that these positive outcomes may have as children mature—it is a well-appreciated fact that many adult diseases have their genesis in childhood, especially those due to high exposure to stress and trauma [128]. In a research review from 2014, Hagen et al. proposed that educational facilities including pre-schools, schools, and community centers offer yoga and mindfulness-based programs for children and adolescents. The authors suggested that these school-based programs may help students improve self-regulation of emotions, stress-coping skills, resiliency and overall mood. They concluded that for young people to start practicing mind-body techniques from an early age may prevent future generations from experiencing more stress in their adult lives. [114].

14. Conclusions

Ongoing research into yoga and mindfulness-based practices continues to reveal and uncover health benefits, supporting its use in health management.

Although there have been many published studies and research trials demonstrating and advocating yoga as a treatment and/or adjunct therapy for multiple disease entities, there are limitations that should be noted for a number of these studies. Many of these studies are single-center trials, have small and/or low-powered sample sizes and use non-standardized methodologies with short follow-up periods. It also should be noted that the field of yoga research encompasses the inherent dilemma of the wide variety of yogic practices used as interventional therapies. Larger, multi-centered studies using standardized yoga programs and uniform methodologies with long-term follow-up and outcomes are needed.

The practice of yoga is not as easy or as quick as taking medication, but mounting evidence suggests it is worth the effort and investment. Yoga helps one to reconnect with oneself. It can help to uncover why and how one's illness may have started, and can work with the body to start the recovery period from the ground up. The practice can help one to see how they may be reacting to the world around them, and may help them learn to respond from a different perspective. Slowing down, quieting our minds and connecting with our inner selves all help to bring one into the present moment. This can ultimately help to relieve one from the pressures and stressors from the hustle and bustle of this very busy world.

References

1. Khalsa, S.B.; Cohen, L.; McCall, T.; Telles, S. *Principles and Practices of Yoga in Health Care*, 1st ed.; Handspring Publishing: Scotland, UK, 2016.
2. Hunter, D.J.; Reddy, K.S. Noncommunicable diseases. *NEJM* **2013**, *369*, 1336–1343. [CrossRef] [PubMed]
3. Miller, J.J.; Fletcher, K.; Kabat-Zinn, J. Three-year follow-up and clinical implications of a mindfulness meditation-based stress reduction intervention in the treatment of anxiety disorders. *Gen. Hosp. Psychiatry* **1995**, *17*, 192–200. [CrossRef]
4. Yadav, R.K.; Sarvottam, K.; Magan, D.; Yadav, R. A two-year follow-up case of chronic fatigue syndrome: substantial improvement in personality following a yoga-based lifestyle intervention. *Altern. Complement. Med.* **2015**, *21*, 246–249. [CrossRef] [PubMed]
5. Klainin-Yobas, P.; Oo, W.N.; Suzanne Yew, P.Y.; Lau, Y. Effects of relaxation interventions on depression and anxiety among older adults: A systematic review. *Aging Ment. Health* **2015**, *19*, 1043–1055. [CrossRef] [PubMed]
6. Amaranath, B.; Nagendra, H.R.; Deshpande, S. Effect of integrated Yoga module on positive and negative emotions in Home Guards in Bengaluru: A wait list randomized control trial. *Int. J. Yoga* **2016**, *9*, 35–43. [CrossRef] [PubMed]
7. DeBruin, E.; Formsma, A.R.; Frijstein, G.; Bogels, S.M. Mindful2Work: Effects of combined physical exercise, yoga and mindfulness meditations for stress relieve in employees. A proof of concept study. *Mindfulness* **2017**, *8*, 204–217. [CrossRef] [PubMed]
8. Danhauer, S.C.; Addington, E.L.; Sohl, S.J.; Chaoul, A.; Cohen, L. Review of yoga therapy during cancer treatment. *Support Care Cancer.* **2017**. [CrossRef] [PubMed]
9. Taimini, I.K. *The Science of Yoga: The Yoga-Sutras of Patanjali in Sanskrit*; Quest Books: New York, NY, USA, 1999.
10. Feuerstein, G. *The Yoga Tradition—Its History, Literature, Philosophy and Practice*; Hohm Press: Chino Valley, AZ, USA, 2008.
11. Penetrating Postures: The Science of Yoga. Available online: https://www.forbes.com/sites/alicegwalton/2011/06/16/penetrating-postures-the-science-of-yoga/?client=safari (accessed on 28 January 2017).

12. How Stress Cripples Your Digestive Health and Three Things to Do about It. Available online: http://www.coreconsciousliving.com/single-post/2015/06/29/How-Stress-Cripples-Your-Digestive-Health-3-Things-To-Do-About-It (accessed on 28 January 2017).
13. Stearns, M.N.; Stearns, R.N. *Yoga for Anxiety—Meditations and Practices for Calming the Body and Mind*; New Harbinger Publications, Inc.: Oakland, CA, USA, 2010.
14. Xiaoyun, L.; Li, H. The Role of Stress Regulation on Neural Plasticity in Pain Chronification. *Neural Plast.* **2016**. [CrossRef]
15. Gerra, G.; Somaini, L.; Manfredini, M.; Raggi, M.; Saracino, M.; Amore, M.; Leonardi, C.; Cortese, E.; Donnini, C. Dysregulated responses to emotions among abstinent heroin users: Correlation with childhood neglect and addiction severity. *Prog. Neuro-Psychopharmacol. Biol. Psychiatry* **2014**, *48*, 220–228. [CrossRef] [PubMed]
16. Mohd, R.S. Life event, stress and illness. *Malays. J. Med. Sci.* **2008**, *15*, 9–18.
17. Nerurkar, A.; Bitton, A.; Davis, R.; Phillips, R.; Yeh, G. When Physicians counsel about stress: Results of a National Study. *JAMA Intern. Med.* **2013**, *173*, 76–77. [CrossRef] [PubMed]
18. Nezi, M.; Mastorakos, G.; Mouslech, Z. *Corticotropin Releasing Hormone and the Immune/Inflammatory Response*; Endotext [Internet]; MDText.com, Inc.: South Dartmouth, MA, USA, 2000.
19. Zhao, J.; Liu, J.; Denney, J.; Li, C.; Li, F.; Chang, F.; Chen, M.; Yin, D. TLR2 Involved in Naive CD4+ T Cells Rescues Stress-Induced Immune Suppression by Regulating Th1/Th2 and Th17. *Neuroimmunomodulation* **2015**, *22*, 328–336. [CrossRef] [PubMed]
20. Morey, J.N.; Boggero, I.A.; Scott, A.B.; Segerstrom, S.C. Current Directions in Stress and Human Immune Function. *Curr. Opin. Psychol.* **2015**, *5*, 13–17. [CrossRef] [PubMed]
21. Steptoe, A.; Hamer, M.; Chida, Y. The effects of acute psychological stress on circulating inflammatory factors in humans: A review and meta-analysis. *Brain Behav. Immun.* **2007**, *21*, 901–912. [CrossRef] [PubMed]
22. Gouin, J.P.; Glaser, R.; Malarkey, W.B.; Beversdorf, D.; Kiecolt-Glaser, J. Chronic stress, daily stressors, and circulating inflammatory markers. *Health Psychol.* **2012**, *31*, 264–268. [CrossRef] [PubMed]
23. Glaser, R.; Kiecolt-Glaser, J.K. Stress-induced immune dysfunction: Implications for health. *Nat. Rev. Immunol.* **2005**, *5*, 243–251. [CrossRef] [PubMed]
24. Dhabhar, F.S. Enhancing versus Suppressive Effects of Stress on Immune Function: Implications for Immunoprotection and Immunopathology. *Neuroimmunomodulation* **2009**, *16*, 300–317. [CrossRef] [PubMed]
25. Carrion, V.G.; Wong, S.S. Can Traumatic Stress Alter the Brain? Understanding the Implications of Early Trauma on Brain Development and Learning. *J. Adolesc. Health* **2012**, *51*, S23–S28. [CrossRef] [PubMed]
26. Tomiyama, A.J.; O'Donovan, A.; Lin, J.; Puterman, E.; Lazaro, A.; Chan, J.; Dhabhar, F.S.; Wolkowitz, O.; Kirschbaum, C.; Blackburn, E.; et al. Does cellular aging relate to patterns of allostasis? An examination of basal and stress reactive HPA axis activity and telomere length. *Physiol. Behav.* **2012**, *106*, 40–45. [CrossRef] [PubMed]
27. Gotlib, I.H.; LeMoult, J.; Colich, N.L.; Foland-Ross, L.C.; Hallmayer, J.; Joormann, J.; Lin, J.; Wolkowitz, O.M. Telomere length and cortisol reactivity in children of depressed mothers. *Mol. Psychiatry* **2015**, *20*, 615–620. [CrossRef] [PubMed]
28. Carrion, V.G.; Weems, C.F.; Richert, K.; Hoffman, B.C.; Reiss, A.L. Decreased prefrontal cortical volume associated with increased bedtime cortisol in traumatized youth. *Biol. Psychiatry* **2010**, *68*, 491–493. [CrossRef] [PubMed]
29. Travis, S.G.; Coupland, N.J.; Hegadoren, K.; Silverstone, P.H.; Huang, Y.; Carter, R.; Fujiwara, E.; Seres, P.; Malykhin, N.V. Effects of cortisol on hippocampal subfields volumes and memory performance in healthy control subjects and patients with major depressive disorder. *J. Affect. Disord.* **2016**, *201*, 34–41. [CrossRef] [PubMed]
30. Reser, J.E. Chronic stress, cortical plasticity and neuroecology. *Behav. Process.* **2016**, *129*, 105–115. [CrossRef] [PubMed]
31. Moreno, G.L.; Bruss, J.; Denburg, N.L. Increased perceived stress is related to decreased prefrontal cortex volumes among older adults. *J. Clin. Exp. Neuropsychol.* **2016**, 1–13. [CrossRef] [PubMed]
32. Holzel, B.K.; Carmody, J.; Evans, K.C.; Hoge, E.A.; Dusek, J.A.; Morgan, L.; Pitman, R.K.; Lazar, S.W. Stress Reduction correlates with structural changes in the amygdala. *SCAN* **2010**, *5*, 11–17. [CrossRef] [PubMed]

33. Choi, J.; Kim, J.E.; Kim, T.K.; Park, J.Y.; Lee, J.E.; Kim, H.; Lee, E.H.; Han, P.L. TRH and TRH receptor system in the basolateral amygdala mediate stress-induced depression-like behaviors. *Neuropharmacology* **2015**, *97*, 346–356. [CrossRef] [PubMed]
34. Kim, T.K.; Han, P.L. Physical Exercise Counteracts Stress-induced Upregulation of Melanin-concentrating Hormone in the Brain and Stress-induced Persisting Anxiety-like Behaviors. *Exp. Neurobiol.* **2016**, *25*, 163–173. [CrossRef] [PubMed]
35. Tafet, G.E.; Nemeroff, C.B. The Links between Stress and Depression: Psychoneuroendocrinological, Genetic, and Environmental Interactions. *J. Neuropsychiatry Clin. Neurosci.* **2016**, *28*, 77–88. [CrossRef] [PubMed]
36. Doll, A.; Hölzel, B.K.; Mulej Bratec, S.; Boucard, C.C.; Xie, X.; Wohlschläger, A.M.; Sorg, C. Mindful attention to breath regulates emotions via increased amygdala-prefrontal cortex connectivity. *Neuroimage* **2016**, *134*, 305–313. [CrossRef] [PubMed]
37. Moriam, S.; Sobhani, M.E. Epigenetic effect of chronic stress on dopamine signaling and depression. *Genet. Epigenet.* **2013**, *5*, 11–16. [CrossRef] [PubMed]
38. Seo, J.S.; Wei, J.; Qin, L.; Kim, Y.; Yan, Z.; Greengard, P. Cellular and molecular basis for stress-induced depression. *Mol. Psychiatry* **2016**. [CrossRef] [PubMed]
39. Souza-Teodoro, L.H.; de Oliveira, C.; Walters, K.; Carvalho, L.A. Higher serum dehydroepiandrosterone sulfate protects against the onset of depression in the elderly: Findings from the English Longitudinal Study of Aging (ELSA). *Psychoneuroendocrinology* **2016**, *64*, 40–46. [CrossRef]
40. Ma, K.; Xu, A.; Cui, S.; Sun, M.R.; Xue, Y.C.; Wang, J.H. Impaired GABA synthesis, uptake and release are associated with depression-like behaviors induced by chronic mild stress. *Transl. Psychiatry* **2016**, *6*, e910. [CrossRef] [PubMed]
41. Dale, E.; Bang-Andersen, B.; Sánchez, C. Emerging mechanisms and treatments for depression beyond SSRIs and SNRIs. *Biochem. Pharmacol.* **2015**, *95*, 81–97. [CrossRef] [PubMed]
42. Usta, M.B.; Tuncel, O.K.; Akbas, S.; Aydin, B.; Say, G.N. Decreased dehydroepiandrosterone sulphate levels in adolescents with post-traumatic stress disorder after single sexual trauma. *Nord. J. Psychiatry* **2016**, *70*, 116–120. [CrossRef] [PubMed]
43. Mizoguchi, K.; Shoji, H.; Ikeda, R.; Tanaka, Y.; Tabira, T. Persistent depressive state after chronic stress in rats is accompanied by HPA axis dysregulation and reduced prefrontal dopaminergic neurotransmission. *Pharmacol. Biochem. Behav.* **2008**, *91*, 170–175. [CrossRef]
44. Shepard, R.; Page, C.E.; Coutellier, L. Sensitivity of the prefrontal GABAergic system to chronic stress in male and female mice: Relevance for sex differences in stress-related disorders. *Neuroscience* **2016**, *332*, 1–12. [CrossRef] [PubMed]
45. McKlveen, J.M.; Morano, R.L.; Fitzgerald, M.; Zoubovsky, S.; Cassella, S.N.; Scheimann, J.R.; Ghosal, S.; Mahbod, P.; Packard, B.A.; Myers, B.; et al. Chronic Stress Increases Prefrontal Inhibition: A Mechanism for Stress-Induced Prefrontal Dysfunction. *Biol. Psychiatry* **2016**, *80*, 754–764. [CrossRef] [PubMed]
46. Payne, P.; Crane-Godreau, M.A. Meditative movement for depression and anxiety. *Front. Psychiatry* **2013**, *4*, 71. [CrossRef] [PubMed]
47. Brown, R.P.; Gerbar, P.L. Sudarshan Kriya yogic breathing in the treatment of stress, anxiety and depression: Part 1—Neurophysiologic model. *J. Altern. Complement. Med.* **2005**, *11*, 189–201. [CrossRef] [PubMed]
48. Telles, S.; Sharma, S.K.; Balkrishna, A. Blood pressure and heart rate variability during yoga-based alternate nostril breathing practice and breath awareness. *Med. Sci. Mont. Basic Res.* **2014**, *20*, 184–193.
49. Torner, L.; Toschi, N.; Nava, G.; Clapp, C.; Neumann, L.D. Incresaed hypothalamic expression of prolactin in lactation: Involvement in behavioural and neuroendocrine stress responses. *Eur. J. Neurosci.* **2002**, *15*, 1381–1389. [CrossRef] [PubMed]
50. Thirthalli, J.; Naveen, G.H.; Rao, M.G.; Varambally, S.; Christopher, R.; Gangadhar, B.N. Cortisol and antidepressant effects of yoga. *Indian J. Psychiatry* **2013**, *55*, S405–S408. [CrossRef] [PubMed]
51. Naveen, G.H.; Varambally, S.; Thirthalli, J.; Rao, M.; Christopher, R.; Gangadhar, B. Serum cortisol and BDNF in patients with major depression-effect of yoga. *Int. Rev. Psychiatry* **2016**, *28*, 273–278. [CrossRef] [PubMed]
52. Riley, K.E.; Park, C.L. How does yoga reduce stress? A systematic review of mechanisms of change and guide to future inquiry. *Health Psychol. Rev.* **2015**, *9*, 379–396. [CrossRef] [PubMed]
53. Davidson, R.; Lutz, A. Buddha's Brain: Neuroplasticity and Meditation. *IEEE Signal Process. Mag.* **2008**, *25*, 176–174. [CrossRef] [PubMed]

54. Davidson, R.; Kabat-Zinn, J.; Schumacher, J.; Rosenkranz, M.; Muller, D.; Santorelli, S.; Urbanowski, F.; Harrington, A.; Bonus, K.; Sheridan, J. Alterations in Brain and Immune Function Produced by Mindfulness Meditation. *Psychosom. Med.* **2003**, *65*, 564–570. [CrossRef] [PubMed]
55. Ricard, M.; Lutz, A.; Davidson, R. Mind of the Meditator. *Sci. Am.* **2014**, *311*, 38–45. [CrossRef] [PubMed]
56. Hernández, S.E.; Suero, J.; Barros, A.; González-Mora, J.L.; Rubia, K. Increased Grey Matter Associated with Long-Term Sahaja Yoga Meditation: A Voxel-Based Morphometry Study. *PLoS ONE* **2016**, *11*, e0150757. [CrossRef] [PubMed]
57. Deepeshwar, S.; Vinchurkar, S.A.; Visweswaraiah, N.K.; Nagendra, H.R. Hemodynamic responses on prefrontal cortex related to meditation and attentional task. *Front. Syst. Neurosci.* **2015**, *8*, 252. [CrossRef] [PubMed]
58. Villemure, C.; Čeko, M.; Cotton, V.A.; Bushnell, M.C. Neuroprotective effects of yoga practice: Age-, experience-, and frequency-dependent plasticity. *Front. Hum. Neurosci.* **2015**, *9*, 281. [CrossRef] [PubMed]
59. Taliaz, D.; Loya, A.; Gersner, R.; Haramati, S.; Chen, A.; Zangen, A. Resilience to chronic stress is mediated by hippocampal brain-derived neurotrophic factor. *J. Neurosci.* **2011**, *31*, 4475–4483. [CrossRef] [PubMed]
60. Hariprasad, V.R.; Varambally, S.; Shivakumar, V.; Kalmady, S.V.; Venkatasubramanian, G.; Gangadhar, B.N. Yoga increases the volume of the hippocampus in elderly subjects. *Indian J. Psychiatry* **2013**, *55*, S394–S396. [PubMed]
61. Engström, M.; Pihlsgård, J.; Lundberg, P.; Söderfeldt, B. Functional magnetic resonance imaging of hippocampal activation during silent mantra meditation. *J. Altern. Complement. Med.* **2010**, *16*, 1253–1258. [CrossRef] [PubMed]
62. Van Rooij, S.J.; Stevens, J.S.; Ely, T.D.; Fani, N.; Smith, A.K.; Kerley, K.A.; Lori, A.; Ressler, K.J.; Jovanovic, T. Childhood Trauma and COMT Genotype Interact to Increase Hippocampal Activation in Resilient Individuals. *Front. Psychiatry* **2016**, *7*, 156. [CrossRef] [PubMed]
63. Desbordes, G.; Negi, L.T.; Pace, T.W.; Wallace, B.A.; Raison, C.L.; Schwartz, E.L. Effects of mindful-attention and compassion meditation training on amygdala response to emotional stimuli in an ordinary, non-meditative state. *Front. Hum. Neurosci.* **2012**, *6*, 292. [CrossRef] [PubMed]
64. Tang, Y.Y.; Hölzel, B.K.; Posner, M.I. The neuroscience of mindfulness meditation. *Nat. Rev. Neurosci.* **2015**, *16*, 213–225. [CrossRef] [PubMed]
65. Hilton, L.; Maher, A.R.; Colaiaco, B.; Apaydin, E.; Sorbero, M.E.; Booth, M.; Shanman, R.M.; Hempel, S. Meditation for Posttraumatic Stress: Systematic Review and Meta-analysis. *Psychol. Trauma* **2016**. [CrossRef] [PubMed]
66. *CADTH Rapid Response Reports. Mindfulness Interventions for the Treatment of Post-Traumatic Stress Disorder, Generalized Anxiety Disorder, Depression, and Substance Use Disorders: A Review of the Clinical Effectiveness and Guidelines*; Canadian Agency for Drugs and Technologies in Health: Ottawa, ON, USA, 2015.
67. Bhavanani, A.B.; Udupa, K.; Madanmohan Ravindra, P. A comparative study of slow and fast suryanamaskar on physiological function. *Int. J. Yoga* **2011**, *4*, 71–76. [CrossRef]
68. Sinha, B.; Ray, U.S.; Pathak, A.; Selvamurthy, W. Energy cost and cardiorespiratory changes during the practice of Surya Namaskar. *Indian J. Physiol. Pharmacol.* **2004**, *48*, 184–190. [PubMed]
69. Godse, A.S.; Shejwal, B.R.; Godse, A.A. Effects of suryanamaskar on relaxation among college students with high stress in Pune, India. *Int. J. Yoga* **2015**, *8*, 15–21. [CrossRef] [PubMed]
70. Harinath, K.; Malhotra, A.S.; Pal, K.; Prasad, R.; Kumar, R.; Kain, T.C.; Rai, L.; Sawhney, R.C. Effects of Hatha yoga and Omkar meditation on cardiorespiratory performance, psychologic profile, and melatonin secretion. *J. Altern. Complement. Med.* **2004**, *10*, 261–268. [CrossRef] [PubMed]
71. Tooley, G.A.; Armstrong, S.M.; Norman, T.R.; Sali, A. Acute increases in night-time plasma melatonin levels following a period of meditation. *Biol. Psychol.* **2000**, *53*, 69–78. [CrossRef]
72. Jayaram, N.; Varambally, S.; Behere, R.V.; Venkatasubramanian, G.; Arasappa, R.; Christopher, R.; Gangadhar, B.N. Effect of yoga therapy on plasma oxytocin and facial emotion recognition deficits in patients of schizophrenia. *Indian J. Psychiatry* **2013**, *55*, S409–S413. [PubMed]
73. Streeter, C.C.; Gerbarg, P.L.; Saper, R.B.; Ciraulo, D.A.; Brown, R.P. Effects of yoga on the autonomic nervous system, gamma-aminobutyric-acid, and allostasis in epilepsy, depression, and post-traumatic stress disorder. *Med. Hypotheses* **2012**, *78*, 571–579. [CrossRef] [PubMed]

74. Lipschitz, D.L.; Kuhn, R.; Kinney, A.Y.; Grewen, K.; Donaldson, G.W.; Nakamura, Y. An Exploratory Study of the Effects of Mind-Body Interventions Targeting Sleep on Salivary Oxytocin Levels in Cancer Survivors. *Integr. Cancer Ther.* **2015**, *14*, 366–380. [CrossRef] [PubMed]
75. Cramer, H. The Efficacy and Safety of Yoga in Managing Hypertension. *Exp. Clin. Endocrinol. Diabetes* **2016**, *124*, 65–70. [CrossRef] [PubMed]
76. Guglietti, C.L.; Daskalakis, Z.J.; Radhu, N.; Fitzgerald, P.B.; Ritvo, P. Meditation-related increases in GABAB modulated cortical inhibition. *Brain Stimul.* **2013**, *6*, 397–402. [CrossRef] [PubMed]
77. Streeter, C.C.; Jensen, J.E.; Perlmutter, R.M.; Cabral, H.J.; Tian, H.; Terhune, D.B.; Ciraulo, D.A.; Renshaw, P.F. Yoga Asana Sessions Increase Brain GABA Levels. *J. Altern. Complement. Med.* **2007**, *13*, 419–426. [CrossRef] [PubMed]
78. Streeter, C.C.; Whitfield, T.H.; Owen, L.; Rein, T.; Karri, S.K.; Yakhkind, A.; Perlmutter, R.; Prescot, A.; Renshaw, P.F.; Ciraulo, D.A.; et al. Effects of yoga versus walking on mood, anxiety, and brain GABA levels: A randomized controlled MRS study. *J. Altern. Complement. Med.* **2010**, *16*, 1145–1152. [CrossRef] [PubMed]
79. Naveen, G.H.; Thirthalli, J.; Rao, M.G.; Varambally, S.; Christopher, R.; Gangadhar, B.N. Positive therapeutic and neurotropic effects of yoga in depression: A comparative study. *Indian J. Psychiatry* **2013**, *55*, S400–S404. [PubMed]
80. Epel, E.S.; Blackburn, E.H.; Lin, J.; Dhabhar, F.S.; Adler, N.E.; Morrow, J.D.; Cawthon, R.M. Accelerated telomere shortening in response to life stress. *Proc. Natl. Acad. Sci. USA* **2004**, *101*, 17312–17315. [CrossRef]
81. Ornish, D.; Lin, J.; Daubenmier, J.; Weidner, G.; Epel, E.; Kemp, C.; Magbanua, M.; Marlin, R.; Yglecias, L.; Carroll, P.; et al. Increased telomerase activity and comprehensive lifestyle changes: A pilot study. *Lancet Oncol.* **2008**, *9*, 1048–1057. [CrossRef]
82. Ornish, D.; Lin, J.; Chan, J.M.; Epel, E.; Kemp, C.; Weidner, G.; Marlin, R.; Frenda, S.J.; Magbanua, M.J.; Daubenmier, J.; et al. Effect of comprehensive lifestyle changes on telomerase activity and telomere length in men with biopsy-proven low-risk prostate cancer: 5-year follow-up of a descriptive pilot study. *Lancet Oncol.* **2013**, *14*, 1112–1120. [CrossRef]
83. Hoge, E.A.; Chen, M.M.; Orr, E.; Metcalf, C.A.; Fischer, L.E.; Pollack, M.H.; de Vivo, I.; Simon, N.M. Loving-Kindness Meditation practice associated with longer telomeres in women. *Brain Behav. Immun.* **2013**, *32*, 159–163. [CrossRef] [PubMed]
84. Ross, A.; Thomas, S. The health benefits of yoga and exercise: A review of comparison studies. *J. Altern. Complement. Med.* **2010**, *16*, 3–12. [CrossRef] [PubMed]
85. Infante, J.R.; Peran, F.; Rayo, J.I.; Serrano, J.; Domínguez, M.L.; Garcia, L.; Duran, C.; Roldan, A. Levels of immune cells in transcendental meditation practitioners. *Int. J. Yoga* **2014**, *7*, 147–151. [CrossRef] [PubMed]
86. Bhargav, H.; Metri, K.; Raghuram, N.; Ramarao, N.H.; Koka, P.S. Enhancement of cancer stem cell susceptibility to conventional treatments through complementary yoga therapy: Possible cellular and molecular mechanisms. *J. Stem Cells* **2012**, *7*, 261–267. [PubMed]
87. Kiecolt-Glaser, J.K.; Christian, L.M.; Andridge, R.; Hwang, B.S.; Malarkey, W.B.; Belury, M.A.; Emery, C.F.; Glaser, R. Adiponectin, leptin, and yoga practice. *Physiol. Behav.* **2012**, *107*, 809–813. [CrossRef] [PubMed]
88. Sarvottam, K.; Magan, D.; Yadav, R.K.; Mehta, N.; Mahapatra, S.C. Adiponectin, interleukin-6, and cardiovascular disease risk factors are modified by a short-term yoga-based lifestyle intervention in overweight and obese men. *J. Altern. Complement. Med.* **2013**, *19*, 397–402. [CrossRef] [PubMed]
89. Yadav, R.K.; Magan, D.; Mehta, N.; Sharma, R.; Mahapatra, S.C. Efficacy of a short-term yoga-based lifestyle intervention in reducing stress and inflammation: Preliminary results. *J. Altern. Complement. Med.* **2012**, *18*, 662–667. [CrossRef] [PubMed]
90. Kiecolt-Glaser, J.K.; Bennett, J.M.; Andridge, R.; Peng, J.; Shapiro, C.L.; Malarkey, W.B.; Emery, C.F.; Layman, R.; Mrozek, E.E.; Glaser, R. Yoga's impact on inflammation, mood, and fatigue in breast cancer survivors: A randomized controlled trial. *J. Clin. Oncol.* **2014**, *32*, 1040–1049. [CrossRef] [PubMed]
91. Hochberg, M.C.; Altman, R.D.; April, K.T.; Benkhalt, M.; Guyatt, G.; McGowan, J.; Towheed, T.; Welch, V.; Wells, G.; Tugwell, P. American College of Rheumatology 2012 Recommendations for the Use of Nonpharmacologic and Pharmacologic Therapies in Osteoarthritis of the Hand, Hip, and Knee. *Arthritis Care Res.* **2012**, *64*, 465–474. [CrossRef]
92. Stenström, C.H.; Minor, M.A. Evidence for the benefit of aerobic and strengthening exercise in rheumatoid arthritis. *Arthritis Care Res.* **2003**, *49*, 428–434. [CrossRef] [PubMed]

93. Exercise and Arthritis. Available online: http://www.rheumatology.org/I-Am-A/Patient-Caregiver/Diseases-Conditions/Living-Well-with-Rheumatic-Disease/Exercise-and-Arthritis#sthash.2dxYmjdw.dpufRA (accessed on 30 January 2017).
94. Holtzman, S.; Beggs, R.T. Yoga for chronic low back pain: A meta-analysis of randomized controlled trials. *Pain Res. Manag.* **2013**, *18*, 267–272. [CrossRef] [PubMed]
95. Tilbrook, H.E.; Cox, H.; Hewitt, C.E.; Kang'ombe, A.R.; Chuang, L.H.; Jayakody, S.; Aplin, J.D.; Semlyen, A.; Trewhela, A.; Watt, I.; et al. Yoga for chronic low back pain: A randomized trial. *Ann. Intern. Med.* **2011**, *155*, 569–578. [CrossRef] [PubMed]
96. Tekur, P.; Nagarathna, R.; Chametcha, S.; Hankey, A.; Nagendra, H.R. A comprehensive yoga programs improves pain, anxiety and depression in chronic low back pain patients more than exercise: An RCT. *Complement. Ther. Med.* **2012**, *20*, 107–118. [CrossRef] [PubMed]
97. Moonaz, S.H.; Bingham, C.O., 3rd; Wissow, L.; Bartlett, S.J. Yoga in Sedentary Adults with Arthritis: Effects of a Randomized Controlled Pragmatic Trial. *J. Rheumatol.* **2015**, *42*, 1194–1202. [CrossRef] [PubMed]
98. Chu, P.; Pandya, A.; Salomon, J.A.; Goldie, S.J.; Hunink, M.G. Comparative Effectiveness of Personalized Lifestyle Management Strategies for Cardiovascular Disease Risk Reduction. *J. Am. Heart Assoc.* **2016**, *5*, e002737. [CrossRef] [PubMed]
99. Manchanda, S.C. Yoga—A promising technique to control cardiovascular disease. *Indian Heat Assoc.* **2014**, *66*, 487–489. [CrossRef] [PubMed]
100. Dzau, V.J.; Antman, E.M.; Black, H.R.; Manson, J.E.; Plutzky, J.; Popma, J.J.; Stevenson, W. The cardiovascular disease continuum validated: Clinical evidence of improved patient outcomes: Part 1: Pathophysiology and clinical trial evidence (risk factors through stable coronary artery disease). *Circulation* **2006**, *114*, 2850–2870. [CrossRef] [PubMed]
101. Yoga and Heart Health. Available online: http://www.heart.org/HEARTORG/HealthyLiving/PhysicalActivity/Yoga-and-Heart-Health_UCM_434966_Article.jsp# (accessed on 31 January 2017).
102. Innes, K.E.; Bourguignon, C.; Taylor, A.G. Risk indices associated with the insulin resistance syndrome, cardiovascular disease, and possible protection with yoga: A systematic review. *J. Am. Board Fam. Med.* **2005**, *18*, 491–519. [CrossRef]
103. Krishna, B.H.; Pal, P.; Pal, G.; Balachander, J.; Jayasettiaseelon, E.; Sreekanth, Y.; Sridhar, M.; Gaur, G. Effect of yoga therapy on heart rate, blood pressure and cardiac autonomic function in heart failure. *J. Clin. Diagn. Res.* **2014**, *8*, 14–16. [PubMed]
104. Thiyagarajan, R.; Pal, P.; Pal, G.K.; Subramanian, S.K.; Trakroo, M.; Bobby, Z.; Das, A.K. Additional benefit of yoga to standard lifestyle modification on blood pressure in prehypertensive subjects: A randomized controlled study. *Hypertens. Res.* **2015**, *38*, 48–55. [CrossRef] [PubMed]
105. Gard, T.; Noggle, J.J.; Park, C.L.; Vago, D.R.; Wilson, A. Potential self-regulatory mechanisms of yoga for psychological health. *Front. Hum. Neurosci.* **2014**, *8*, 770. [CrossRef] [PubMed]
106. Alexander, G.K.; Innes, K.E.; Selfe, T.K.; Brown, C.J. "More than I expected"; perceived benefits of yoga practice among older adults at risk for cardiovascular disease. *Complement. Ther. Med.* **2013**, *21*, 14–28. [CrossRef] [PubMed]
107. Hagins, M.; States, R.; Selfe, T.; Innes, K. Effectiveness of Yoga for Hypertension: Systematic Review and Meta-Analysis. *Evid. Based Complement. Altern. Med.* **2013**. [CrossRef] [PubMed]
108. Lakkireddy, D.; Atkins, D.; Pillarisetti, J.; Ryschon, K.; Bommana, S.; Drisko, J.; Vanga, S.; Dawn, B. Effect of yoga on arrhythmia burden, anxiety, depression, and quality of life in paroxysmal atrial fibrillation: The YOGA My Heart Study. *Am. Coll. Cardiol.* **2013**, *61*, 1177–1182. [CrossRef] [PubMed]
109. Mearns, B.M. Arrhythmias: Benefits of yoga in patients with atrial fibrillation. *Nat. Rev. Cardiol.* **2013**, *10*, 182. [CrossRef] [PubMed]
110. Sifferlin, A. The Most Stressed-Out Generation? Young Adults (2013). Available online: http://healthland.time.com/2013/02/07/the-most-stressed-out-generation-young-adults/ (accessed on 25 January 2017).
111. Yoga for Kids: How to Calm Little Minds. Available online: http://www.todaysparent.com/family/family-health/yoga-for-kids-how-to-calm-little-minds/ (accessed on 21 December 2016).
112. The Benefits of Yoga for Kids, One Downward Dog at a Time. Available online: http://www.good2grow.com/healthy-living-library/the-benefits-of-yoga-for-kids-one-downward-dog-at-a-time#sthash.2nc91QVF.dpuf (accessed on 21 December 2016).

113. Rosen, L.; French, A.; Sullivan, G. Complementary, Holistic, and Integrative. *Pediatr. Rev.* **2015**, *36*, 468. [CrossRef] [PubMed]
114. Hagen, I.; Nayar, U.S. Yoga for Children and Young People's Mental Health and Well-Being: Research Review and Reflections on the Mental Health Potentials of Yoga. *Front. Psychiatry* **2014**, *5*, 35. [CrossRef] [PubMed]
115. Khalsa, S.B.S. Yoga in Schools Research: Improving Mental and Emotional Health. In Proceedings of the Second International Conference on Yoga for Health and Social Transformation, Haridwar, India, 7–10 January 2013.
116. Khalsa, S.B.; Butzer, B. Yoga in school settings: A research review. *Ann. N. Y. Acad. Sci.* **2016**, *1373*, 45–55. [CrossRef] [PubMed]
117. Vohra, S.; McClafferty, H. Mind-Body Therapies in Children and Youth, Section on integrative medicine. *Pediatrics* **2016**, *138*, e20161896.
118. Tsao, J.C.; Meldrum, M.; Kim, S.C.; Jacob, M.C.; Zeltzer, L.K. Treatment preferences for CAM in children with chronic pain. *Evid. Based Complement. Altern. Med.* **2007**, *4*, 367–374. [CrossRef] [PubMed]
119. Birdee, G.S.; Yeh, G.Y.; Wayne, P.M.; Phillips, R.S.; Davis, R.B.; Gardiner, P. Clinical Applications of Yoga for the Pediatric Population: A Systematic Review. *Acad. Pediatr.* **2009**, *9*, 212–220. [CrossRef] [PubMed]
120. Galantino, M.L.; Galbavy, R.; Quinn, L. Therapeutic effects of yoga for children: A systematic review of the literature. *Pediatr. Phys. Ther.* **2008**, *20*, 66–80. [CrossRef]
121. Cramer, H.; Lauche, R.; Dobos, G. Characteristics of randomized controlled trials of yoga: A bibliometric analysis. *BMC Complement. Altern. Med.* **2014**, *14*, 328. [CrossRef] [PubMed]
122. Kaley-Isley, L.C.; Peterson, J.; Fischer, C.; Peterson, E. Yoga as a Complementary Therapy for Children and Adolescents: A Guide for Clinicians. *Psychiatry* **2010**, *7*, 20–32. [PubMed]
123. Balasubramaniam, M.; Telles, S.; Doraiswamy, P.M. Yoga on Our Minds: A Systematic Review of Yoga for Neuropsychiatric Disorders. *Front. Psychiatry* **2012**, *3*, 117. [CrossRef] [PubMed]
124. Jensen, P.S.; Kenny, D.T. The effects of yoga on the attention and behavior of boys with Attention-Deficit/ hyperactivity Disorder (ADHD). *J. Atten. Disord.* **2004**, *7*, 205–216. [CrossRef] [PubMed]
125. Haffner, J.; Roos, J.; Goldstein, N.; Parzer, P.; Resch, F. The effectiveness of body-oriented methods of therapy in the treatment of attention-deficit hyperactivity disorder (ADHD): Results of a controlled pilot study. *Z. Kinder Jugendpsychiatr. Psychother.* **2006**, *34*, 37–47. [CrossRef] [PubMed]
126. Khalsa, S.B.; Hickey-Schultz, L.; Cohen, D.; Steiner, N.; Cope, S. Evaluation of the mental health benefits of yoga in a secondary school: A preliminary randomized controlled trial. *J. Behav. Health Serv. Res.* **2012**, *39*, 80–90. [CrossRef] [PubMed]
127. Mendelson, T.; Greenberg, M.; Dariotis, J.; Feagans Gould, L.; Rhoades, B.; Leaf, P. Feasibility and Preliminary Outcomes of a School-Based Mindfulness Intervention for Urban Youth. *J. Abnorm. Child Psychol.* **2010**, *38*, 985–994. [CrossRef] [PubMed]
128. Sibinga, E.; Webb, L.; Ghazarian, S.; Ellen, J. School-Based Mindfulness Instruction: An RCT. *Pediatrics* **2016**, *137*. [CrossRef] [PubMed]

8

Applied Pediatric Integrative Medicine: What We Can Learn from the Ancient Teachings of Sebastian Kneipp in a Kindergarten Setting

Marion Eckert [1,*] and Melanie Anheyer [2]

[1] Kinderkrankenhaus St. Marien, 84036 Landshut, Germany
[2] Elisabeth Krankenhaus, 45138 Essen, Germany; m.anheyer@contilia.de
* Correspondence: dr-eckert@t-online.de

Abstract: Pediatric integrative medicine focuses on the whole child and the environment in which the child grows up during the treatment of a child's illness. Nowadays, many different treatment modalities are applied even in children, and doctors need to know about them and, ideally, be able to apply different approaches in the process of treating a child themselves. The program Pediatric Integrative Medicine in Residency (PIMR) already provides residents with several tools to provide this kind of service for the child. In our PIMR pilot program in Germany, we chose to diversify our knowledge about treatment and prevention options by visiting a Kneipp-certified kindergarten in Germany. The philosophy of Sebastian Kneipp focuses on five pillars of health, which incorporate aspects of prevention, self-awareness, self-responsibility, and consciousness of health by means of hydrotherapy, herbal medicine, exercise, nutrition, and lifestyle-medicine. These are being taught to the children during the early years they spend in kindergarten, and represent integral parts of integrative medicine. Integration of Kneipp-based health programs within a kindergarten setting can work well and provides an effective means of early prevention education in childhood.

Keywords: Kneipp; kindergarten; PIMR

---

1. Introduction

In Germany, there has been a long tradition of naturopathic medicine. Hildegard von Bingen (1098–1179), a Benedictine abbess, is considered the founder of natural history and her work still greatly influences modern naturopathic medicine movements. One of the more recent forefathers of the naturopathic movement was the priest, Sebastian Kneipp (1821–1897), who is most commonly associated with hydrotherapy and the "Kneipp-Cure", which he claimed had therapeutic or healing effects. But, it was not only hydrotherapy that he based his principles of achieving and maintaining health on. In fact, he proposed an entire system of healing, which rested on five pillars: Hydrotherapy, herbal medicine, exercise, nutrition, and lifestyle-medicine (order and balance) [1]. Even nowadays, his teachings and philosophy are a part of many naturopathic teachings in Germany, being represented in national and regional Kneipp-associations who certify a wide variety of qualified facilities with the "Kneipp certificate", such as schools and kindergartens as well as health resorts and spas, campgrounds, and guest houses, who must fulfill certain requirements according to the Kneipp philosophy. As Kneipp's principles form the basis for European traditional naturopathic medicine, they are an essential part of the curriculum offered for physicians in Germany who want to become legally certified naturopathic doctors. The pillars of Kneipp can also be found in modern and international integrative and naturopathic medicine and teaching curriculums [2,3], which makes them an essential part of knowledge for the integrative physician.

Integrative medicine in pediatrics focuses on the whole child and the environment in which the child grows up. Currently, obesity in children and allergies as well as stress related disorders are on the rise. An immediate reward principle, with everything readily available and a focus outside of oneself, is an increasing phenomenon. Therefore, prevention aspects, as well as self-awareness and mindfulness in life and health, have become important aspects of modern medicine. Especially, children need tools to grow up healthy in this kind of environment. Nowadays, many treatment modalities are being applied in integrative medicine and in the field of pediatrics [2]. The teaching program, "Pediatric Integrative Medicine in Residency (PIMR)" [3], provides residents with the knowledge about a wide variety of complementary healing approaches. In Germany, the PIMR program was used as a pilot program at three different childrens' hospitals. To deepen and diversify their knowledge about integrative medicine approaches, the group explored the principles of a Kneipp-certified kindergarten in Germany as an extracurricular activity. As described above, the philosophy of Sebastian Kneipp focuses on five pillars of health, which incorporate prevention, self-awareness, self-responsibility, and consciousness of health. These principles are being taught to the children during the years they spend in kindergarten.

2. Visit of the Kneipp Kindergarten

2.1. General Information

The kindergarten, St. Stephanus, in Essen, Germany, is one of 400 Kneipp-certified child daycare facilities in Germany. Certification by the Kneipp-Bund requires the offer of a multitude of self-awareness and self-experience opportunities that lie within the Kneipp principles to attain the ability of prevention in everyday life. In the case of a kindergarten, at least 50% of the teachers are required to attend an advanced 30-h training in health concepts according to Kneipp, and must attend yearly refresher courses. For implementation in daily life, a set of guidelines has been laid out, which must be fulfilled by the kindergarten to be certified [4]. These guidelines incorporate adequate outdoor and physical activity spaces, integration of parents, balance of life (e.g., daily routine, time for sleep and rest), offer of physical activities in- and outdoors, healthy nutrition, use of herbs, and, finally, daily water treatments according to Kneipp. After 18 months of gaining experience, certification of the facility ensues.

In the facility of St. Stephanus, the children are divided into three groups, with a total of 54 children. Two of the groups have children aged 3–6 years and one group is for children aged 0.3 months–3 years of age. The children can stay in the kindergarten either 35 h (7:00 a.m. through 2:00 p.m.) or 45 h (7:00 a.m. through 4:30 p.m.) per week. Still, there are many intergroup activities so children experience a greater variety of experiences and decision processes. There is a total of six teachers, one pediatric nurse, one childcare assistant, and the director of the facility. Children have two group rooms, two side rooms, a big common room, two wash rooms, a sleep room, one activity room, and a wide outdoor area at their disposal. They can play in all weather conditions, as the facility considers itself an all-weather kindergarten.

This kindergarten is closely associated with the local catholic community. Religious work is characterized by the appreciation of others and their beliefs, so acceptance and tolerance of different religions is actively lived. St. Stephanus is under the administration union of the "KiTa Zweckverband", a union of child daycare facilities in the Bishopric of Essen, and is financed partly by the union, the parents, and the city of Essen.

St. Stephanus is situated amidst one of the most densely populated parts of the city of Essen, namely Essen Holsterhausen, with close to 27,000 inhabitants. This part of Essen is characterized by a mixed population of all social classes where many single parents are in need of long hours of care for their child. The kindergarten is well accessible by car, bus, and is in walking distance of the surrounding residential areas.

2.2. Conceptual Design

Life in the kindergarten, St. Stephanus, has been lived according to the principles of Sebastian Kneipp since April 2013, when the kindergarten was officially certified by the "Kneipp-Bund".

As soon as you enter the facility the spirit of Kneipp's principles becomes evident: Binders in different colours and decorated stones representing the five pillars welcome the visitor. Throughout the kindergarten, it is obvious how deeply the Kneipp concept is integrated into everyday life. The following examples show how each of the five pillars of hydrotherapy, phytotherapy, physical activity, nutrition, and lifestyle-medicine is lived and applied by the children and their teachers.

Hydrotherapy is applied in many ways: The children learn through the effects of cold- or warm water washings or brushings how to calm themselves down or energize themselves. Every child has their own washcloth or brush and learns how to use it. There are tubs for arm-baths and foot-baths. In winter, children with warm feet go for a short walk in the snow, and, in spring and summer, the dew on the lawn is used for the "dew cure". This is one of the more than 120 forms of hydrotherapies of Kneipp, where a barefoot walk with initially warm feet in the fresh morning grass is performed for 2–5 min to boost the circulation, and strengthen the immune system and foot muscles. Water basins with cold water are used for water treading, the most well-known water application of Sebastian Kneipp. Always, the individual child, its health condition, body temperature etc. is considered so the child learns to listen to signs of their own body to determine what is good for them and what can be potentially harmful. Therefore, a self-determined and responsible care for their own health and body condition is taught to the children.

Herbs also play a central role in the kindergarten. An outdoor herb garden is used for planting and identifying herbs with the children. They pick and dry them and use them for making herb sachets and herbal teas as well as reference books. Also, aroma-oil diffusions are done in the group rooms, and herbal inhalations in a tent under supervision of a teacher. This way the children learn about the properties of the herbs and how they can be applied. Herbs used are common traditional European medicinal plants, for example chamomile, fennel, peppermint, anise, and lavender. Throughout the kindergarten, herbs and information sheets on how to use them are displayed for parents. This provides the families and children with respect and knowledge about nature as well as with tools for their own health.

Physical activity is also an important module in the kindergarten as well as promoting feeling and sensing the own body. Hence, there is a movement room in which children can move freely, climb, and be wild. To promote sensation, all is done barefoot. Also, the large outdoor area of the kindergarten gives the children the opportunity to move around outdoors in all weather conditions. With a feeling parcours, on which they also walk barefoot, children learn the different feeling of grass, asphalt, rocks, snow etc. in a mindful way. Thus, the children's innate joy of movement can be considered. The aim is to promote this in a sustainable way, which also shapes the social and emotional development of the children.

In early childhood, the foundations for a consciousness of healthy nutrition and way of eating can be built and shaped. Nutrition in the kindergarten is according to the recommendations of the Germany society for nutrition, incorporating seasonal and regional foods as well as whole grain products. A healthy diet is promoted through a daily changing breakfast buffet from which children can choose, serve themselves, and thereby determine what it is they want to eat. The lunch menu is selected each week by a different group of children. This way the children learn to listen to their body's needs while being able to choose from a healthy buffet.

The principle of order and balance is taught by the rules of Papilio for children as well as through daily and seasonal rituals, which promote a feeling of safety and assurance for the children. Balance between sleep and activity during the day, and a regulated day with fixed meal and play times is as important as lunch rituals, sleep rituals, birthday rituals, etc. Papilio is a program for the primary prevention of behavioral problems and for supporting the socio-emotional competencies of children. It has been designed for three different age groups and aims for the prevention of addictions and violence. The program is based on scientific studies and the effects have been proven by a controlled longitudinal study [5]. The kindergarten uses the program designed for children aged 3–6 years. According to the principles of Papilio, children learn how to interact with themselves and others in a respectful way, how to contribute their own matters, and how to be considerate of others.

The first principle is: Learn how to play with others and how to make yourself happy without the use of specific toys. Therefore, one day per week there is a "toys are on vacation day" where children only work with natural materials or must come up with own interactive ideas for playing.

The second principle is learning social rules and awareness of others in a playful way. Daily rules are made up together with the children, and one child always makes sure the rules are kept. For example, "I let others finish their sentence", "I listen to what others are saying", and "I put toys away after I'm finished playing with them".

The third principle is about teaching the children about emotions, so that they learn to recognize these in themselves and others, and, this way, learn how to deal with them. Puppets, in the form of emotion-goblins, displaying the major emotions of anger, happiness, sadness, and fear are applied in various ways. The happiness-goblin always smiles and cannot understand that anyone could feel different, the anger-goblin could explode upon every opportunity, the crying-goblin is always sad, and the fright-goblin is always afraid because something bad could happen at any time. The children learn how to recognize their own feelings as well as the feelings of others, and develop an understanding for the feelings of someone else. This is an important task in the development of a personality.

3. Discussion

In the kindergarten of St. Stephanus, the children live the principles of Kneipp in everyday life. In a playful way, they learn the basics for a healthy lifestyle, not only about "what can make me sick", but, even more so, "what keeps me healthy". Health-conscious behaviors and attitudes are being learned and practiced so that they become natural to the child and can provide the basis for a better consciousness of health and a healthier lifestyle later in life.

Despite health problems being a rising phenomenon in children, health education is usually not a teaching subject in schools and kindergartens. Different concepts of education can be found in kindergartens in Germany, yet, a concept based on physical and mental health education is unique to a Kneipp kindergarten.

The principle of order and balance forms the basis for the other four pillars according to the principles of Kneipp. It helps and supports children in implementing health-promoting attitudes into their daily life. In the kindergarten, this is achieved by the rules according to Papilio, as well as rituals, so that children can orient themselves and have a sense of stability. Thus, they can acquire skills that help them to find the balance between resources and everyday requirements.

There are no studies that have been performed specifically on Kneipp kindergarten children. However, studies done on children in various ages and adults show that water treatments lead to active training of blood vessels. Cold and warm water treatments increase blood flow and result in the training of blood vessels, which leads to a stabilization of the immune system [6]. A variety of benefits have been described, including a lowering of the frequency of coughing in respiratory tract infections and various immunological modulations [7–11]. As most children love water, washings, arm- and foot-baths, and walking in dew, snow, and water are perfect ways to playfully help in the prevention of common colds [7]. By directly experiencing their bodily reactions to the water-stimuli, they can learn to develop a better awareness of their own body.

Herbs, which the children grow in their own herb garden, are an essential component of complementary medicine as well as an integral part of the Kneipp philosophy. The direct contact with nature teaches the children respect and lays the foundation of an understanding of the benefits and damages of nature. The child recognizes the involvement of the human being in its environment. The sense of responsibility towards the environment and one's own body is supported and promoted.

Physical activity is a fundamental need and an integral part in the mental and physical development and well-being of children. In the kindergarten of St. Stephanus, the children are allowed to follow their daily urge to move. The focus is on elementary forms of movement and combines movement with positive experiences. This can prevent physical inactivity, which is associated with various diseases, such as metabolic syndrome and back pain.

Sebastian Kneipp recognized that many diseases occur due to the wrong type of nutrition. Therefore, he promoted a simple, natural diet with enough calories to support the functions of the organs and the body. Nutrition has also gained importance in conventional medicine, as the influence of malnutrition and over-nutrition on the development of civilization diseases is widely recognized nowadays. In St. Stephanus, the children receive a healthy, balanced diet, which is as natural and seasonal as possible. This can help establish a healthy eating pattern in the children. As parents are integrated into the activities of the kindergarten, this is also transported into the homes and families of the children.

Many publications show that despite huge medical advances, many children suffer from lifestyle (obesity, stress related disorders), chronic, and severe diseases [12–15]. Therefore, the promotion of health and wellness in childhood is essential. Kneipp had already recognized, in the 19th century, that the relationship between the body, mind, and soul plays a pivotal role in health and disease. Accordingly, he placed the whole human being, with its physical, psychological, and social needs, in the center of his prevention and therapy system, just like modern integrative medicine is dedicated to. He demanded responsibility for one's own health, including an active participation in one's own lifestyle and social relationships. Apart from a certain way and order of life, he claimed that physical activity, nutrition, and the use of herbs can be used to prevent and treat sickness. Those aspects are an integral part of modern integrative and complementary medicine, and are also represented in the curriculum of the PIMR [3].

The fact that this can already effectively be applied to children makes the Kneipp concept an ideal target for kindergartens and early priming for a healthy lifestyle. Most children are open and curious and love to learn [16,17]. This provides an excellent ground for laying new and lasting foundations regarding their own health. Teaching them Kneipp's prevention and treatment tools in a fun way at an early age provides an effective way to make those principles a palpable experience for children and allows for a holistic childhood education.

The limitation of applying some of Kneipp's principles in a kindergarten lies in the fact that treatments of sick children cannot be performed by teachers or nurses due to legal issues. Therefore, the use of Kneipp is limited to prevention aspects in this setting.

In Germany, no curriculum for a certification in naturopathic or integrative pediatrics exists. To obtain the certification of a naturopathic physician, only doctors can go through a curriculum designed for adult patients. In this curriculum, the principles according to Kneipp are an essential part and even a specific certification as a Kneipp physician exists. Visiting a Kneipp certified kindergarten helps pediatric residents and physicians to directly gain knowledge about the application of those principles to children so that they can use that knowledge in their care of children and transfer theory into practice. In this way, they can advise parents or educate kindergartens and schools in the application of Kneipp's principles and, therefore, support the inclusion of health promoting activities (both physical and social-emotional) in educational settings. Also, certain modalities, like hydrotherapy, can be introduced by adept doctors into pediatric hospitals interested in holistic healthcare approaches.

4. Conclusions

It has been shown that even in early childhood basic attitudes and patterns regarding one's own health and healing can be developed. Kneipp's system of healing, with its pillars of hydrotherapy, phytotherapy, exercise, and nutrition as well as order and balance, can be well integrated within a kindergarten setting and are perfectly suitable for teaching children about responsibility and connectedness towards self, others, and nature. In this way, the Kneipp principles can provide holistic support for the development of personality and health-conscious behaviors of the child. An awareness of individual health resources and avoidance of risk factors are promoted, as well as the development of a natural feeling for physical and emotional health, respect for others and the environment, mindfulness towards one's own resources, self-empowerment, and self-responsibility for health and emotional competencies.

A significant proportion of children worldwide suffer from health problems and with an increasing age the risk of civilizational diseases rises. A healthy lifestyle can prevent diseases or diminish their progression. Child day care facilities offer an ideal setting to introduce children to a health-promoting and health-conscious way of living: For one, children are curious, and their behavioral patterns can still be shaped. Secondly, kindergarten is a universal area of life for pre-school children, which makes it possible to reach children and parents from all social backgrounds. Even though there are currently no studies existing that give evidence about the advantages of a Kneipp based education in kindergarten, the principles of Kneipp are integral parts of modern integrative and naturopathic medicine. Kneipp based educational systems for children provide a good opportunity for physicians to observe and promote self-care strategies applied in children.

Author Contributions: M.E. is primarily responsible for the conception and design of this article. M.E. and M.A. drafted the text. Both authors provided evaluation and revision of the manuscript and have given final approval of the manuscript.

Acknowledgments: The authors thank Gustav Dobos, without whom this project and article would not exist. We thank the Weil Foundation for their funding of the pilot program PIMR in Germany and Birgit Drückler for the visit in the Kindergarten and her support regarding this publication. Thank you, Dennis Anheyer, for your input during the writing of this article and Mr. Brand for his overall support of our project.

References

1. Locher, C.; Pforr, C. The legacy of Sebastian Kneipp: Linking wellness, naturopathic, and allopathic medicine. *J. Altern. Complement. Med.* **2014**, *20*, 521–526. [CrossRef] [PubMed]
2. Vohra, S.; Surette, S.; Mittra, D.; Rosen, L.D.; Gardiner, P.; Kemper, K.J. Pediatric integrative medicine: Pediatrics' newest subspecialty? *BMC Pediatr.* **2012**, *12*, 123. [CrossRef] [PubMed]
3. McClafferty, H.; Dodds, S.; Brooks, A.J.; Brenner, M.G.; Brown, M.L.; Frazer, P.; Mark, J.D.; Weydert, J.A.; Wilcox, G.M.G.; Lebensohn, P.; et al. Pediatric Integrative Medicine in Residency (PIMR): Description of a New Online Educational Curriculum. *Children* **2015**, *2*, 98–107. [CrossRef] [PubMed]
4. Kneipp-Bund e.V. Available online: https://www.kneippbund.de/fileadmin/user_upload/kneipp-bund/dokumente/guetesiegel_zertifizierung/Richtlinien_2014/Richtlinien_Kitas_2014.pdf (accessed on 8 June 2018).
5. Scheithauer, H.; Bondü, R.; Niebank, K.; Mayer, H. Prävention von Verhaltensproblemen und Förderung prosozialen Verhaltens bei Hoch-und Niedrig-Risikokindern im Kindergarten: Erste Ergebnisse der Augsburger Längsschnittstudie zur Evaluation des Programms Papilio®(ALEPP). *Praxis der Rechtspsychologie* **2007**, *17*, 376–391.
6. Mooventhan, A.; Nivethitha, L. Scientific evidence-based effects of hydrotherapy on various systems of the body. *N. Am. J. Med. Sci.* **2014**, *6*, 199–209. [CrossRef] [PubMed]
7. Goedsche, K.; Förster, M.; Kroegel, C.; Uhlemann, C. Repeated cold water stimulations (hydrotherapy according to Kneipp) in patients with COPD. *Forsch. Komplementmed.* **2007**, *14*, 158–166. [PubMed]
8. Ring, J.; Teichmann, W. Immunological changes during hydrotherapy. *Dtsch. Med. Wochenschr.* **1977**, *102*, 1625–1630. [CrossRef] [PubMed]
9. Grüber, C.; Riesberg, A.; Mansmann, U.; Knipschild, P.; Wahn, U.; Bühring, M. The effect of hydrotherapy on the incidence of common cold episodes in children: A randomised clinical trial. *Eur. J. Pediatr.* **2003**, *162*, 168–176. [CrossRef] [PubMed]

10. Pilch, W.; Pokora, I.; Szyguła, Z.; Pałka, T.; Pilch, P.; Cisoń, T.; Malik, L.; Wiecha, S. Effect of a single finnish sauna session on white blood cell profile and cortisol levels in athletes and non-athletes. *J. Hum. Kinet* **2013**, *39*, 127–135. [CrossRef] [PubMed]
11. Werner, G.T.; Drinovac, V.; Penz, M.G. Immunologic testing on the effects of hydrotherapy according to Kneipp. *Münch. Med. Wochenschr.* **1998**, *140*, 566–569.
12. Miller, G.F.; Coffield, E.; Leroy, Z.; Wallin, R. Prevalence and Costs of Five Chronic Conditions in Children. *J. Sch. Nurs.* **2016**, *32*, 357–364. [CrossRef] [PubMed]
13. Burns, K.H.; Casey, P.H.; Lyle, R.E.; Bird, T.M.; Fussell, J.J.; Robbins, J.M. Increasing prevalence of medically complex children in US hospitals. *Pediatrics* **2010**, *126*, 638–646. [CrossRef] [PubMed]
14. Juonala, M.; Magnussen, C.G.; Berenson, G.S.; Venn, A.; Burns, T.L.; Sabin, M.A.; Srinivasan, S.R.; Daniels, S.R.; Davis, P.H.; Chen, W.; et al. Childhood adiposity, adult adiposity, and cardiovascular risk factors. *N. Engl. J. Med.* **2011**, *365*, 1876–1885. [CrossRef] [PubMed]
15. Messerli-Burgy, N.; Kakebeeke, T.H.; Arhab, A.; Stülb, K.; Zysset, A.E.; Leeger-Aschmann, C.S.; Schmutz, E.A.; Fares, F.; Meyer, A.H.; Munsch, S.; et al. The Swiss Preschoolers' health study (SPLASHY): Objectives and design of a prospective multi-site cohort study assessing psychological and physiological health in young children. *BMC Pediatr.* **2016**, *16*, 85. [CrossRef] [PubMed]
16. Perry, B.D. Why Young Children Are Curious. Available online: https://www.scholastic.com/teachers/articles/teaching-content/why-young-children-are-curious/ (accessed on 8 June 2018).
17. Kiser, B. Early child development: Body of knowledge. *Nature* **2015**, *523*, 286–289. [PubMed]

9

Incorporating Hypnosis into Pediatric Clinical Encounters

Robert A. Pendergrast Jr.

Department of Pediatrics, Medical College of Georgia, Augusta University, 1120 15th Street, Augusta, GA 30912, USA; rpenderg@augusta.edu

Abstract: Increasing numbers of licensed health professionals who care for children have been trained in clinical hypnosis. The evidence base for the safety and efficacy of this therapeutic approach in a wide variety of conditions is also growing. Pediatricians and other health professionals who have received training may wish to apply these skills in appropriate clinical scenarios but still may be unsure of the practical matters of how to incorporate this skill-set into day to day practice. Moreover, the practical application of such skills will take very different forms depending on the practice setting, types of acute or chronic conditions, patient and family preferences, and the developmental stages of the child or teen. This article reviews the application of pediatric clinical hypnosis skills by describing the use of hypnotic language outside of formal trance induction, by describing natural trance states that occur in children and teens in healthcare settings, and by describing the process of planning a clinical hypnosis encounter. It is assumed that this article does not constitute training in hypnosis or qualify its readers for the application of such skills; rather, it may serve as a practical guide for those professionals who have been so trained, and may serve to inform other professionals what to expect when referring a patient for hypnotherapy. The reader is referred to specific training opportunities and organizations.

Keywords: hypnosis; pediatric hypnosis; pediatric skills development; self-hypnosis; primary care; therapeutic use of language; hypnosis consult; practice style

---

1. Introduction

Though called by different names, there has been interest in the concept of clinical hypnosis by health professionals caring for children at least as far into Western history as the 18th century. This has been reviewed briefly by Kohen and Kaiser [1] and in more detail in Kohen and Olness' Hypnosis and Hypnotherapy in Children [2]. Since the 1960s, there has been a rapid expansion of dissemination of knowledge in the field, numbers of professionals receiving training and certification, and the development of a specifically pediatric curriculum. Since 1987, annual pediatric training workshops have been offered, initially under the auspices of the Society for Developmental and Behavioral Pediatrics, and since 2010 by the National Pediatric Hypnosis Training Institute, both American organizations. In Germany, the Kindertagung (the largest child hypnosis congress in the world) has been held periodically since 1990, with thousands of participants and an international faculty. There are excellent textbooks in the field, including Hypnosis and Hypnotherapy in Children [2], and Therapeutic Hypnosis with Children and Adolescents [3]. The American Journal of Clinical Hypnosis has published special issues on pediatric specific themes [4]. However, despite increasingly rich training and education resources, the number of licensed health professionals regularly utilizing hypnosis in practice is relatively small compared, say, to other similar skill sets such as active listening, motivational interviewing, or mindfulness training for example. Even after training, a practitioner may face the difficulty of local access to mentoring or modeling of the practical matters of incorporating hypnosis into pediatric clinical encounters. While not a substitute for training, this article will review some of those matters of practical application, the use of language, and may demystify the hypnosis referral process for other professionals.

2. Utilizing and Planning

A clinician who wishes to be purposeful in utilizing hypnosis in clinical encounters can begin by simply noticing the number of ways that children demonstrate spontaneous trance, or display behaviors that may be interpreted or understood as spontaneous self-hypnosis skills. While these are not quite conscious or intentional, they are nonetheless common in the context of everyday clinical encounters [5]. These quite natural states may take the form of imaginative language or play during a clinical encounter, intense focus or concentration on an activity, game, book, or puzzle, intense (and even fearful) focus on a physical sensation or injury, or distracted daydreaming that serves the purpose of adaptive dissociation for the child in an otherwise unpleasant situation. The fact that natural trance states occur so frequently in children in healthcare settings leads to the inescapable conclusion that *all* clinicians, whether trained in hypnosis or not, must be very careful with word choices around children. During any trance state, a person is much more likely to accept a suggestion as true (and act upon it); even unintentional suggestions or developmentally misinterpreted statements may have a larger than expected impact on a child [6]. For example, a clinician attempting humor with a 5-year-old with a wrist fracture may say something like "it's OK, you won't miss using that arm for a while . . . ." While an adult would be able to process such language as jest, a child in the trance of pain and injury may hear those words as suggestions for disuse or loss of the arm. Both children and adults interpret suggestions made during a trance state very literally and concretely. The concept of "trance logic" implies that during trance, a person may have very limited reality testing and would likely accept and act upon whatever suggestion is offered [7]. A natural trance state may be generated by a variety of healthcare encounters, such as an illness visit, awaiting an immunization, pre-operative preparation, or hearing an interpretation of lab tests or radiology results. Clinicians in these settings must think carefully about their choice of words and the effect of unintentional suggestions.

Conversely, natural trance states give clinicians the opportunity to decide when and how to utilize the child's demonstrated strengths by the purposeful use of language to build positive expectancy and positive outcomes. Thoughtful use of hypnotic language includes choice of words, tone of voice, and reflective listening. The decision to utilize the child's own natural self-hypnosis may be implemented immediately (e.g. "I'm impressed by how you are helping yourself right now" for a child with Tourette's who is not having tics in the office), or implemented later when appropriate in the conversation (e.g., "remember a few minutes ago when you were enjoying your new book? Did you know *you can do that* while the nurse is giving you medicine in your arm so it doesn't have to *bother* you so much?").

Natural trance states in children can be understood as the child's spontaneous and subconscious attempt to organize their experiences (especially novel and perhaps frightening experiences) and make new connections in four areas of self-regulation: cognitive, affective/emotional, physiologic, and behavioral. When clinicians are attentive and prepared, they can notice and then facilitate the child's nascent self-regulatory capacity by "being hypnotic" in a clinical conversation. For example, an observant clinician dealing with a child with a delayed sleep onset disorder may be watching for a child's attempts at emotional self-regulation and learning about how the child might self-soothe from anxiety symptoms. Based on moment-to-moment observation of the child, the clinical interview might include something like "I notice you took a nice deep breath just now . . . I wonder why/how your brain chose *right now* to do that?" Or to access the child's ability for physiologic self-regulation, a clinician could ask "what have you done in the past to help that tummy feel better when stress or worry had made it uncomfortable?" This approach is quite different from one that would take a clinical history, view all of that as devoid of trance or hypnotic phenomena, and then verbally move into a new section of the appointment understood or even labeled as "doing hypnosis." The concept of utilizing children's trance as a way of enhancing self-regulatory skills has been expertly reviewed by Kaiser [8].

This approach to enhancing children's self-regulatory capacity by utilizing hypnotic language without "doing hypnosis" can be characterized as noticing and cultivating the natural hypnotic state, or "using the hypnosis" in the encounter. It usually occurs in the context of taking a clinical history. But the history taking process can and should be more of a conversation than a question and answer checklist, in which clinical questions and open-ended reflection are designed to help the child begin to reframe their experiences, expand their cognitive capacity by attaching new labels to experience, and expand their emotional fluency and self-awareness. The clinician can be extremely helpful to children and teens by simply using reflective listening skills to enhance self-awareness, knowing that self-awareness is a foundational first step to self-regulation. For example, a child may present to the medical office with both chronic abdominal pain and separation anxiety, but has never comprehended the connection between the two. The clinical conversation helps the child to make sense of his or her disconnected experiences and understand that they are not separate phenomena. Because of curiosity and novelty, this conversation is often hypnotic, but is not "doing hypnosis" in the sense that there is a formal sequence of invitation, induction or any script. It is important in this type of clinical conversation for the clinician to provide observations of the co-incidence of phenomena in the child's life, but in the end each patient must make the connections for themselves by responding to questions like "tell me what you make of that . . . ."

Complementary to the concept of utilizing natural trance states, it is equally important for clinicians to be deliberate in planning or designing hypnotic encounters, especially before entering a consult in which the reason for the appointment is already known. This implies intentional planning, a carefully crafted encounter with a patient that is more likely to have been thought out ahead of time, reviewing a clinical history that is (mostly) known and planning the structure and content of an appointment, including the type of induction and the metaphors/suggestions that would be most appropriate based on the clinical history. It may be helpful for the clinician to outline in writing some expected steps of the appointment, following a predicted sequence: interim history, today's therapeutic goals, induction technique, intensification strategy, suggestions/metaphors, post-hypnotic suggestions, alerting and ratification, and follow-up plan. It involves giving therapeutic, specific suggestions related to specific goals for that particular clinical encounter. (Induction and intensification techniques and the specific use of hypnotic suggestion and therapeutic metaphor are beyond the scope of this article.) Thoughtful planning of each of the expected steps of the appointment can make a positive outcome more likely. Still, even when carefully planned and conceived ahead of time, in any given appointment a clinician must be prepared to flexibly follow cues from the child, adapting strategies based on how the child demonstrates readiness for help in cultivating these skills.

Whether "doing hypnosis" or "noticing and utilizing and being hypnotic", clinicians must recognize in this model that patients, especially children, bring trance with them into the setting without being aware of it. Trance is what the brain does naturally when it encounters something for the first time, giving attention to novelty: "I never saw that before," "I never thought of it that way before," "I never met anyone quite like you before," or even "I never had a pain quite like this before." Trance can be elevating and activating (like a 6-month old reaching for a cardboard picture book), or it can be terrible like the fight or flight response of someone who encounters a phobic object. Within that trance, there is often an openness to change, a readiness to see and experience the world differently, that is, to learn. That may occur with or without the patient having any cultivated self-hypnosis skills, but the attentive clinician will often find that children and teens arrive at appointments with some skills they have already discovered for themselves in this area.

Thus, whether the encounter is spontaneous or planned, clinicians bring their own skill sets and attentiveness to the encounter, ready to cultivate change for the patient, but only when and if the child or teen allows that to happen. In any encounter where the clinician is doing something formally or informally planned to be hypnotic or to evoke hypnosis in the patient, nothing happens at all unless the patient is willing and open to this. In this model, one may see hypnosis as an interpersonal interaction by which the clinician cultivates a trance that the patient makes accessible, for the purpose of a specific health related outcome.

3. Primary Care Pediatrics

In the primary care pediatric setting, there are four areas in which a clinician's choice of words can intersect with a child's curiosity and become a spontaneously hypnotic encounter that facilitates positive outcomes. They are: developmental mastery, positive expectation, behavior change/motivation, and discovering self-regulation.

Developmental mastery: Even during well-child checkups for infants and toddlers, a clinician can reinforce the child's own growing sense of competence or the maternal-infant dyad's resilience by making the screening history conversational. For example, pointing out to a new mother how alert and attentive a nursing infant is, talking with parents about how their newborn is constantly learning, commenting on how focused is the 6-month old reaching for a cardboard picture book (demonstrating trance, encountering novelty). In these settings, the mother is often also in trance focusing on her child, so these are opportune moments for positive comments and suggestions regarding the multitude of opportunities that parents and caregivers have to interact with the child in ways that build resilience and developmental mastery.

Pediatric practitioners have daily opportunities to reinforce the child's growing developmental competence. The verbal content of the well-child history changes with age and developmental stages, but at each age, the words that a clinician chooses can be powerfully reinforcing. The child's natural trance state in the healthcare encounter creates an opportunity for purposeful suggestions that are specific to the developmental stage of the child or teen. Any pediatric health provider wishing to apply clinical hypnosis must first become fluent in the normal stages of child development and learn how to connect with children in a developmentally appropriate way [9]. For example, a 3-year-old (in Erikson's stage of autonomy versus shame and doubt) would have his/her developmental mastery reinforced by a comment like, "look how well you climbed onto the exam table *by yourself*! When you were a baby you couldn't do that!," or during a checkup saying to a 10-year-old (stage of industry versus inferiority, where competence is the key strength to be developed) "You're good at lots of things! I wonder how many things you'll learn to be good at by this time next year?."

Positive expectation: Setting positive expectations for children in pediatric healthcare settings is an important and often neglected challenge. Immunizations, phlebotomy, or the uncertainty and anxiety regarding the physical examination all create strongly negative expectations for children and teens in medical offices. Using distraction and other hypnotic approaches to reduce children's discomfort in medical offices is a very important subject in its own right and will not be covered in detail in this paper [10]. A growing body of literature supports the idea that measures to reduce pain of immunizations and procedures in children are both important and achievable [11]. Even without structured office interventions to reduce discomfort, each clinician can help children and teens feel more comfortable, physically and emotionally, by careful choice of words. Because children and teens are often in a natural trance state (albeit a negative one full of intense focus on a feared event) in the medical office, a carefully crafted statement that reframes the experience and opens the child to new expectations can be powerful. For example, "I don't really know just what it will feel like for you, but I do know that you may be surprised at how little it will have to bother you, and how easy it may be for you just to pay attention to something else while the nurse takes good care of that arm over there . . . ." On the other hand, suggestions such as "it's not going to *hurt*," can be pro-nociceptive. A child's thoughts will invariably focus on the word "hurt" and ignore the word "not." Finding ways to use words to substitute for "pain" and "hurt" is important. Use "bother" in place of "hurt," and "discomfort" instead of "pain".

Behavior change/motivation: Any primary care office caring for adolescents will present daily opportunities to use hypnotic language to promote behavior change. In this context, there is a large overlap between the use of hypnotic language and the principles of motivational interviewing [12,13]. One of the core concepts of motivational interviewing is Developing Discrepancy. This is the process in which the clinician facilitates the patient's awareness of his/her current state versus a desired future state. A respectful and empathetic conversation that provokes the teen to think deeply about this discrepancy can often lead to spontaneous trance experiences in the patient. For example, asking a teen, "I wonder what sort of things you picture or think about when you think about yourself one year from now . . . " can be followed by an expectant silence, in which trance phenomena may be observed. This can be a very useful way to gauge readiness to change. Another key concept of motivational interviewing is that of Exploring Ambivalence. A question such as "will you miss the extra weight when it is gone?" is an implied hypnotic suggestion that the weight will in fact be gone at some future time. Second, it implies that the patient may be ambivalent about it and can (perhaps in spontaneous trance induced by such a novel question) explore the pros and cons of continuing current behaviors versus changing. One can also explore other motivational interviewing domains while the patient is in trance, either from a formal hypnotic induction or spontaneous. A suggestion for future visualization of the self (either with the positive health behavior change or not) can assist the patient in exploring his/her readiness to change, and in affirming his/her own goals. For example, "while these thoughts are on your mind, take a moment to picture yourself, as if on a 'future TV screen' and get a sense of what you like about that picture, what you don't like about that picture, and what choices you can make now that affect that future." This clinical encounter may be in the mental health office or in the primary care office around issues of health behavior.

Self-regulation: Another important way in which purposeful language in outpatient settings can be hypnotic is in facilitating discovery of psychophysiological self-regulation (e.g., breath awareness). Many opportunities for this in clinical care. For example, a brief intervention in the office for a child with anxiety can start with a question like, "Can you put your hand on the place where that worry shows up most in your body?" Most children will readily identify the site of the most troubling somatic symptoms related to stress. A follow-up question can immediately follow: "Would it be OK to learn how to help yourself feel better there?" Teaching the child or teen simple techniques of abdominal breathing and then noticing how they feel differently can be a powerful first step in enhanced self-regulation. It is also important during the clinical encounter to encourage the child or teen to reflect on how they may have already discovered their own methods of physiologic self-regulation. It is not uncommon for a patient to disclose their own techniques to the clinician, such as "I already use my imagination and breathing when I am nervous at bedtime." The clinician's task then is to reinforce and ratify the child's own strengths with statements like "helping you learn to help yourself is going to be easier than I thought, since you are *already good at changing things*".

4. Hospital and Acute Care Settings

Hypnotic language can often be utilized in hospital settings or in preparation for medical procedures [14]. This can be very informal, without a formal induction, and may occur in the routine course of daily work for a pediatric hospitalist or a Child Life professional. A clinician may also set a longer appointment time for more formal hypnotherapy to prepare for an anticipated procedure. Fundamentally, this involves rehearsing the procedure in trance and creating positive expectations. However, any such intervention must be developmentally appropriate, and expecting a preschooler to sit quietly and visualize is not developmentally on target. Such a child could be encouraged to bring a doll or favorite toy with them, and a playful conversation about how well the doll can experience the upcoming procedure may be sufficient, as long as the child is engaged in the imaginative experience. More formal trance induction in an older child could be followed by imaginal desensitization (the "future TV of me") using imagery and suggestions that reframe and change the child or teen's expectations. In urgent care and emergency settings, clinicians have opportunities to help children in crisis. The negative trance that children and teens bring with them into that circumstance in fact makes the use of hypnotic language easier, and is also a reminder of the critical importance of choice of words in acute care settings. Our language in such settings is important, because the children are already in a highly suggestible state. During evaluation of an acute injury, it is possible to embed hypnotic suggestions such as "I can tell it hurts, and you know it may keep on keep on hurting until it feels better, or until it doesn't need to any more . . . ." The likelihood is that the words that "stick" in the child's consciousness are the words "it feels better," which is, after all, the desired outcome. Reframing is possible as well, such as "isn't it nice that your body knows how to use all that good healthy blood to clean out the cut?"

5. The Hypnotherapy Consult

Clinicians who are trained and develop their clinical hypnosis practice will invariably be consulted by other clinicians, usually regarding patients who remain symptomatic despite all the usual diagnostic and therapeutic approaches of more conventional pediatric medicine. For such appointments, it is wise to block a longer extended appointment time, at least 45 min, in order to establish rapport, gather the clinical history, explain hypnosis and self-hypnosis to the child and parent(s), clarify the rationale for using hypnotherapy for the troubling symptoms, reassure the parents (more than the child) that a referral for hypnotherapy does not imply that anyone believes the symptoms are not "real," and then (perhaps) to begin self-hypnosis coaching for the child or teen. Often there is not sufficient time in a first appointment to give adequate attention to the actual use of hypnotherapy, and a quick return appointment is expected.

There are a number of ways that hypnotic language shows up in these appointments even well before anything that looks like hypnosis, and should start during the process of gathering the medical history. The clinician should be alert to signs of trance in the child, and then reflecting their own trance state back to them in several ways. First, find out what they do well, and what resources they have already discovered for wellness and self-regulation. Short phrases that can be useful include:

Tell me about something you do so well, and is so much fun, that you often or usually forget most everything else . . .

What was going on the last time you felt really good?

Can we talk about that time when you felt really worried but didn't (throw-up, have a headache, etc.)?

This process always involves the clinician noticing what the patient is saying, how s/he is saying it, the moments which appear to be moments of trance in which s/he is attempting to make sense of connections and novel ideas, and then offering new interpretations of what s/he has said, as a way of opening possibilities to change based on what s/he already knows.

Words and phrases that can help as therapeutic reflection of child's own trance, specifically planned to cultivate and nurture the child's own curiosity include:

How do YOU think is the best way to learn that?

You have lots of skills (in whatever areas already discussed)*, are you ready to learn some new things or new ways to help yourself solve that problem with . . . ?*

How does your bladder know to keep the gate shut while you are sitting in school during the day?

Is there a time when pain can be useful?

Do you know about the pain switches?

I wonder how soon you will be able to turn off the pain switch when it's not needed . . .

How did you do that?

Preparation is critical for these consult appointments. The prepared clinician will review prior medical records, referral documents, and his/her own notes for return appointments. This implies that one should keep very detailed notes of appointments. Write down in the medical record the child's own words that describe their situation; record the history from the parents' perspective; record observations of the child's demeanor during the appointment and how that may have changed over the course of the appointment; record their likes and dislikes, things they do well, who they live with, how they are doing in school, and any special circumstances of the family, such as military deployments for example. When the child returns for the second appointment, the prepared clinician has already reviewed these notes in order to build on that rapport and to remember what worked well and what did not work well.

During the appointment, it is advisable to direct most of the conversation to the child, not to the parent. One can explicitly say to the child at the outset that s/he is important, what s/he thinks is important, what s/he says is important, *and* that the parent will also have a turn to talk, because *s/he has some important things to say too*, but that can wait.

This deliberately child-centric posture is, in all likelihood, completely different from any prior experience this child has had with medical professionals, who tend to talk *about* them *to* their parents, but not talking *with* them and acting respectful of what they have to say. This implies to the child that one is confident in them to articulate and express their own wishes and desires. It builds their trust in the clinician, and it most certainly builds their curiosity in what is about to happen because it breaks previously held expectations about conversations with doctors. It creates the space and opportunity to transform old cognitive, emotional, physiologic, or behavioral patterns of self-regulation. It implies a belief that they *themselves* can be an effective change agent for their own issues. This conversation with the child must always be done in a developmentally appropriate way, remembering to talk with a 7-year-old *very* differently than with a 14-year-old.

After planning and preparation is done, the clinician's behavior toward the patient is that of leading with permission. Leading implies that one has a skill set to use in order to show the patient in a collaborative way *how* they can get to their goals. The patient came to the appointment with a need and did not know on their own how to meet that need; it is the clinician's job to lead them there. Equally as important, it is the clinician's job to recognize that all of this happens only if the patient wants it to happen. That is true not just of the hypnotherapy itself, but also of the appointment in general. A useful introductory comment is that "things happen in hypnosis because you want them to happen, not because I want them to happen." This "leading with permission" posture and behavior continues even during hypnosis, so that the language of suggestions is not prescriptive (e.g., "you will have the pain down to zero by the time I count down from 10"), but permissive (e.g., "I wonder how soon you will find that old pain completely gone . . . let me know when you get it down to zero . . . ").

There are pros and cons of keeping parents in the consult room while working with a child or teen [15]. Many clinicians keep the parent in the room for most if not all of the first appointment, enhancing insights into the parent-child interaction and whether it may be a strength or a liability; it can also help to get two different perspectives on the issues at hand. At subsequent appointments, it may not be advisable to keep a parent in the room during hypnotherapy, as a parent can be distracting and cause the child to "perform" in a way that they believe their parents would expect rather than exercising their own autonomy and mastery. Similar to the child's performance expectations with parents watching, the clinician may also become overly self-conscious with parents watching. A clinician who is personally attached to creating a certain outcome in the clinical encounter or who is consciously or unconsciously trying to please a parent is not likely to give his or her best energy to creating a therapeutic alliance with the child or teen. This can inadvertently sabotage the very clinical outcome the clinician is anxious to demonstrate to the parent. A clinician who is anxious about what a parent is thinking about him or her is not likely to be clinically effective. If a child is very anxious, one may more strongly consider keeping the parent in the room, hoping to gradually wean the child from that anxious attachment to facilitate their mastery of new skills in self-regulation.

Audio recordings of hypnotherapy sessions can be very helpful as a tool to help the child/teen practice at home, and most families now have a smart phone with a voice recorder app, making recording almost effortless. One may want to introduce the idea of using the recording at home with a comment like "you can find this a helpful way to start practicing, until you don't need the audio anymore."

On return appointments, the interim history will reveal if things have gone well or not. If the patient's experience was positive or neutral, they will expect to have a repeat hypnotherapy session with more guidance for self-hypnosis practice at home. It may be advisable on the second visit to use the same hypnotic induction as at the first appointment in order to help reinforce what may still be a fragile practice of self-hypnosis at home. On future appointments with a patient who is making progress, it can be a good idea to teach them a new type of self-induction for themselves at home, to build skills and the opportunity for new types of self-discovery.

If parents or children report that things did not go well after the first appointment, the clinician must gather all the details about what happened in the interim, and re-assess the child/teen's interest and willingness to use such techniques to feel better. All that may be required is a different approach, along with continued optimism that a child who is motivated to feel well will discover (with expert guidance) a way to enhance their own self-regulatory ability in order to resolve an issue.

6. Resources and Training

It is incumbent on all professionals who care for children in healthcare settings to be aware of the power of words in affecting the mental and physical health of children, for better or for worse. Experienced and thoughtful pediatric clinicians are aware of this even without specific training in clinical hypnosis. Over time, most clinicians become more careful in how they speak during clinical encounters, helping children become more comfortable in healthcare settings. However, many of the concepts described in this paper are quite different from widespread practice patterns. A thoughtful clinician wanting to interact with children and teens in such new ways will soon realize that specific and more concentrated training is needed. The annual training workshops conducted by the National Pediatric Hypnosis Training Institute (NPHTI, a United States registered non-profit 501(c)(3) corporation) are directed by experienced clinician educators and achieve consistently high ratings from attendees. More information is available [16]. The American Society of Clinical Hypnosis (ASCH) conducts annual meetings, national and regional workshops, and is the certifying body for health professionals in the United States who have had clinical hypnosis training. There is a small but consistent presence of pediatric offerings the annual workshops by ASCH [17]. Professionals in Europe can avail themselves of the resources and training events from the European Society of Hypnosis [18]. And while one does not become skilled in clinical hypnosis by reading articles or books, there are seminal readings which should form the foundation of basic knowledge of any pediatric clinician. These include Michael Yapko's book, Trancework [19], and the more specific pediatric titles Hypnosis and Hypnotherapy in Children [2], and Therapeutic Hypnosis with Children and Adolescents [3]. ASCH publishes pediatric specific articles frequently to keep professionals abreast with progress in the field [4]. With frequent attendance at hypnosis training workshops and meetings, a commitment to reading core books and articles, a thoughtful pediatric clinician can not only facilitate transformation for his or her patients, but also transform his or her own professional life and satisfaction.

Acknowledgments: I am grateful to my colleagues and mentors in the National Pediatric Hypnosis Training Institute and to the children and families with whom I am privileged to work.

References

1. Kohen, D.P.; Kaiser, P. Clinical Hypnosis with Children and Adolescents—What? Why? How? Origins, Applications, and Efficacy. *Children* **2014**, *1*, 74–98. [CrossRef] [PubMed]
2. Kohen, D.P.; Olness, K.N. *Hypnosis and Hypnotherapy with Children*, 4th ed.; Routledge Publications: New York, NY, USA, 2011.

3. Wester, W.; Sugarman, L.I. *Therapeutic Hypnosis with Children and Adolescents*; Crown House Publishing: Carmarthen, Wales, UK, 2007.
4. Anbar, R.D. Guest Editorial: Clinical Pearls Gleaned from Pediatric Hypnosis. *Am. J. Clin. Hypn.* **2011**, *54*, 3–4. [CrossRef] [PubMed]
5. Olness, K.N.; Gardner, G.G. Some Guidelines for uses of hypnotherapy in pediatrics. *Pediatrics* **1978**, *62*, 228. [PubMed]
6. Kohen, D.P.; Olness, K.N. *Hypnosis and Hypnotherapy with Children*, 4th ed.; Routledge Publications: New York, NY, USA, 2011; pp. 109–112.
7. Yapko, M. *Trancework*, 4th ed.; Routledge Publications: New York, NY, USA, 2012; pp. 185–186.
8. Kaiser, P. Childhood anxiety, worry and fear: Individualizing hypnosis goals and suggestions for self-regulation. *Am. J. Clin. Hypn.* **2011**, *54*, 16–31. [CrossRef] [PubMed]
9. *Growth and crises of the "healthy personality"*; Erikson, E.H.; Senn, M.J.E. (Eds.) Symposium on the healthy personality; Josiah Macy Jr. Foundation: Oxford, England, 1950; pp. 91–146.
10. Berberich, F.R.; Landman, Z. Reducing immunization discomfort in 4 to 6 year old children: A randomized clinical trial. *Pediatrics* **2009**, *124*, e203–e209. [CrossRef] [PubMed]
11. Lee, G.Y.; Yamada, J.; Shorkey, A.; Stevens, B. Pediatric Clinical Practice Guidelines for Acute Procedural Pain: A Systematic Review. *Pediatrics* **2014**, *133*, 1–16. [CrossRef] [PubMed]
12. Miller, W.R.; Rollnick, S. *Motivational Interviewing: Helping People Change*, 3rd ed.; Guilford Press: New York, NY, USA, 2013.
13. Barnes, A.J.; Gold, M.A. Promoting Healthy Behaviors in Pediatrics. *Pediatr. Rev.* **2012**, *33*, e57–e68. [CrossRef] [PubMed]
14. Kuttner, L. Management of young children's acute pain and anxiety during invasive medical procedures. *Pediatrician* **1989**, *16*, 39–45. [PubMed]
15. Linden, J. Hypnosis and Parents: Pattern interruptus. *Am. J. Clin. Hypn.* **2011**, *54*, 70–81. [CrossRef] [PubMed]
16. National Pediatric Hypnosis Training Institute. Available online: www.nphti.org (accessed on 14 March 2017).
17. American Society of Clinical Hypnosis. Available online: www.asch.net (accessed on 14 March 2017).
18. European Society of Hypnosis. Available online: http://esh-hypnosis.eu (accessed on 14 March 2017).
19. Yapko, M. *Trancework*, 4th ed.; Routledge Publications: New York, NY, USA, 2012.

10

Review of Randomized Controlled Trials of Massage in Preterm Infants

Anna-Kaisa Niemi

Department of Pediatrics, Division of Neonatal & Developmental Medicine, Stanford University, Palo Alto, CA 94304, USA; annakaisa.niemi@gmail.com

Abstract: Preterm birth affects about 10% of infants born in the United States. Massage therapy is being used in some neonatal intensive care units for its potential beneficial effects on preterm infants. This article reviews published randomized controlled trials on the effects of massage in preterm infants. Most studies evaluating the effect of massage in weight gain in premature infants suggest a positive effect on weight gain. Increase in vagal tone has been reported in infants who receive massage and has been suggested as a possible mechanism for improved weight gain. More studies are needed on the underlying mechanisms of the effects of massage therapy on weight gain in preterm infants. While some trials suggest improvements in developmental scores, decreased stress behavior, positive effects on immune system, improved pain tolerance and earlier discharge from the hospital, the number of such studies is small and further evidence is needed. Further studies, including randomized controlled trials, are needed on the effects of massage in preterm infants.

Keywords: infant massage; preterm; premature; newborn; neonate; weight gain; hyperbilirubinemia; mind–body; randomized controlled trial; tactile-kinesthetic stimulation

---

1. Introduction

Preterm birth (birth at <37 weeks of gestation) affects about 10% of infants born in the USA [1]. Premature infants often spend weeks or months in intensive care unit due to immaturity and need for intensive medical care, with hospital stay often prolonged by feeding immaturity and slow weight gain. Massage therapy is being used in some neonatal intensive care units for its possible beneficial effects with minimal side effects. This article reviews published randomized controlled trials on the effects of massage in preterm infants.

A PubMed search was performed for randomized controlled trials (RCTs) of massage in preterm infants. RCTs in English and indexed in PubMed by January 2017 were included. Studies assessing the effects of massage on caregivers only were excluded. A total of 34 randomized controlled trials on the effects of massage in preterm infants are reviewed [2–35].

2. Results

The outcome most commonly assessed on randomized controlled trials of massage in preterm infants (Table 1) was weight gain, either as primary or secondary outcome [2,5,8–10,12,15–19,21,26,28–31,33–35]. Other outcomes assessed in RCTs of massage in preterm infants include levels of transcutaneous bilirubin [3], sleep [4,26], calorie intake [5,17,19,30,33–35], vagal activity [5,19,24,26,29,30], gastric motility or number of stools [3,24,30], heart rate variability (HRV) [6,7,19,24,30], immunologic parameters [12], bone metabolism [11,32], changes in electroencephalogram (EEG) [13], behavior and/or neurodevelopment [14,15,23,26,28,29,31,34,35], pain [25], length of hospital stay [12,16,18] and levels of serum markers such as insulin-like growth factor I (IGF-1) [8,19], adiponectin [8], and serum triglycerides [9,27,31].

Most randomized controlled trials compared massage to standard care [2–4,6–9,11–14,16–35], while some compared oil massage to massage without oil [10], tactile massage to kinesthetic stimulation [5] and massage to light still touch [15]. While the type of massage used varied between studies, most studies assessed the effects of the tactile-kinesthetic stimulation (TKS) type of infant massage originally described by Field et al. in 1986 [36] or a modified version of TKS (Table 1). Modifications of TKS included shorter or longer duration of massage as well as elimination of kinesthetic range of movement exercise with only tactile stimulation provided. Other massage types evaluated include oil massage combined with either TKS or other standardized technique [2,9,10,27,28,31], Vimala massage [17] and acupressure and meridian massage [21].

In the following sections the outcomes of these studies as well as limitations are briefly reviewed. For number of study participants, gestational age, age at the time of study entry, and duration of massage intervention see Table 1.

2.1. Weight Gain

Weight gain, either as primary or secondary outcome is the most commonly assessed outcome in randomized controlled trials of massage in preterm infants [2,5,8–10,12,15–19,21,26,28–31,33–35]. Most studies have demonstrated a significantly greater daily or overall weight gain during the study period in massage group compared to control group [2,9,10,12,17,19,21,26,28,30,33–35] while some studies did not show a statistically significant difference in weight gain between groups [5,8,15,16,18,29,31]. Massaro et al. [16] evaluated the effects of massage or massage + kinesthetic stimulation on weight gain and length of hospital stay in a study of 59 infants who were randomized to massage only (n = 19), massage and kinesthetic stimulation (n = 20) or control group (n = 20). After controlling for covariates (birth weight, gestational age, caloric intake, etc.) the infants whose birth weight was >1000 g benefited from massage with a significantly higher average daily weight gain with more pronounced effects in infants who received massage + kinesthetic stimulation ($p = 0.012$) [16]. To study the possible contribution to weight gain of medium chain triglyceride (MCT) oil used in massage therapy (via absorption of oil through the skin) Saeidi et al. compared the effects of massage with MCT oil to massage without oil and controls (with no massage) and demonstrated a significanly higher weight gain during the 7-day study in the group that received massage with MCT oil compared to massage only ($p = 0.002$) and controls ($p = 0.000$) [2]. The mean weight gain during the study period in the MCT oil massage group was 105 $\pm$ 1.3 grams compared to a gain of 52 $\pm$ 0.1 grams in the massage only group and loss of 54 $\pm$ 1.3 grams in the control group [2].

2.2. Caloric Intake and Expenditure

Some studies have evaluated the effects of massage on caloric intake [5,8,17,19,30,33–35] and its possible connection to weight gain in preterm infants. Most studies did not show a difference in caloric intake between infants who received massage compared controls despite statistically significant higher weight gains in infants who received massage [8,17,19,30,33,34]. A study by Diego et al. showed increased calorie intake in infants who received kinesthetic stimulation compared to those who received tactile stimulation only, no difference in weight gain between the two groups [5]. Scafidi et al. evaluated factors that predict higher weight gain in infants who receive massage and a higher caloric intake was one of the factors that predicted weight gain [35]. One study evaluated energy expenditure in preterm infants, which was reported to be lower after a 5-day study period in infants who received massage compared to controls [22] suggesting that a decrease in energy expenditure may be in part responsible for the enhanced growth caused by massage therapy.

Table 1. Randomized controlled trials of massage in preterm infants.

Year	First Author	Number of Infants (Cases, Controls)	Gestational Age (Age at the Time of Study)	Massage Type	Intervention	Outcomes Measured	Results
2015	Basiri-Moghadam [3]	40 (20 massage, 20 controls)	34–36 weeks (<1 week)	N/A	20 min of massage twice daily for 4 days	Number of defecations Transcutaneous bilirubin level	Massage group had higher number of defecations ($p = 0.002$) and lower levels of transcutaneous bilirubin ($p = 0.003$)
2015	Saeadi [2]	121 (40 oil massage, 40 massage, 41 controls)	<37 weeks (<28 days)	N/A	5 min of massage 4 times a day for 7 days	Weight gain	The MCT oil-massage group gained more weight than massage ($p = 0.002$) and control groups ($p = 0.000$)
2014	Yates [4]	23 (cross-over study)	28–37 weeks (34–48 PMA)	TKS (modified, no kinesthetic component)	13 infants received a massage on day 1 and no massage on day 2 (10 infants received a massage on day 2)	Sleep efficiency Number of infants asleep at the end of massage	No significant difference in sleep efficiency ($p = 0.13$)
2014	Diego [5]	30 (15 tactile, 15 kinesthetic stimulation)	28–32 weeks; (15–60 days)	TKS (tactile or kinesthetic stimulation)	15 infants received tactile and 15 received kinesthetic stimulation 10 min a day for 5 days (no control group without massage)	Weight gain Calorie intake Vagal activity	No difference in weight gain. Increased calorie intake in kinesthetic group ($p < 0.05$). Increased vagal tone in tactile group ($p = 0.01$), decreased vagal tone in kinesthetic group.
2013	Fallah [10]	54 (17 oil massage, 17 massage alone) LBW infants	33–37 weeks (<10 days)	Moderate pressure	17 received moderate pressure massage alone, 17 received massage with sunflower oil 3 times a day for 14 days (no control group without massage)	Weight gain at 14 days, 1 month, 2 months	The oil massage group had a higher mean weight at ages 1 month ($p = 0.04$) and 2 months ($p = 0.005$) than the massage alone group.
2013	Smith [6]	21 (10 massage, 11 controls)	28–33 weeks (mean 31 weeks PMA)	Moderate pressure strokes with kinesthetic movement of extremities	20 min of massage twice daily for 4 weeks	Heart rate variability (HRV)	Significant group × time × sex interaction effect ($p < 0.05$) with male infants who received massage demonstrating higher HRV indicating increased vagal tone.
2013	Smith [7]	37 (17 massage, 20 control)	29–32 weeks	Soft-tissue compression strokes with following range of motion to arms and legs	20 min massage twice daily for 4 weeks	HRV	HRV improved in massage group but not in controls ($p < 0.05$). Male infants who received massage had a greater improvement in HRV than females ($p < 0.05$).

Table 1. *Cont.*

Year	First Author	Number of Infants (Cases, Controls)	Gestational Age (Age at the Time of Study)	Massage Type	Intervention	Outcomes Measured	Results
2013	Moyer-Mileur [8]	44 (22 massage, 22 controls)	29–32 weeks (32–33 weeks PMA)	Soft-tissue strokes with following range of motion to arms and legs	Twice-daily massage 6 days a week for 4 weeks	Energy and protein intake, body circumference, weight, length, ponderal index (PI), skinfold thickness (triceps, mid-thigh, subscapular), and IGF-1, leptin and adiponectin levels	Male infants in the massage group had smaller PI and skinfold thickness than control males ($p < 0.05$). Females in the massage group had larger subscapular skin fold increase than control females ($p < 0.05$). Adiponectin increased in control males ($p < 0.01$) and correlated to PI ($r = 0.39$, $p < 0.01$).
2013	Kumar [9]	48 (25 oil massage, 23 controls)	<35 weeks (<48 h)	20 strokes in: shoulders starting from neck with baby prone, upper back to the waist. Then limbs in supine position	10 min 4 times a day for 28 days	Weight, length, head circumference, serum triglyceride levels	At 7 days the massage group had less weight loss compared to controls ($p = 0.003$). At 28 days massage group had greater weight compared to controls ($p < 0.05$). No significant difference in serum triglycerides and other measured parameters.
2012	Haley [11]	40 (20 massage, 20 controls)	29–32 weeks, (mean 32 weeks PMA)	TKS	20 min twice daily, 6 days a week for 15 days	Tibial speed of sound (tSOS), urine markers of bone metabolism (pyridinium crosslinks and urinary osteocalcins (OC) U-MidOC and unOC)	Massage group had less decrease in tSOS than controls ($p < 0.05$). Urinary pyridinium crosslinks decreased in both massage and controls ($p < 0.005$). Massage group had greater increases in urinary osteocalcin (U-MidOC, $p < 0.001$ and unOC, $p < 0.05$) suggesting improved mineralization.
2012	Ang [12]	120 (58 massage, 62 controls)	Mean 30 weeks, range 25–33 (mean 32 weeks PMA, range 28–33)	TKS	5 days a week until hospital discharge for a maximum of 4 weeks	Immunologic parameters (absolute natural killer (NK) cells, T and B cells, T cell subsets, NK cytotoxicity), weight, number of infections, length of hospital stay	NK cytotoxicity was higher in the massage group, particularly in those who received ≥ 5 consecutive days of massage ($p = 0.04$). Infants in the massage group weighed more ($p = 0.05$) and had greater daily weight gain ($p = 0.01$) compared to controls. Other parameters, did not differ between the groups.
2011	Guzzetta [13]	20 (10 massage, 10 controls)	30–33 weeks (10 days)	TKS	10 min of massage 3 times a day for 12 days during a 2-week period	Changes in EEG spectral activity (before and after study period)	Significant difference in EEG spectral power.
2010	Procianoy [14]	73 (35 massage, 38 controls)	<32 weeks (48 h of life)	TKS (modified)	Massage and skin to skin care 15 min 4 times a day during hospital stay (skin to skin only)	Neurodevelopment (PDI, MDI) and growth at 2 years of corrected age	Massage group had higher MDI scores ($p = 0.035$), PDI scores and growth did not differ significantly.

Table 1. *Cont.*

Year	First Author	Number of Infants (Cases, Controls)	Gestational Age (Age at the Time of Study)	Massage Type	Intervention	Outcomes Measured	Results
2010	Ho [15]	24 (12 massage, 12 controls) VLBW infants	<34 weeks (34 weeks PMA)	TKS (modified)	15 min of massage daily, 5 days/week for 4 weeks (light still touch)	Test of Infant Motor Performance (TIMP) score gain, weight gain, post-conceptional age at discharge	No significant difference in TIMP score gain and weight gain when all subjects were analyzed. Those who had below-average pre-massage TIMP score and received massage had higher TIMP score gain ($p = 0.043$) and earlier discharge ($p = 0.045$) than controls.
2009	Massaro [16]	60 (20 massage with kinesthetic stimulation, 20 massage, 20 controls)	<32 weeks, mean 29 weeks for massage groups, 27 weeks for controls (30 weeks PMA)	TKS	15 min of massage ± kinesthetic stimulation (KS) twice daily from study enrollment until discharge	Weight gain Length of stay (LOS)	Average daily weight gain and LOS did not differ between the groups except for infants with BW > 1000 g, in whom average daily weight gain was higher in massage + KS group compared to control.
2009	Gonzalez [17]	60 (30 massage, 30 controls)	<35 weeks, mean 31 weeks (30–35 weeks PMA, mean 33)	Vimala massage	15–20 min twice daily massage for 10 days	Weight, head circumference, caloric intake, nutritional method, hospital stay	Massage group had higher weight gain ($p < 0.001$) and shorter hospital stay ($p = 0.03$) than controls.
2008	Field [19]	42 (N/A)	Mean 29–30 weeks (mean 34.8 weeks PMA)	TKS	15 min per day for 5 days	Weight gain, caloric consumption, vagal activity (high frequency component of HRV), serum insulin and IGF-1	Vagal activity increased during massage ($p < 0.001$). Massage group had greater increase in weight gain ($p = 0.02$), insulin ($p = 0.001$) and IGF-1 ($p = 0.05$). No difference in caloric consumption was noted between groups.
2008	Mendes [18]	104 (52 massage, 52 controls) VLBW infants	<32 weeks, mean 29 weeks (48 h)	TKS (modified)	15 min 4 times a day until discharge	Length of hospital stay (primary). Other outcomes: weight, length, head circumference, growth rate, ponderal index, age of partial and total enteral feeding, age of partial and total oral feeding, incidence of late onset sepsis, necrotizing enterocolitis (NEC), bronchopulmonary dysplasia (BPD)	Massage group had a higher probability of earlier hospital discharge ($p = 0.023$). Incidence of late-onset sepsis was lower in the massage group ($p = 0.005$).
2008	Chen [21]	40 (20 massage, 20 controls)	<34 weeks (>7 days)	Acupressure and meridian massage	15 min 3 times a day for 10 days	Weight gain	During 14-day study period the massage group gained more weight ($p = 0.038$) There was no significant difference in weight gain in the first week ($p = 0.384$). In the second week, the massage group had had higher weight gain than controls ($p = 0.035$).

Table 1. *Cont.*

Year	First Author	Number of Infants (Cases, Controls)	Gestational Age (Age at the Time of Study)	Massage Type	Intervention	Outcomes Measured	Results
2008	Diego [20]	72 (abstract) or 48 (methods)(N/A)	Mean 29 weeks (N/A)	TKS	15 min of massage once	Temperature (15 min before, during massage and 15 min after)	Massage group had a greater increase in temperature
2007	Lahat [22]	10 (cross over)	Mean 32 weeks (29–34 weeks PMA, mean 3 weeks)	TKS (modified)	15 min 3 times a day for 5 days (5 infants received a massage for 5 days and no massage for 5 days, opposite sequence for 5 infants)	Energy expenditure by indirect calorimetry	Energy expenditure was lower in infants after the 5 days massage therapy than after the period with no massage ($p = 0.05$).
2007	Diego [24]	70 (36 massage, 34 controls)	Mean 29 weeks (mean 30 days)	TKS	15 min 3 times a day for 5 days	Vagal activity (HRV). Gastric motility (by EGG) measurements performed on days 1 and 5 of study 15 min before, during and 15 min after massage	Group-by-time analysis revealed significant increase in vagal activity that peaked during massage ($p < 0.001$); a significant increase in gastric motility that peaked 15 min after massage ($p < 0.01$) in the massage group. No changes in basal vagal activity or gastric motility were noted.
2007	Hernandez-Reif [23]	32 (16 massage, 16 controls)	28–32 weeks (15–60 days)	TKS	15 min 3 times a day for 5 days	Stress behavior (crying, grimacing, yawning, jerky arm or leg movement, sneezing, startles, finger flaring). Activity (movement of the limbs, torso or gross body movement of any kind)	Group-by-time analysis showed reduction in duration of stress behaviors in massage group ($p < 0.05$) and reduction in overall movement for the massage group ($p < 0.05$). No change in controls in these parameters were observed.
2006	Field [26]	68 (N/A)	28–32 weeks, mean 30 weeks (15–60 days, mean 23)	TKS	15 min 3 times a day for 5 days of moderate vs. light pressure massage (no control group without massage)	Behavior state, stress behaviors, heart rate, weight gain	Moderate pressure massage group had a higher increase in weight gain ($p < 0.02$), less decrease in deep sleep ($p < 0.05$), less increase in active sleep ($p < 0.02$), less increase in fussing ($p < 0.01$), less increase in crying ($p < 0.02$), less increase in gross movement ($p < 0.05$), less increase in stress behavior ($p < 0.01$), greater decrease in heart rate ($p < 0.01$), and greater increase in vagal tone ($p < 0.05$).
2006	Jain [25]	23 (crossover)	<37 weeks (1–7 days)	Slow massage of outer aspect of the leg	2-min massage of the ipsilateral leg prior to heel stick (n = 13) and no massage prior to next heel stick 2–7 days later (10 infants had reverse order)	Neonatal Infant Pain Scale NIPS (primary outcome) Heart rate, respiratory rate, oxygen saturation	NIPS ($p < 0.001$) and heart rate ($p = 0.03$) were higher after a heel stick with no massage.

Table 1. *Cont.*

Year	First Author	Number of Infants (Cases, Controls)	Gestational Age (Age at the Time of Study)	Massage Type	Intervention	Outcomes Measured	Results
2005	Arora [31]	69 (23 oil massage, 23 massage, 23 controls) VLBW infants	<37 weeks	Standardized technique for the study as described in article	10 min 4 times a day	Weight gain at 28 days after enrolment (primary), length, head circumference triceps skin fold thickness, neurobehavior (NBAS), serum triglycerides.	No significant differences in any of the measured parameters. Trend for increased weight gain/day in massage group ($p = 0.07$).
2005	Sankaranara-yanan [28]	112 (38 coconut oil, 37 mineral oil, 37 controls)	Mean 34.8 weeks (day 2 of life)	TKS	Four times a day for 31 days.	Weight gain velocity over the first 31 days of life (primary), length gain velocity, head growth, neuro-behavioral outcome, incidence of adverse events	Coconut oil massage group had a greater weight gain velocity compared to mineral oil ($p < 0.05$) and control groups ($p < 0.05$). Infants receiving coconut oil massage also showed a greater length gain velocity compared to controls ($p < 0.05$). No significant difference in other measures.
2005	Diego [30]	48 (16 massage, 16 light pressure sham massage, 16 controls)	22–37 weeks, mean ~30 (9–76 days, mean 29–34, no significant N difference between groups)	TKS	15 min 3 times a day for 5 days	Weight gain, vagal activity (HRV), gastric motility (EGG), days to discharge, caloric intake	Massage group had greater weight gain ($p < 0.01$), increased vagal tone ($p < 0.05$) and increased gastric motility ($p < 0.01$) during and after treatment. Weight gain was significantly related to gastric motility ($p < 0.01$) and vagal tone ($p < 0.01$). No differences in other parameters.
2005	Lee [29]	26 (13 massage, 13 controls)	< 36 weeks (second day after starting enteral feeds)	TKS	15 min massage twice daily for 10 days	Weight, vagal tone, heart rate, oxygen saturation, and behavioral responses (behavioral states, motor activity, behavioral distress)	Massage group had significantly higher vagal tone after massage ($p = 0.05$) no change in controls. Massage group had higher scores for awake state ($p = 0.000$), fidgeting or crying ($p = 0.04$), and motor activity ($p = 0.04$) than controls.
2005	Solanki [27]	120 (40 coconut oil, 40 safflower oil, 40 no oil)	Three groups: GA < 34 weeks, GA 34–37 weeks, GA > 37 weeks	Not specified	5 mL of oil massaged for 10 min 4 times a day for 5 days	Serum triglycerides, serum fatty acid profile (linoleic, arachidonic, alpha linolenic acid, docosahexaenoic acids and saturated fats)	Serum triglyceride values were significantly higher after massage in all groups compared to baseline (coconut oil $p < 0.001$, safflower oil $p < 0.001$, controls $p < 0.05$). There was a significant rise in linoleic and arachidonic acid in the safflower oil group ($p < 0.001$) and saturated fats in coconut oil group ($p < 0.001$).

Table 1. *Cont.*

Year	First Author	Number of Infants (Cases, Controls)	Gestational Age (Age at the Time of Study)	Massage Type	Intervention	Outcomes Measured	Results
2004	Aly [32]	30 (15 massage, 15 controls)	28–35 weeks (< 2 weeks)	TKS	Daily massage until infant reached 1.8 kg of weight.	Serum type I collagen C-terminal propeptide (PICP) and urinary pyridinoline crosslinks of collagen (Pyd)	Serum PICP increased in massage group ($p < 0.01$) and decreased in control group ($p < 0.01$) compared to baseline, and this change differed significantly between massage group and controls ($p = 0.0001$). Urinary Pyd increased in both groups compared to baseline ($p < 0.01$ for both) but did not differ between the groups.
2002	Ferber [33]	57 (21 massage by mother, 17 massage by professional, 19 controls)	26–34 weeks, mean 31 weeks (mean 12–17 days)	TKS (modified)	15 min massage 3 times a day for 10 days	Weight gain Calorie intake	Infants massaged by either their mother or professional gained more weight than controls ($p = 0.03$). No significant difference in caloric intake.
1993	Wheeden [34]	30 (15 massage, 15 controls) All cocaine exposed infants	<37 weeks, mean 30 weeks (mean 16 days in controls, 20 days in massage group, NS)	TKS	15 min massage 3 times a day for 10 days	Weight gain, calorie intake, stress behavior, behavior (NBAS)	Massage group had greater weight gain per day ($p = 0.009$) than controls. There was no difference in feed type or caloric intake. Massage group had fewer postnatal complications ($p = 0.005$) and stress behaviors ($p = 0.05$) and more mature motor behaviors at the end of the 10-day study period ($p = 0.02$) than controls.
1993	Scafidi [35]	93 (50 massage, 43 controls)	26–36 weeks, mean 30 weeks (mean 15 days)	TKS	15 min massage 3 times a day for 10 days	Weight gain, calorie intake, stress behavior, behavior (NBAS)	Massage group had greater average daily weight gain ($p < 0.01$) than controls. Factors that predicted higher weight gain were history of obstetric complications, higher caloric intake and longer stay in intermediate nursery.

Controls received standard care unless otherwise noted. Statistically significant differences are noted in "Results" column, for other outcomes measured the difference was not statistically significant. BW = birth weight, EEG = electroencephalogram, EGG = electrogastrogram, GA = gestational age, HRV = heart rate variability, IGF-1 = insulin-like growth factor I, LBW = low birth weight, MCT = medium chain triglycerides, MDI = mental development index, NBAS = Brazelton's neonatal behavior assessment scale, NS = , PDI = Psychomotor Development Index, PMA = post-menstrual age, TKS = tactile/kinesthetic stimulation, a massage technique originally described by Field in 1986 [36], U-MidOC = urine osteocalcin midfragments, unOC = undercarboxylated form of osteocalcin, VLBW = very low birth weight.

2.3. Vagal Tone

Increased vagal activity induced by massage has been suggested as one potential mechanism for higher weight gain in infants who receive massage therapy. Vagal activity in most studies is assessed by measuring heart rate variability (HRV) with increased high frequency (HF) variability indicating higher vagal tone [37]. All studies that evaluated vagal activity demonstrated an increase in vagal tone in infants who receive massage [5–7,19,24,26,29,30]. However, in two studies, the increased vagal effect was more pronounced in male infants [6] or was demonstrated only in males [7]. In a study by Diego et al. comparing the effects of tactile to kinesthetic stimulation (the two components of TKS massage [36]), an increase in vagal tone measured by HRV was only noted in in the tactile group in group-by-time analysis ($p = 0.01$), whereas a decreased vagal tone was noted in infants receiving kinesthetic range of motion excercises only [5].

2.4. Gastric Motility

Massage-induced increases in vagal activity may lead to increased gastric motility, which has also been suggested as a possible mechanism for increased weight gain in infants who receive massage therapy. Gastric motility or number of stools have been assessed in three studies [3,24,30]. In infants who received massage therapy, significantly increased gastric motility during and immediately after massage and decreased tachygastria has been reported [24,30]. This increase in gastric motility was significantly correlated with increased weight gain and vagal tone [24,30]. During a 4-day study which evaluated the effects of massage on transcutaneous bilirubin levels and stool frequency, a significantly increased stool frequency was reported in the massage group compared to controls during the entire study period (day 1: $p = 0.001$, day 2: $p = 0.02$, day 3: $p = 0.01$ and day 4: $p = 0.04$) [3].

2.5. Immunological Effects

Two randomized controlled studies have reported on the effects of massage in immunological parameters and incidence of infections in preterm infants [12,18]. Absolute number of natural killer (NK) cells, white blood cells, B and T cells, and T-cell subsets were not statistically different between the groups. Number of infections did not differ between the groups. While the mean absolute NK cell number was not statistically different between the massage and control group, the adjusted mean NK cell cytotoxicity was higher in the massage group ($p = 0.05$) [12]. Mendes et al. reported on significantly lower incidence of late-onset sepsis in massage group ($p = 0.005$) [18]. The incidence of late-onset sepsis was 38.3% (18/47 infants) in controls compared to 10.9% (5/46 infants) in massage group. No serum immunological markers were reported in this latter study.

2.6. Bone Metabolism

Preterm infants have increased morbidity from osteopenia [38]. Physical activity stimulates bone formation. Two studies have evaluated the effects of massage therapy with physical activity on bone metabolism in preterm infants (Table 1) [11,32]. Physical activity was defined either as kinesthetic movement part of TKS massage [11] or a similar daily range of motion exercise, with gentle compression and extension/flexion to both upper and lower extremities [32]. Aly et al. reported an increase in serum type I collagen C-terminal propeptide (PICP, marker of bone formation) in the massage group ($p < 0.01$) compared to baseline, while PICP decreased in controls group ($p < 0.01$). This change differed significantly between the groups ($p = 0.0001$), suggesting increased bone formation in massage group. Furthermore, serum parathyroid hormone (PTH) level increased in the massage group while it decreased in the control group ($p < 0.001$).

2.7. Behavior, Sleep and Neurodevelopment

Yates et al. studied the effects of TKS massage on sleep efficiency in preterm infants in a crossover study [4] and found no significant difference between groups for sleep efficiency ($p = 0.13$). More infants were reported to sleep on the non-massage day ($p = 0.026$) [4]. Several studies have assessed the effects of massage on behavior and/or neurodevelopment of preterm infants [14,15,23,26,28,29,31,34,35]. Most studies have reported on immediate behavioral effects of massage [15,23,26,28,29,31,34,35] and only one randomized controlled trial has reported on long term neurodevelopmental outcome [14]. Massage groups were reported to have significantly less stress-related behaviors (crying, fidgeting) than controls in three studies [23,26,34], no difference between the groups in two [28,31], and one study reported increased crying and fidgeting in infants who received massage [29]. Ho et al. reported on a higher gain in motor performance score (Test of Infant Motor Performance, TIMP) in very low birth weight (VLBW) infants who received massage and who had a below-average pre-study score compared to a control group who received light touch ($p = 0.043$) suggesting that massage may have positive effects in motor outcomes in a subgroup of VLBW infants who have low motor performance [15]. Procianoy et al. compared neurodevelopmental outcomes (Psychomotor Development Index, PDI and Mental Development Index, MDI) at 2 years of age between preterm infants who had received massage intervention during hospital stay and controls [14]. Infants who had been randomly assigned to massage therapy group or control group during their hospital stay both received skin-to-skin care. Growth and neurodevelopmental outcome were evaluated in both groups at 2 years corrected age. Growth at 2 years corrected age did not differ between the groups. The massage group had slightly but not significantly higher PDI score ($p = 0.072$) and significantly higher MDI scores ($p = 0.035$) than controls [14].

2.8. Length of Hospital Stay

Length of hospital stay (LOS) was reported to be similar in the massage group and controls in one study [12], and in one there was a significant difference between groups [16] but this difference disappeared after controlling for gestational age, gender, sepsis and birth weight. Two studies have reported shorter duration of hospitalization in infants who received massage compared to controls [17,18]. A study by Gonzalez et al. evaluating the effects of Vimala massage in preterm infants reported a shorter hospital stay in infants of massage group (15.36 $\pm$ 5.41 days) compared to controls (19.33 $\pm$ 7.92 days ($p = 0.03$) [17]. A study by Mendez et al. on VLBW infants reported that those who received massage had a 1.85 times higher (95% confidence interval (CI): 1.09 to 3.13; $p = 0.023$) probability of earlier hospital discharge than control group [18].

2.9. Serum Markers

Levels of serum markers of growth and metabolism such as IGF-1 [8,19], adiponectin [8], serum triglycerides [9,27,31] have been studied in small randomized controlled trials. Moyer-Mileur et al. studied IGF-1, leptin, and adiponectin levels in infants who received massage and controls and correlated them with skin fold thickness, weight gain and ponderal index (PI) [8]. Serum leptin levels correlated significantly with weight gain, PI, triceps skin-fold thickness and mid-thigh skin-fold thickness [8]. Serum adiponectin level correlated with PI. There was no difference in weight gain however in this study between massage and control groups. In a study by Field et al. the massage group had a greater increase in weight gain ($p = 0.02$), and a greater increase in both insulin ($p = 0.001$) and IGF-1 ($p = 0.05$) levels [19] and weight gain correlated with increased insulin ($p = 0.05$) and IGF-1 ($p = 0.02$) levels [19]. Three randomized controlled trials have evaluated the effects of oil massage on serum triglycerides [9,27,31]. The primary objective of Solanki et al. was to assess transcutaneous absorption of massage oils by assessing serum lipid profiles in infants assigned to a massage without oil, or with safflower oil (rich in essential fatty acids, EFAs) or coconut oil (rich in saturated fats and medium chain triglycerides, MCTs) [27]. No weight gain was measured in this study. Serum triglyceride levels were significantly higher after massage compared to baseline in all groups (coconut oil $p < 0.001$, safflower oil $p < 0.001$, controls $p < 0.05$) though the rise was significantly higher in oil groups compared to controls ($p < 0.05$). In infants randomized to massage with safflower oil, a significant rise was seen in the essential fatty acids linoleic and arachidonic acid ($p < 0.001$) after massage. In those who received a massage with coconut oil an increase in serum saturated fats was reported ($p < 0.001$). In the control group who received a massage without oil a small but significant increase in serum linoleic ($p < 0.05$) and total saturated fats was seen ($p < 0.05$) [27]. The other two studies that assessed serum triglyceride levels used sunflower oil in the massage group evaluated serum triglyceride levels as a secondary outcome and reported no significant difference between massage group and controls [9,31].

2.10. Bilirubin levels, markers of brain maturation, pain

Basiri-Moghadam et al. reported significantly lower transcutaneous bilirubin levels ($p = 0.003$) in the massage group compared to controls after four days of massage [3]. Guzzetta et al. reported differences in EEG spectral power (an index of brain maturation) in massaged infants compared to controls suggesting a process of brain maturation in those who received massage [13]. Jain et al. reported in a cross-over study higher scores in Neonatal Infant Pain Scale (primary outcome) ($p < 0.001$) and heart rate ($p = 0.03$) in infants who had a blood sampling via a heel stick without a preceding 2-min massage of the ipsilateral leg compared to infants who had a massage prior to heel stick [25]. Respiratory rate, oxygen saturation and serum cortisol levels did not differ [25].

3. Discussion

Preterm birth (birth at <37 weeks of gestational age) is the leading cause of neonatal morbidity and mortality in the United States [39,40] and affects 10% of infants born in the USA [1]. Slow weight gain and poor oral-motor ability to feed are common factors delaying discharge from hospital in infants born prematurely. Interventions that improve either weight gain or oral-motor function may lead to shorter hospital stay and cost savings. Improved weight gain is the most commonly and consistently reported effect of massage in preterm infants with significantly greater daily or overall weight gain found in infants who received massage compared to controls [2,9,10,12,17,19,21,26,28,30,33–35]. While one study reported increased gain in an infant motor performance score in VLBW infants who received massage suggesting positive effects on motor development [15], oral–motor coordination and ability to feed was not evaluated. To date there are no randomized controlled trials evaluating the effects of massage on oral–motor coordination or feeding ability offering an area of future studies.

A recent meta-analysis by Wang et al. concluded that massage improved daily weight gain by 5.32 g (95% CI 4.15, 6.49 g, $p < 0.00001$) and reduced length of hospital stay by 4.41 days (95% CI 2.81, 6.02 days, $p < 0.00001$) [41]. A Cochrane systematic review by Vickers et al. also concluded that massage improved daily weight gain by 5.1 g (95% CI 3.5, 6.7 g) and appeared to reduce length of hospital stay by 4.5 days (95% CI 2.4, 6.5 days) [42], consistent with meta-analysis by Wang et al. [41]. Furthermore, a review by Field et al also suggested that infant massage leads to 3–6 days shorter length of hospital stay and, consequently, significant cost-savings up to $10,000 per infant [43].

The mechanism by which massage improves weight gain in preterm infants is not well understood. One suggested mechanism is that massage leads to higher consumption of calories. However, studies have not shown a difference in caloric intake between infants who received massage compared controls [8,17,19,30,33,34]. Another possible mechanism is increased vagal tone which may promote food absorption and anabolism. Increase in vagal activity has indeed been consistently reported in infants who receive massage in all randomized controlled trials that evaluated vagal tone [5–7,19,24,26,29,30]. Levels of serum anabolic hormones insulin and IGF-1 have been reported to be higher in infants who had received massage and correlated with weight gain [19] suggesting a possible anabolic effect. Field et al. postulate in more detail potential mechanisms for improved weight gain in preterm infants who received massage, including increased vagal tone and IGF-1 levels [44].

Furthermore, increased weight gain in preterm infants who receive massage with oil may be due to transcutaneous absorption of oils and contribution to caloric intake. While Solanki et al. reported a significant increase in serum essential fatty acids and saturated fats in infants massaged with safflower and coconut oil, respectively, their study did not assess weight gain [27]. Thus, the possible effects of transcutaneous absorption of oil in weight gain could not be evaluated. Study by Saeidi et al. did demonstrate a significantly higher weight gain in infants who received massage with MCT oil compared to massage only or controls [2] suggesting that MCT oil, possibly via transcutaneous absorption, may partly contribute to weight gain.

Improved weight gain and decreased length of hospital stay are important measures on the effects of massage in preterm infants and may lead to significantly lower health care costs [43]. Yet little is known about the long-term effects of early massage on infant development. Only one small study (n = 73) has assessed the long-term effects of massage given during neonatal hospital stay and compared neurodevelopmental scores between infants who received massage therapy to controls [14] and reported on a slightly higher PDI score and significantly higher MDI scores in the massage group, suggesting massage may induce long-term effects in neural modeling and neurodevelopment.

Overall, several studies as well as meta-analyses have suggested beneficial effects of massage in preterm infants with regards to improved weight gain and shortening the length of hospital, the latter of which has potential for significant cost-savings. Limitations and challenges of current randomized controlled trials on the effects of massage in preterm infants include small sample size in most studies, lack of studies in extremely premature infants, and lack of studies in infants with congenital anomalies or congenital heart disease who often have poor weight gain. The provider of the massage is also not consistent between studies. Massage has been variably provided by licensed massage therapists, trained nurses, or by a mother trained in massage technique. Although one study assessed the effects of massage in weight gain in infants massaged by either the mother or a professional gained and reported more weight gain in both groups compared to controls ($p = 0.03$) suggesting that different providers provide equally effective massage. There is limited information available on side effects of massage therapy with most of the studies not reporting side effects or quoting massage as "safe" or "relatively safe". However, given lack of reported side effects it is likely safe to conclude that massage is "relatively safe" in the infant groups in which it has been studied. There is not enough evidence to recommend massage for all preterm infants but it may be beneficial in selected clinically-stable preterm infants with slow weight gain.

4. Conclusions

In summary, randomized controlled trials on the effects of massage in preterm infants suggest improved weight gain and shortened length of hospital stay. Improved weight gain may be mediated through increase in vagal tone but more studies are needed on the underlying mechanisms of the effects of massage. Further randomized controlled studies are needed on the effects of massage on outcomes such as neurodevelopment, stress behavior, immune system, and pain tolerance.

References

1. Hamilton, B.E.; Martin, J.A.; Osterman, M.J.; Curtin, S.C.; Matthews, T.J. Births: Final data for 2014. *Natl. Vital Stat. Rep.* **2015**, *64*, 1–64. [PubMed]
2. Saeadi, R.; Ghorbani, Z.; Shapouri Moghaddam, A. The effect of massage with medium-chain triglyceride oil on weight gain in premature neonates. *Acta Med. Iran.* **2015**, *53*, 134–138. [PubMed]
3. Basiri-Moghadam, M.; Basiri-Moghadam, K.; Kianmehr, M.; Jani, S. The effect of massage on neonatal jaundice in stable preterm newborn infants: A randomized controlled trial. *J. Pak. Med. Assoc.* **2015**, *65*, 602–606. [PubMed]
4. Yates, C.C.; Mitchell, A.J.; Booth, M.Y.; Williams, D.K.; Lowe, L.M.; Whit Hall, R. The effects of massage therapy to induce sleep in infants born preterm. *Pediatr. Phys. Ther.* **2014**, *26*, 405–410. [CrossRef] [PubMed]
5. Diego, M.A.; Field, T.; Hernandez-Reif, M. Preterm infant weight gain is increased by massage therapy and exercise via different underlying mechanisms. *Early Hum. Dev.* **2014**, *90*, 137–140. [CrossRef] [PubMed]
6. Smith, S.L.; Lux, R.; Haley, S.; Slater, H.; Beachy, J.; Moyer-Mileur, L.J. The effect of massage on heart rate variability in preterm infants. *J. Perinatol.* **2013**, *33*, 59–64. [CrossRef] [PubMed]

7. Smith, S.L.; Haley, S.; Slater, H.; Moyer-Mileur, L.J. Heart rate variability during caregiving and sleep after massage therapy in preterm infants. *Early Hum. Dev.* **2013**, *89*, 525–529. [CrossRef] [PubMed]
8. Moyer-Mileur, L.J.; Haley, S.; Slater, H.; Beachy, J.; Smith, S.L. Massage improves growth quality by decreasing body fat deposition in male preterm infants. *J. Pediatr.* **2013**, *162*, 490–495. [CrossRef] [PubMed]
9. Kumar, J.; Upadhyay, A.; Dwivedi, A.K.; Gothwal, S.; Jaiswal, V.; Aggarwal, S. Effect of oil massage on growth in preterm neonates less than 1800 g: A randomized control trial. *Indian J. Pediatr.* **2013**, *80*, 465–469. [CrossRef] [PubMed]
10. Fallah, R.; Akhavan Karbasi, S.; Golestan, M.; Fromandi, M. Sunflower oil versus no oil moderate pressure massage leads to greater increases in weight in preterm neonates who are low birth weight. *Early Hum. Dev.* **2013**, *89*, 769–772. [CrossRef] [PubMed]
11. Haley, S.; Beachy, J.; Ivaska, K.K.; Slater, H.; Smith, S.; Moyer-Mileur, L.J. Tactile/kinesthetic stimulation (TKS) increases tibial speed of sound and urinary osteocalcin (U-MidOC and unOC) in premature infants (29–32 weeks PMA). *Bone* **2012**, *51*, 661–666. [CrossRef] [PubMed]
12. Ang, J.Y.; Lua, J.L.; Mathur, A.; Thomas, R.; Asmar, B.I.; Savasan, S.; Buck, S.; Long, M.; Shankaran, S. A randomized placebo-controlled trial of massage therapy on the immune system of preterm infants. *Pediatrics* **2012**, *130*, e1549–e1558. [CrossRef] [PubMed]
13. Guzzetta, A.; D'Acunto, M.G.; Carotenuto, M.; Berardi, N.; Bancale, A.; Biagioni, E.; Boldrini, A.; Ghirri, P.; Maffei, L.; Cioni, G. The effects of preterm infant massage on brain electrical activity. *Dev. Med. Child Neurol.* **2011**, *53* (Suppl. 4), 46–51. [CrossRef] [PubMed]
14. Procianoy, R.S.; Mendes, E.W.; Silveira, R.C. Massage therapy improves neurodevelopment outcome at two years corrected age for very low birth weight infants. *Early Hum. Dev.* **2010**, *86*, 7–11. [CrossRef] [PubMed]
15. Ho, Y.B.; Lee, R.S.; Chow, C.B.; Pang, M.Y. Impact of massage therapy on motor outcomes in very low-birthweight infants: Randomized controlled pilot study. *Pediatr. Int.* **2010**, *52*, 378–385. [CrossRef] [PubMed]
16. Massaro, A.N.; Hammad, T.A.; Jazzo, B.; Aly, H. Massage with kinesthetic stimulation improves weight gain in preterm infants. *J. Perinatol.* **2009**, *29*, 352–357. [CrossRef] [PubMed]
17. Gonzalez, A.P.; Vasquez-Mendoza, G.; Garcia-Vela, A.; Guzman-Ramirez, A.; Salazar-Torres, M.; Romero-Gutierrez, G. Weight gain in preterm infants following parent-administered vimala massage: A randomized controlled trial. *Am. J. Perinatol.* **2009**, *26*, 247–252. [CrossRef] [PubMed]
18. Mendes, E.W.; Procianoy, R.S. Massage therapy reduces hospital stay and occurrence of late-onset sepsis in very preterm neonates. *J. Perinatol.* **2008**, *28*, 815–820. [CrossRef] [PubMed]
19. Field, T.; Diego, M.; Hernandez-Reif, M.; Dieter, J.N.; Kumar, A.M.; Schanberg, S.; Kuhn, C. Insulin and insulin-like growth factor-1 increased in preterm neonates following massage therapy. *J. Dev. Behav. Pediatr.* **2008**, *29*, 463–466. [CrossRef] [PubMed]
20. Diego, M.A.; Field, T.; Hernandez-Reif, M. Temperature increases in preterm infants during massage therapy. *Infant Behav. Dev.* **2008**, *31*, 149–152. [CrossRef] [PubMed]
21. Chen, L.L.; Su, Y.C.; Su, C.H.; Lin, H.C.; Kuo, H.W. Acupressure and meridian massage: Combined effects on increasing body weight in premature infants. *J. Clin. Nurs.* **2008**, *17*, 1174–1181. [CrossRef] [PubMed]
22. Lahat, S.; Mimouni, F.B.; Ashbel, G.; Dollberg, S. Energy expenditure in growing preterm infants receiving massage therapy. *J. Am. Coll. Nutr.* **2007**, *26*, 356–359. [CrossRef] [PubMed]
23. Hernandez-Reif, M.; Diego, M.; Field, T. Preterm infants show reduced stress behaviors and activity after 5 days of massage therapy. *Infant Behav. Dev.* **2007**, *30*, 557–561. [CrossRef] [PubMed]
24. Diego, M.A.; Field, T.; Hernandez-Reif, M.; Deeds, O.; Ascencio, A.; Begert, G. Preterm infant massage elicits consistent increases in vagal activity and gastric motility that are associated with greater weight gain. *Acta Paediatr.* **2007**, *96*, 1588–1591. [CrossRef] [PubMed]
25. Jain, S.; Kumar, P.; McMillan, D.D. Prior leg massage decreases pain responses to heel stick in preterm babies. *J. Paediatr. Child Health* **2006**, *42*, 505–508. [CrossRef] [PubMed]
26. Field, T.; Diego, M.A.; Hernandez-Reif, M.; Deeds, O.; Figuereido, B. Moderate versus light pressure massage therapy leads to greater weight gain in preterm infants. *Infant Behav. Dev.* **2006**, *29*, 574–578. [CrossRef] [PubMed]
27. Solanki, K.; Matnani, M.; Kale, M.; Joshi, K.; Bavdekar, A.; Bhave, S.; Pandit, A. Transcutaneous absorption of topically massaged oil in neonates. *Indian Pediatr.* **2005**, *42*, 998–1005. [PubMed]

28. Sankaranarayanan, K.; Mondkar, J.A.; Chauhan, M.M.; Mascarenhas, B.M.; Mainkar, A.R.; Salvi, R.Y. Oil massage in neonates: An open randomized controlled study of coconut versus mineral oil. *Indian Pediatr.* **2005**, *42*, 877–884. [PubMed]
29. Lee, H.K. The effect of infant massage on weight gain, physiological and behavioral responses in premature infants. *Taehan Kanho Hakhoe Chi* **2005**, *35*, 1451–1460. [CrossRef] [PubMed]
30. Diego, M.A.; Field, T.; Hernandez-Reif, M. Vagal activity, gastric motility, and weight gain in massaged preterm neonates. *J. Pediatr.* **2005**, *147*, 50–55. [CrossRef] [PubMed]
31. Arora, J.; Kumar, A.; Ramji, S. Effect of oil massage on growth and neurobehavior in very low birth weight preterm neonates. *Indian Pediatr.* **2005**, *42*, 1092–1100. [PubMed]
32. Aly, H.; Moustafa, M.F.; Hassanein, S.M.; Massaro, A.N.; Amer, H.A.; Patel, K. Physical activity combined with massage improves bone mineralization in premature infants: A randomized trial. *J. Perinatol.* **2004**, *24*, 305–309. [CrossRef] [PubMed]
33. Ferber, S.G.; Kuint, J.; Weller, A.; Feldman, R.; Dollberg, S.; Arbel, E.; Kohelet, D. Massage therapy by mothers and trained professionals enhances weight gain in preterm infants. *Early Hum. Dev.* **2002**, *67*, 37–45. [CrossRef]
34. Wheeden, A.; Scafidi, F.A.; Field, T.; Ironson, G.; Valdeon, C.; Bandstra, E. Massage effects on cocaine-exposed preterm neonates. *J. Dev. Behav. Pediatr.* **1993**, *14*, 318–322. [CrossRef] [PubMed]
35. Scafidi, F.A.; Field, T.; Schanberg, S.M. Factors that predict which preterm infants benefit most from massage therapy. *J. Dev. Behav. Pediatr.* **1993**, *14*, 176–180. [CrossRef] [PubMed]
36. Field, T.M.; Schanberg, S.M.; Scafidi, F.; Bauer, C.R.; Vega-Lahr, N.; Garcia, R.; Nystrom, J.; Kuhn, C.M. Tactile/kinesthetic stimulation effects on preterm neonates. *Pediatrics* **1986**, *77*, 654–658. [PubMed]
37. Task Force of the European Society of Cardiology and the North American Society of Pacing and Electrophysiology. Heart rate variability: Standards of measurement, physiological interpretation and clinical use. *Circulation* **1996**, *93*, 1043–1065.
38. American Academy of Pediatrics, Committee on Nutrition. Nutritional needs of low-birth-weight infants. *Pediatrics* **1985**, *75*, 976–986.
39. Manuck, T.A.; Rice, M.M.; Bailit, J.L.; Grobman, W.A.; Reddy, U.M.; Wapner, R.J.; Thorp, J.M.; Caritis, S.N.; Prasad, M.; Tita, A.T.; et al. Preterm neonatal morbidity and mortality by gestational age: A contemporary cohort. *Am. J. Obstet. Gynecol.* **2016**, *215*, 103.e1–103.e14. [CrossRef] [PubMed]
40. Stoll, B.J.; Hansen, N.I.; Bell, E.F.; Walsh, M.C.; Carlo, W.A.; Shankaran, S.; Laptook, A.R.; Sanchez, P.J.; Van Meurs, K.P.; Wyckoff, M.; et al. Trends in care practices, morbidity, and mortality of extremely preterm neonates, 1993–2012. *JAMA* **2015**, *314*, 1039–1051. [CrossRef] [PubMed]
41. Wang, L.; He, J.L.; Zhang, X.H. The efficacy of massage on preterm infants: A meta-analysis. *Am. J. Perinatol.* **2013**, *30*, 731–738. [PubMed]
42. Vickers, A.; Ohlsson, A.; Lacy, J.B.; Horsley, A. Massage for promoting growth and development of preterm and/or low birth-weight infants. *Cochrane Database Syst. Rev.* **2004**, *2014*, CD000390.
43. Field, T.; Diego, M.; Hernandez-Reif, M. Preterm infant massage therapy research: A review. *Infant Behav. Dev.* **2010**, *33*, 115–124. [CrossRef] [PubMed]
44. Field, T.; Diego, M.; Hernandez-Reif, M. Potential underlying mechanisms for greater weight gain in massaged preterm infants. *Infant Behav. Dev.* **2011**, *34*, 383–389. [CrossRef] [PubMed]

11

Pediatric Integrative Medicine in Academia: Stanford Children's Experience

Gautam Ramesh [1], Dana Gerstbacher [2], Jenna Arruda [3], Brenda Golianu [4], John Mark [5] and Ann Ming Yeh [6,*]

1 School of Medicine, University of California, San Diego, La Jolla, CA 92093, USA; gramesh@ucsd.edu
2 Division of Rheumatology, Department of Pediatrics, School of Medicine, Stanford University, Palo Alto, CA 94304, USA; gerstl@stanford.edu
3 Department of Pediatrics, School of Medicine, Stanford University, Palo Alto, CA 94304, USA; jarruda@stanford.edu
4 Division of Pediatric Anesthesia and Pain Medicine, Department of Anesthesiology, Perioperative and Pain Medicine, School of Medicine, Stanford University, Palo Alto, CA 94304, USA; bgolianu@stanford.edu
5 Division of Pulmonary Medicine, Department of Pediatrics, School of Medicine, Stanford University, Palo Alto, CA 94304, USA; jmark@stanford.edu
6 Division of Gastroenterology, Hepatology and Nutrition, Department of Pediatrics, School of Medicine, Stanford University, Palo Alto, CA 94304, USA
* Correspondence: annming@stanford.edu

Abstract: Pediatric integrative medicine is an emerging field which, to date, has not been described in detail in academic medical centers in the United States. Early research of pediatric integrative medicine modalities shows promise for the treatment of common pediatric conditions such as irritable bowel syndrome, acute and chronic pain, headache, and allergy, among others. In light of the growing prevalence of pediatric illnesses and patient complexity, it is crucial to emphasize the patient's overall well-being. As academic centers around the world start to develop pediatric integrative medicine programs, the aim of this manuscript is to briefly highlight evidence of effective integrative treatments in pediatric subspecialties, to describe the establishment of our integrative medicine program, to summarize its early efforts, and to discuss potential barriers and keys to success.

Keywords: pediatric; integrative medicine; academic medicine

---

1. Background

Integrative medicine (IM) is a patient-centric, evidence-based, therapeutic paradigm that coordinates the integration of all pertinent conventional and complementary approaches to achieve patient health. Integrative medicine incorporates all appropriate therapies, emphasizes the patient–provider relationship, and utilizes lifestyle changes to holistically optimize health and healing [1]. It addresses the biologic, psychosocial, spiritual, and environmental aspects of patient wellbeing. Integrative modalities range from mind–body interventions to nutrition. While current biomedical practices have made great strides in the treatment of many conditions, the addition of IM principles and practices can help restore the patient to a state of personal wellbeing and optimal function [2,3].

The National Center for Complementary and Integrative Health clarifies definitions frequently used with integrative medicine: complementary medicine refers to using non-allopathic medicine in conjunction with conventional allopathic medical treatment, and alternative medicine refers to utilizing a non-allopathic therapy instead of a conventional allopathic treatment. These two approaches are commonly referred to as complementary and alternative medicine (CAM) [4]. Throughout this article, the term "integrative medicine" (IM) or "IM practices" will be employed to refer to the concurrent use of CAM therapies in conjunction with traditional allopathic practice, in order to highlight this emerging practice paradigm in pediatric practice, except where the articles quoted have specifically employed the terminology of the terms "complementary" or "alternative" medicine.

The National Health Interview Survey results from 2012 show that 33% of adults and 12% of children used complementary health approaches [5,6]. Children with chronic illnesses are significantly more likely to use IM therapies than healthy children [7,8]. Integrative medicine is used by more than 50% of pediatric patients with chronic disease [2].

In the pediatric population, IM practices have enormous potential to reduce healthcare costs and ensure a healthier future for children by emphasizing prevention and promoting wellness [9]. The literature over the last two decades has confirmed the clinical efficacy of certain IM therapies and has demonstrated improved patient outcomes (e.g., improved quality of life, decreased cardiovascular risk factors), symptom relief, and patient satisfaction [10,11]. Large systematic reviews indicate potential cost-effectiveness and even cost savings for IM modalities in adult populations, though higher quality studies are needed [10]. Similar studies have not yet been published for pediatric patients but are currently underway [12].

By promoting healthy lifestyle practices early in the child's life, pediatric IM sets a high standard for a lifetime of disease prevention behaviors. In many instances these therapies are simple and inexpensive to implement (e.g., improved sleep hygiene, exercise) and may provide long-lasting wellbeing. Exercise and lifestyle changes can treat depression, coronary heart disease, and type II diabetes [13–18]. Consuming a myriad of fruits, vegetables, spices, and extracts have shown preventative and treatment potential [19–27]. Mindfulness meditation has undergone extensive study utilizing functional magnetic resonance imaging (fMRI), and is emerging as an effective therapy for pain, anxiety, and depression [28–33].

The majority of integrative medicine users, however, do not report usage to their primary care physician; only 34–50% disclose use to their provider [34,35]. This number is likely even lower in certain ethnic and socioeconomic groups [1]. Parents and patients may feel intimidated by clinicians' perceived negative attitudes towards alternative therapies, even though three in four pediatricians believe that parents would disclose this information [35]. Improved communication regarding IM therapies would allow for physicians to (1) understand patients' and families' priorities and values in health and illness, and (2) help avoid treatment interactions between CAM and conventional therapies [36].

It is important for pediatricians to have knowledge and facility with integrative medicine in order to initiate conversation about CAM utilization [37]. Helpful to the cause, guidelines for advising patients seeking CAM have been published [38,39]. Although clinicians have an ethical obligation to discuss treatment alternatives [40], the overwhelming majority of pediatric providers do not feel comfortable discussing CAM with their patients. Both Kemper and O'Connor [41] and Sawni and Thomas [42] found that less than 37% of pediatricians inquire regarding CAM use while taking a routine medical history; any dialogue regarding CAM is typically initiated by the family. Pediatricians have a positive attitude towards CAM, but desire further education to adequately address patient concerns [2,41]. In a national study of 648 pediatricians, less than one in five reported any formal training in CAM, and 84% of respondents desired a continuing medical education curriculum, exhibiting self-awareness of their low familiarity with the topic [3,41–43].

To meet the growing needs of patients and practitioners alike, representatives from eight institutions (including Stanford) met in Kalamazoo, Michigan in July 1999. The outcome of this conference was the creation of the Academic Consortium for Integrative Medicine and Health. The vision of this group was to support leaders in integrative medicine in their advocacy, expand familiarity with the field, and develop a scientific knowledge base and research opportunities. Most importantly, it aimed to establish a community of providers in this rapidly growing field of medicine. A survey in 2007 indicated that 16 of 143 North American medical schools had dedicated academic pediatric IM programs [44]. The growth of dedicated academic departments and training programs in IM highlight institutional interest and support for IM.

2. Pediatric Integrative Subspecialties in Academia

Academic medical centers are often the hub where education, research, and clinical care meet innovation to improve medical care. The field of pediatric integrative medicine thrives in this setting, which allows for collaboration across disciplines and the opportunity to treat medically complex patients across all socioeconomic and cultural backgrounds. Further, academic centers are conducive to the inception of novel scholarship and training initiatives.

The 2005 Institute of Medicine report recommended CAM education for all training levels in health professions schools [45]. From an educational standpoint, training in pediatric IM was spearheaded by the University of Arizona Center for Integrative Medicine. The 100-h online Pediatric Integrative Medicine in Residency (PIMR) program was designed to address the lack of IM training available to pediatric trainees [46]. The PIMR program teaches residents habits for their own personal wellness alongside an introduction to evidence-based IM principles. This program was adopted by five pediatric residency programs in 2012 as a pilot program. Inclusion of a curriculum on physician wellness in the PIMR program was intentional and necessary. Physician burnout and fatigue is associated with major medical errors and decreased productivity. Furthermore, it has been shown that healthy physicians are more likely to advise patients to follow healthy lifestyle habits and are more effective at motivating patients [47–54]. Embedding integrative medicine education in a pediatric academic setting has the additional advantage of increasing institution-wide exposure and comfort with IM modalities.

Pediatric IM is a much-needed subspecialty, emerging to meet the needs of today's children. From a research standpoint, rigorous studies evaluating the safety, efficacy, and cost effectiveness of IM approaches in pediatrics are needed to justify usage [3]. Research into the efficacy of a pediatric integrative care model is often conducted at academic medical centers where patient diversity and research support are available. Due, in part, to increased research, IM approaches are being integrated into the fields of pediatric gastroenterology, pain, neurology, oncology, and pulmonology, among others. Frequently, the multidisciplinary approach afforded by IM can effectively treat symptoms, decrease polypharmacy, and enhance overall wellness in pediatric illness.

2.1. Gastroenterology

Pediatric gastroenterology (GI) patients have a high frequency of CAM usage; studies estimate utilization to be between 36% and 72% [55,56]. Herbal medicines, dietary supplements, and special diets are the most prevalent therapies utilized [57]. The strongest predictor of CAM use was prior or feared side effects of conventional medicine [55].

Integrative approaches for inflammatory bowel disease (IBD) include dietary assessment to identify food intolerances, dietary and herbal supplements, and mind–body therapies (relaxation techniques, meditation, and aromatherapy) [58]. Some studies have suggested a modest effect of probiotics, curcumin, and acupuncture in promoting remission in patients with IBD [59–62]. Mind–body interventions also have a limited body of evidence showing benefit in adolescents with IBD. A 2010 study of 67 adolescents with IBD described frequent utilization of prayer (62%), relaxation (40%), and imagery (21%) for disease management [63,64].

In patients with irritable bowel syndrome (IBS), there exists increasing evidence for the bidirectional connection between the mind, body, and gut. Gut-directed hypnotherapy (both in-person and home-based exercises) is also showing promise for pediatric IBS symptom relief [65–67]. Small studies on enteric coated peppermint oil have also demonstrated improvement of pediatric IBS symptoms [68].

2.2. Pain/Perioperative

Complementary and alternative medicine therapies for pediatric pain management are becoming increasingly accessible. A 2005 survey of 43 pediatric anesthesia fellowship programs approved by the Accreditation Council for Graduate Medical Education (ACGME) showed that nearly 90% of institutions had CAM therapies available for pediatric pain management. Common available modalities included biofeedback (65%), guided imagery (49%), and hypnosis (44%) [69].

Children and adolescents experience both acute and chronic pain, and each requires a different clinical approach. Nearly 40% of children with chronic pain experience persistent or recurrent pain at least once weekly, with common diagnoses being headaches, abdominal pain, and musculoskeletal pain [70]. Chronic pain can negatively impact a patient's school functioning, sleep, and parent burden (e.g., financial obligations, missed work) [71]. Treating chronic pain requires a multidisciplinary approach. The complex interplay between the patient's effective coping skills, parental reinforcement of pain behavior, and patient's mood can all alter and affect patient functioning [71]. This patient demographic is, reassuringly, open to an integrative approach to their care. According to a study of 110 pediatric patients with chronic pain (headache, abdominal pain, and musculoskeletal pain) presenting at an academic integrative clinic, 100% of families were interested in additional counseling regarding diet, exercise, sleep, or stress management [70]. Further, evidence is emerging for non-pharmacologic treatments for pain. For instance, physical therapy (stretching, trigger point physiotherapy, massage) can relieve headaches, musculoskeletal pain, and chronic regional pain syndrome (CRPS) [72–74]. Cotton et al. found that after massage therapy, mean pain scores decreased in over 500 hospitalized children with chronic pain and anxiety [75]. Acupuncture and mindful meditation have been shown to be an effective treatment for chronic pain and can decrease opioid usage, but more robust randomized control trials (RCTs) are needed [29,76].

Acute pain in children can be experienced in acute illness, during procedures (including venipuncture or immunization), or post-operatively. Acute pain can also evolve into a chronic pain condition, requiring flexibility in diagnosis and management. Integrative modalities have been successfully used in the treatment of acute pain. For instance, acupuncture, clinical hypnosis, and breathing techniques have all been shown to improve pain scores in children with acute pain from illness or procedures [77–79]. Newer technologies, such as virtual reality devices, show significant promise in minimizing discomfort with vascular access and minor procedures [80,81].

2.3. Neurology/Neurodevelopmental Pediatrics

Pediatric patients with a wide variety of neurologic and neurodevelopmental conditions utilize CAM to alleviate symptoms and supplement conventional therapy. The use of CAM among pediatric neurology patients ranges from 24% to 78% [82,83]. In a survey of 327 pediatric neurology patients at the Mayo Clinic, over 40% used CAM, and melatonin for sleep disorders was the most commonly used therapy [84]. A 2014 survey of 206 pediatric neurology patients in a Canadian children's hospital diagnosed with epilepsy, headache, and cerebral palsy illustrated high use of multivitamins, massage, and chiropractic therapies (89.9%, 47.1%, and 36.8%, respectively); most practices were reported as helpful [85]. Among children with autism spectrum disorder (ASD), special diets are the most common form of CAM utilized according to eight independent studies [57,86].

In pediatric headache patients, headache frequency and intensity has been shown to improve with magnesium and riboflavin (vitamin B2) [87,88]. Furthermore, screening and treating comorbid sleep disorders such as sleep apnea, bruxism, insomnia, and restless leg syndrome can indirectly improve headache [89]. Neurofeedback has documented potential in treatment of epilepsy and headache [90,91]. Meditation, breath work, and relaxation activities have reduced school absences in patients with headaches, migraines, and seizures [83].

2.4. Pediatric Oncology

Between 1977 and 2011, 31 studies on the use of IM practices in pediatric oncology patients listed spirituality/prayer, positive mental imagery, and natural health products (multivitamins, megavitamins and herbals) as common interventions [57]. Mind–body therapies are readily accessible and low risk, with several trials showing decreased side effects of cancer therapy, increased patient self-confidence, and improved coping skills [92]. The largest study of pediatric oncology patients (1063 patients) found that 71% utilized IM modalities and only 4% reported adverse events [93]. The most common reasons cited by patients for using IM were to aid in treating cancer, symptomatic relief, support of conventional treatment, and management of side effects [94,95].

Integrative modalities may also play a role in long-term cancer risk reduction. Patient lifestyle factors such as stress, cigarette smoking, poor diet, alcohol consumption, and a sedentary lifestyle are revealed and discussed with greater frequency in the IM approach. Research has suggested numerous cancers to be primarily nutrition-responsive and preventable by dietary [96,97] and lifestyle changes [98,99]. The mechanism responsible may be by aliment-induced reversible epigenetic modification or the protective effects conferred by a diet high in fiber and antioxidants [20,100,101]. Establishing healthy habits in children to focus on healthy nutrition, mind–body interventions for stress reduction, quality sleep, and generous physical activity may be paramount in decreasing overall risk of some cancers (colon, lung, breast, and prostate) in later life [102].

2.5. Asthma and Allergy

Pediatric asthma is another area where an integrative approach may provide benefit. Elimination diets and those emphasizing core facets of the Mediterranean diet (high in fruits, vegetables, and legumes) have been shown to protect children from asthma and allergies [103–105]. A systematic review and meta-analysis by Cramer et al. in 2014 highlighted yoga as a supplementary intervention for asthma patients to improve symptoms and quality of life [106]. Breathing exercises and breath retraining techniques such as Buteyko breathing, yoga/pranayama, and physiotherapy have decreased bronchodilator usage [107,108]. Mark describes a multitude of integrative therapies as effective for pediatric asthma, including: (1) mind–body therapies to reduce anxiety and stress, lowering immune response and sympathetic activity; (2) proper prenatal and childhood nutrition that is high in fruits and vegetables; and (3) exercise and yoga to improve regimen adherence and decrease anxiety [109,110].

2.6. Other Subspecialties

There is a role for an integrative approach within many subspecialties. We know, for instance, that diet and exercise management can halt or reverse cardiovascular disease, diabetes, and obesity [10,13,23,111–113]. Integrative cardiology targets high body mass index (BMI) and poor nutrition using mind–body therapies to influence caloric consumption, sedentary or stressful lifestyles, and depression-associated symptoms [114]. Cognitive behavioral therapy has been used as an adjuvant in pediatric obesity management [115]. Mindfulness-based cognitive therapy has shown preliminary efficacy in youths with anxiety disorder and mindfulness based stress reduction programs in urban youth have improved psychological functioning and decreased negative effects of stress [33,116]. Furthermore, a recent study has proposed mechanistic pathways of action of acupuncture in alleviating cardiovascular disease [117–120].

As the evidence base to support the use of integrative approaches in each pediatric subspecialty grows, the use of CAM in pediatrics will increase. In light of this, clinical practices and academic centers are starting to integrate CAM modalities. Existing models of care can provide a foundation for future growth and utilization of integrative approaches for children.

3. Integrative Medicine at Stanford Children's Health

This section presents the historical development of Pediatric Integrative Medicine at Stanford Children's Health with the intent to afford inspiration and perspective for future programs in pediatric IM.

3.1. Program Background and History

Lucile Packard Children's Hospital and Stanford University School of Medicine are located in Palo Alto, California and serve the broader region of the San Francisco Bay area. The inpatient children's hospital houses 361 beds and outpatient clinics serve over 500,000 visits annually. Families travel from

50 states and 40 countries for care. Fifty-two percent of families have private insurance, while 45% have public health insurance.

The Pediatric Integrative Medicine (PIM) program was established at Stanford Children's Health in 2011 with support from the pediatric department leadership. The program was developed in recognition of the growing interests of patients and their families in the use, benefits, and potential complications of complementary therapies. The program's first activity was to survey all Stanford Children's Health medical providers (including nurse practitioners, residents, fellows, and attending physicians) and measure their knowledge of and interest in IM. The survey revealed that a majority of practitioners (over 75%) wished to learn more about IM. Reasons for wanting further education included: (1) a desire to learn more about different CAM therapies to better advise their patients and families about safety and efficacy of supplements and mind–body approaches (which they were already using); and (2) a need to knowledgably introduce evidence-based pediatric IM practices into patient care.

The PIM faculty prepared a business plan to ensure the new program's sustainability and improve access for families seeking expertise in these therapies. The business plan included: proposed faculty, support staff allocation (0.5 days per week), and projected revenue from clinical services. Rather than creating a separate PIM clinic, the four faculty members centered the integrative clinics within four established specialty clinics: pain, gastroenterology (GI), pulmonary, and rheumatology. This model aimed to decrease overhead cost (space, staff, supplies) and make PIM clinics easily accessible. This model was fiscally sustainable as it allowed continued financial support of the faculty for conventional work in their respective subspecialty in addition to the subspecialty PIM clinics. The anecdotal response to this model by patients, families, and institutional leadership was positive. Patients and families expressed satisfaction (e.g., >80% provider satisfaction scores on yearly Press Ganey reports) and gratitude for finding pediatric subspecialists that were knowledgeable in both mainstream treatments and integrative modalities. As the program grew, institutional leadership and division chiefs continued to support the program, allowing the IM faculty to shift more time toward integrative clinics. In addition, as pediatric providers in the community learned of the PIM faculty's expertise, they began referring families for consultation. Community providers were welcomed to educational sessions offered by the program leaders and began incorporating evidence-based IM practices into their own specialties. Figure 1 is a diagram of the program's accomplishments.

3.2. Clinical Work

The four subspecialty integrative clinics (staffed by four IM-trained faculties in the pulmonary, rheumatology, pain medicine, and gastroenterology fields), continue to grow. Clinical volume has increased significantly since inception in 2012. In 2016, there were 160 visits for integrative medicine, and by 2017 that number had nearly doubled to over 300 annual visits. The greatest growth was noted in integrative pain and gastroenterology clinics. Referrals have come from community alternative care providers (e.g., Chinese medicine practitioners and naturopathic practitioners), community pediatricians, providers within Stanford Children's Health, and self-referrals. Approximately 25% of encounters are new patient visits and the rest are follow-up visits.

Prior to an initial visit with a PIM provider, insurance authorization is obtained. If the visit is with an acupuncture provider, patients interested in acupuncture are given current procedure terminology (CPT) codes and instructed to determine insurance benefits and out-of-pocket costs. Many insurances in California do cover acupuncture services for certain indications. Authorization is also required for pain psychology services through the IM pain clinic. An insurance authorization team is available to assist in this process.

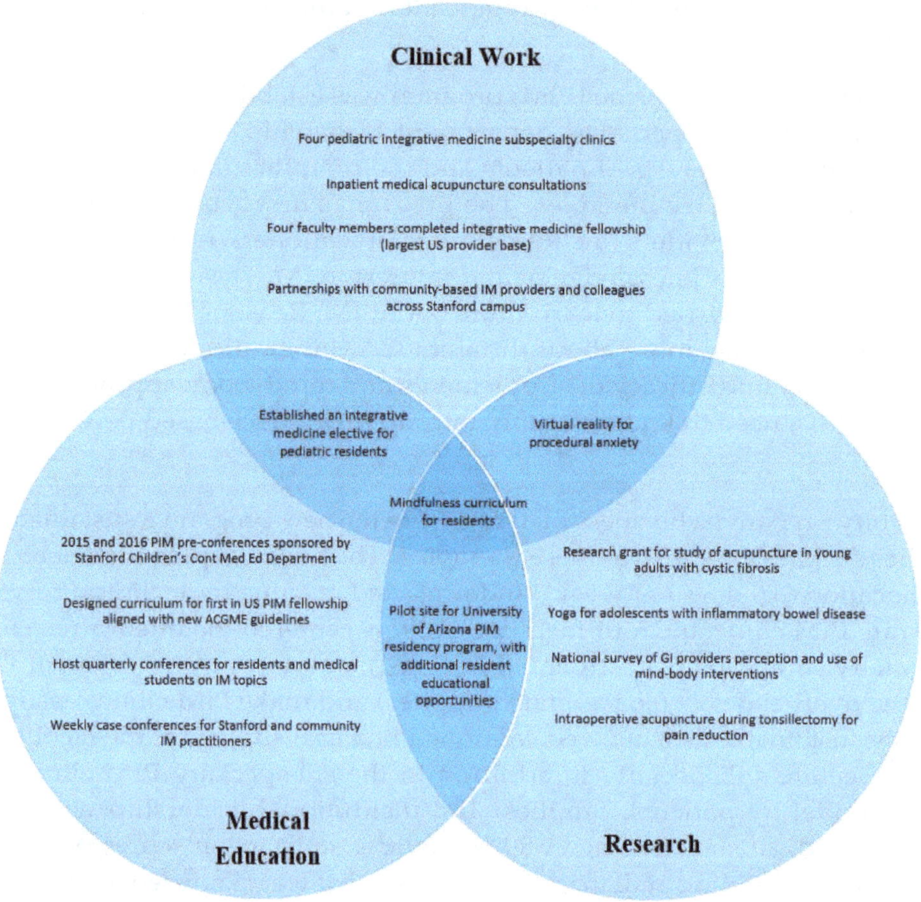

Figure 1. Program accomplishments. IM: integrative medicine; PIM: pediatric IM; GI: gastrointestinal; ACGME: Accreditation Council for Graduate Medical Education.

Each subspecialty clinic has a slightly different staffing structure. The integrative pain clinic includes a comprehensive initial pain evaluation for each new patient with the pain physician, nurse practitioner (NP), and pain psychologist. Depending on patient's needs, subsequent follow-up visits are with the pain medical doctor (MD)/NP and either the Stanford pain psychologist or community psychologist. Pain clinic NPs are also medical acupuncture-trained and therefore can continue treatment plans started by the acupuncture-trained physician. New patient visits in IM GI, pulmonary, and rheumatology clinics are for 90 min with an IM physician and follow-up visits are for 45 min. After a through intake evaluation, a comprehensive treatment plan is developed. The modalities offered depend largely on the individual training of the providers. The range of integrative treatment modalities include: nutrition recommendations, mind–body interventions, acupuncture, botanical or supplement review, and recommendations. The integrative GI clinic and integrative pulmonary clinic both have access to a registered dietician and social worker directly within the clinic. Pediatric IM providers will often refer to Stanford colleagues in the fields of nutrition, occupational therapy, psychiatry, child and pain psychology, and physical therapy. Frequency of referral to these services depends somewhat on the subspecialty, but the highest utilized services include psychology and occupational therapy for biofeedback. Further, the IM faculty will refer to community providers outside of the institution in acupuncture, massage, physical therapy, biofeedback, clinical hypnosis, mindfulness, and yoga. Community referrals are especially common when a patient lives a far distance from the Stanford campus and needs a particular therapy frequently (for example, weekly acupuncture for a patient who lives three hours away).

In the inpatient setting, a few IM modalities are available to inpatients through existing clinical departments. For example, the inpatient pain service provides acupressure and acupuncture. The child life department provides mind–body therapies, including guided imagery and virtual reality. The child psychology service provides clinical hypnosis as one of their treatment interventions. At this point there is not a dedicated PIM inpatient service but rather a meshwork of services offered by individual departments. For the future, an inpatient IM consultation service is a planned area for program expansion.

3.3. Research

Research for many integrative modalities is lacking, especially for pediatric patients. The Stanford faculties have produced a variety of publications including narrative reviews, book chapters, prospective pilot studies, retrospective studies of clinic outcomes, and position statements. Three faculty members are in the clinician educator track which does not afford protected research time. One faculty member is in the physician scientist track and has a dedicated 0.25 full time equivalent (FTE) of research time. Several generous foundation grants (Lawlor Foundation and Mayday Foundation) have allowed for support of the faculty and research assistants. Notable scholarly work includes faculty collaboration with PIM thought leaders to produce an Academy of Pediatrics (AAP) position statement on pediatric integrative medicine [3] and detailed results from the Pediatric Integrative Medicine in Residency (PIMR) pilot program [46,121]. A recent study found immersive virtual reality safe and effective for treating complex regional pain syndrome [80,122]. This has prompted further research on using virtual reality for other types of chronic, acute, and procedural pain. Intraoperative acupuncture for patients undergoing tonsillectomy and adenoidectomy was found to be feasible, decreased postoperative pain, and increased return of diet [77]. A pilot study on yoga for adolescents with inflammatory bowel disease found yoga to be widely acceptable, feasible, and safe [123]. For further details and a summary on research productivity and ongoing projects please see Table 1.

Challenges to studying the PIM program as a whole is that program providers often recommend a comprehensive treatment plan instead of a single intervention. This mirrors the wide array of interventions offered at other programs around the country (particularly for pain clinics) [69,124]. Therefore, developing research techniques to study multimodal interventions is needed to adequately study the integrative medicine approach as a whole [125]. This may include examining cost effectiveness and resource utilization (emergency visits, urgent care visits, and hospitalizations) in patients seen in a PIM program versus standard care.

Table 1. Summary of Published Scholarly Work on Integrative Medicine.

Category	Name of Study	Study Type	Findings	Funding
Pediatric integrative medicine	Pediatric Integrative Medicine [3]	Position Statement	Position Statement of Pediatric Integrative Medicine	N/A
Medical education	Pediatric Integrative Medicine in Residency (PIMR): Description of a New Online Educational Curriculum [46]	Retrospective review	Online curriculum targets integrative medicine (IM) knowledge gaps in pediatric residents	Funding received from foundation grants outside of Stanford
	Pediatric Integrative Medicine in Residency Program: Relationship between Lifestyle Behaviors and Burnout and Wellbeing Measures in First-Year Residents [121]	Retrospective review	Details burnout wellbeing in PIMR participants	Funding received from foundation grants outside of Stanford

Table 1. *Cont.*

Category	Name of Study	Study Type	Findings	Funding
Pediatric pulmonary	Complementary and Alternative Medicine in Pulmonology [126]	Literature review	Examines complementary and integrative medicine (CAM) use and effectiveness in children with pulmonary disorders	N/A
	Integrative Medicine in Asthma [127]	Literature review	Details integrative approach for children with asthma	N/A
	Nutrition in Pediatric Cystic Fibrosis [128]	Book chapter	Details evidence of nutritional therapies in children with cystic fibrosis	N/A
	Integrated Medicine and Asthma [129]	Book chapter	Details evidence of integrative approach to asthma	N/A
Pediatric gastroenterology	Yoga as adjunct therapy for adolescents with inflammatory bowel disease: A pilot clinical trial [127]	Prospective pilot	Yoga is acceptable, safe and feasible for adolescents with IBD	Tracie Lawlor Foundation, prAna
	Mind-Body Interventions for Pediatric Inflammatory Bowel Disease [130]	Literature review	Review of evidence on mind-body interventions for IBD	N/A
	Integrative Treatment of Reflux and Functional Dyspepsia in Children [130]	Case study and literature review	Describes integrative approach to children with reflux and functional dyspepsia	N/A
	Acupuncture and Integrative Medicine for Pediatric Gastroesophageal Reflux and Functional Dyspepsia [131]	Retrospective case series	Describes effect of acupuncture on children with GERD and functional dyspepsia	Stanford Medical Scholars Program
Pediatric neurology	Integrative Medicine in Child Neurology: what do providers think and what do they need to learn? [132]	National survey	Describes results of a national survey of IM modalities used in pediatric neurology	N/A
Pediatric pain	The Impact of Massage and Reading on Children's Pain and Anxiety After Cardiovascular Surgery: A Pilot Study [133]	Randomized prospective trial	Massage was safe and feasible for children undergoing cardiac surgery. Massage decreased anxiety scores and lowered exposure to benzodiazepines.	N/A
	Immersive Virtual Reality for Pediatric Pain [80]	Literature review	Review of evidence on using virtual reality for acute, chronic, and procedural pain	Mayday Foundation
	Two Virtual Reality Pilot Studies for the Treatment of Pediatric CRPS [122]	Prospective pilots	Virtual Reality feasible and effective for treating pediatric CRPS	Mayday Foundation
	Non-Pharmacological Techniques for Pain Management in Neonates [134]	Literature review	Details evidence of non-pharmacologic techniques to treat neonatal pain	N/A
Acupuncture	Acupuncture as an Anesthetic Adjuvant for Pediatric Orthopedic Patients: A Pilot Study and Protocol Description [79]	Prospective pilot	Acupuncture was associated with low pain scores and levels of nausea in patients undergoing orthopedic surgery	N/A
	Does Acupuncture Reduce Stress Over Time? A Clinical Heart Rate Variability Study in Hypertensive Patients [135]	Retrospective case study	Acupuncture increased heart rate variability after acupuncture treatment in adults undergoing treatment for hypertension	N/A
	Does Noninvasive Electrical Stimulation of Acupuncture Points Reduce Heelstick Pain in Neonates [136]	Randomized prospective trial	Noninvasive electrical stimulation at acupuncture points was not effective to decrease heelstick pain in neonates	Mayday Foundation
	Intraoperative acupuncture for post-tonsillectomy pain: a randomized, double-blind, placebo-controlled trial. [77]	Randomized prospective trial	Intraoperative acupuncture is feasible, well tolerated, and results in improved pain and earlier return of diet after tonsillectomy.	Stanford Medical Scholars Program, Howard Hughes Medical Institute Medical Fellows Program, Stanford Children's Health Research Institute Akiko Yamazaki and Jerry Yang Faculty Scholar

3.4. Medical Education

Stanford pediatric residents began participating in the University of Arizona's Pediatric Integrative Medicine Residency (PIMR) pilot online training curriculum in 2014. Trainee participation in this curriculum was a pivotal step towards formalizing PIM medical education efforts at Stanford Children's. In addition to providing a foundation in PIM knowledge, the curriculum enabled residents to improve their own lifestyle and wellness behaviors during the pilot [121]. To supplement the online curriculum offered by PIMR, the faculty developed a pediatric integrative medicine and wellness elective for pediatric residents who wanted in-depth exposure to integrative medicine in practice. The elective is currently offered as either a two-week or four-week in-person rotation. Residents taking the elective participate in the subspecialty PIM clinics (average four to five half-day clinic sessions per two-week rotation). Required readings and hands-on didactic sessions (average 4 h per two-week rotation) include lectures about plant-based nutrition and mind–body medicine. A field trip to a natural foods store provides the venue for a hands-on discussion of herbs and supplements. Residents are also asked to choose one integrative modality to experience for themselves to improve their own health. Meditation, massage, acupuncture, and yoga have been the most popular modalities that residents explore. Residents enrolled in the four-week elective are required to complete the 100-h PIMR online curriculum in addition to the above activities. The PIM elective at Stanford Children's has become one of the most popular electives, with approximately 20% of the 76 categorical pediatric residents participating annually.

At the fellow physician level, a new wellness curriculum has been developed by the Stanford Children's faculty, including the PIM faculty. The Fellowship WellBeing Program (FWP) focuses on fatigue mitigation, self-care, resiliency, and stress mitigation for over 100 pediatric fellows. This seven-hour curriculum emphasizes the use of breathing, movement, mindfulness and nutrition to help physician trainees find and maintain wellness.

In 2018, Stanford Children's launched the first one-year clinical fellowship in pediatric integrative medicine to formally train pediatricians in integrative medicine. The PIM fellowship includes partnership with the University of Arizona Fellowship in Integrative Medicine, a 1000-h, two-year distance learning program with three, week-long, hands-on training sessions. The fellow has a dedicated general pediatrics IM clinic precepted by the PIM faculty (average two half-day clinics per week) and also works alongside faculty members in their respective subspecialty PIM clinics (average two half-day clinics per week). Curriculum intensives—one to three-week mini courses—were developed by the PIM and adjunct faculty members to cover the important PIM topics of nutrition, mind–body medicine, botanical medicine, and inpatient consultation. The fellow may also work with non-Stanford affiliated community integrative medicine pediatric providers on an elective basis for niche skill development and clinical exposure. The fellow is also required to teach pediatric residents formally in several conferences per year and informally when residents are on the PIM elective. The fellowship curriculum includes weekly didactic and case conferences in the style of "Professor's Rounds" where a patient case is discussed with providers from various medical backgrounds and training expertise. The conferences are attended by community integrative medicine general pediatricians, PIM subspecialty providers (GI, pulmonary, pain, rheumatology), massage therapists, acupuncturists, psychologists, mind–body intervention providers, and nutritionists. After each case presentation, attendees offer their treatment recommendations (from their own unique perspectives), and these recommendations are provided to the patient at clinic follow-up.

Sample Case Presentation (Identifying Details Changed for Patient Privacy)

A 15-year-old girl presented to the outpatient pediatric integrative medicine clinic with chief complaint of abdominal pain for three years which had been diagnosed as abdominal migraines. A comprehensive history was taken regarding her pain including an evaluation of life stressors, a detailed diet history, and her extensive medication list.

Pertinent findings included a past medical history of anxiety and release of a tethered cord at nine months of age. Her prescription medications included duloxetine, cariprazine, amitriptyline, topiramate, polyethylene glycol, and a combined estrogen–progesterone oral contraceptive pill daily. She took clonazepam, ondansetron, sumatriptan, cyproheptadine, and simethicone on an as-needed basis for symptoms related to abdominal migraine. She did not find any of these as needed medications particularly helpful in treating her abdominal migraine episodes. Supplements included melatonin nightly and peppermint oil by mouth as needed for abdominal pain. She was an only child of her mother and father. She was starting the 10th grade and achieved good grades. Her bedtime was 22:00 h nightly and she fell asleep easily. She reported occasional overnight awakenings and feeling tired on waking at 06:00 h daily. She described herself as a worrier but also as willful and ambitious. Her favorite color was teal, and her favorite season was winter. She preferred salty foods. Both mom and patient readily offered that the patient's desire to please her teachers often led to high anxiety and tears if she felt like she was not working to her potential due to illness. Her self-reported personal strength was relating to other people, including classmates. She stated she was weak in mathematics. Her physical activity included biking to school or walking to the school bus stop. She was planning to join the school speech and debate team at the time of the visit.

On physical exam her weight was in the 73rd percentile and her height was in the 38th percentile. Her body mass index was 22. She was talkative and engaged. Abdominal exam was significant for hyperesthesia with light touch of all abdominal quadrants with significant epigastric tenderness. There was no palpable stool burden. The remainder of her physical exam was normal. Prior negative workup for her abdominal pain included infectious stool studies, *Helicobacter pylori*, fecal calprotectin, complete blood count with differential, and a comprehensive metabolic panel including liver function testing, amylase, lipase, sedimentation rate, lipids, tissue transglutaminase immunoglobulin A, ceruloplasmin, and thyroid stimulation hormone. The results of these studies were normal.

The patient's comprehensive treatment plan included mind–body, lifestyle, and diet recommendations. Mind–body therapies were discussed, and the patient elected to start attending a free yoga class at her primary medical center. She continued to see her outpatient psychiatrist for weekly psychotherapy including cognitive behavioral therapy. From a lifestyle perspective, she was recommended to increase physical activity and offered that she would start walking a few evenings per week with her mother. A therapy plan for acute abdominal discomfort was formulated, and, in addition to her current pharmaceutical regimen, included: acupressure massage, enteric coated peppermint oil, and aromatherapy.

At her first follow-up the patient reported acupressure massage helpful, and she and the family asked for further instruction on in-home use of acupressure massage. At the third visit, approximately six weeks later, the patient emphatically reported she had aborted two abdominal migraines using acupressure beads with massage—something she had never achieved before. She started receiving biweekly acupuncture. She continued yoga once per week. She also found benefit from using a mind–body application on her mobile phone for daily meditation to augment anxiety treatment. She weaned off amitriptyline and topiramate without incident and reserved only ondansetron and clonazepam on an as needed basis for acute discomfort. In the first three months of treatment the patient aborted abdominal migraines twice and experienced only two breakthrough episodes. Additionally, she missed fewer days of school due to abdominal pain. She continues to follow-up in the integrative medicine clinic every two–three weeks for acupuncture treatments.

4. Discussion

4.1. Pediatric Integrative Medicine in Academia

Pediatric Integrative Medicine is an emerging subspecialty that provides the foundation for whole-patient and whole-child preventative care and lifestyle medicine [44]. Within children's hospitals, patients are acutely sick, and in the outpatient setting, the incidence of children with complex and chronic medical problems has grown. According to a national survey performed by the Centers for Disease Control, in 2009, 15.1% of all children in the United States had special health care needs, up from 12.8% in 2001 [137]. These children often have multiple subspecialties involved in their care and their subsequent care coordination and communication between multiple consultants can be challenging. Specialists tend to focus on their organ system of interest, and the holistic approach to the care and healing of the child may be overlooked. Integrative medicine may help bring together all aspects of care since PIM is a blend of mainstream therapies with the other aspects of wellness. Further, our PIM faculty members are trained in both a pediatric subspecialty and integrative medicine. This affords a unique opportunity for specialized clinical care, education, and research in these integrative pediatric subspecialties.

4.2. Drivers for Success

A primary reason for our program's initial success was due to institutional support, strong leadership, and a financial model of embedding the integrative clinics within subspecialty divisions. Institutional leadership recognized that the PIM program is an attractive feature that is "uniquely Stanford" and serves the local San Francisco Bay Area community and beyond.

In addition, recruiting and collaborating with the well-respected existing faculty within the institution to provide consultations (rather than hiring or contracting with external providers) established trust, garnered respect for the program, and continued collegiality amongst providers. This mirrors an important key to success among other established non-pediatric integrative medicine centers around the world [44,138]. Given that integrative medicine at times can include treatment modalities that may not be well known to mainstream medicine, the faculty group also emphasizes evidence-informed treatment modalities to the extent available and emphasizes patient safety. Lifestyle recommendations that have minimal side effects such as good nutrition, sleep hygiene, physical activity, and mind–body modalities are often cornerstones of each treatment plan. When research on treatment efficacy in a pediatric population may not be available, providers extrapolate data from adult populations and utilize shared-decision making with families, and use the safety-effectiveness rubric to discuss and document efficacy [139]. Every effort is made to utilize available resources to ensure the safety of a treatment recommendation, especially in regard to botanicals or supplements. Further, pharmacy consultations are sometimes required in patients who have significant polypharmacy.

The medical education initiatives jumpstarted awareness of integrative medicine throughout the children's hospital faculty and leadership. The resident PIMR pilot and subsequent PIM elective required residency leadership approval of the residency curriculum change. The elective also increased resident exposure and engagement with the integrative medicine faculty, which led to several resident-initiated scholarly works [123,132]. The novel conception of the pediatric integrative medicine fellowship has additionally increased clinical services and education efforts. The weekly didactic conference (available in person and by webinar) had the unanticipated benefit of bringing together PIM providers within Stanford and the larger community. Continuing education courses for the pediatric community also stimulated community building and aided in patient referrals. As students, residents, and other community providers increase their exposure to and knowledge of integrative modalities, these treatment options become part of the norm, and then truly "integrated" into conventional care. Therefore, medical education and teaching are important keys to success.

Finally, the educational and research programs would not exist without generous philanthropic support—both in the form of private donations and research grants. These funds aided to establish funding for the program's research and have allowed the pediatric integrative medicine fellow to attend the Arizona Center for Integrative Medicine's distance learning fellowship.

4.3. Challenges and Financial Considerations

The program has faced several challenges. From a financial standpoint, integrative medicine bills using time-based evaluation and management codes, behavioral health codes, and acupuncture

CPT codes. Although we have not had significant challenges having physician billing codes covered, preventative services in the current fee-for-service model do not reimburse equally when more time is spent with the patient (compared to seeing several patients in the same time period). Currently, the PIM faculty members work in their respective pediatric subspecialties to offset some of the costs of the PIM clinic. A separate bill center was created to track financial progress and will add insight to this challenge. As newer models of care such as accountable care organizations (ACOs) are adopted in adult primary care fields [140], this will hopefully translate to novel prevention models for pediatrics.

While children from underserved populations are still able to be seen by PIM providers at our institution, additional services such as acupuncture, biofeedback, psychology, and nutrition may not be as readily covered. Further, these patients may not be able to afford additional supplements and suggested dietary changes. This continues to pose a significant challenge for our underserved population and deserves significant and sustained advocacy and philanthropy.

While the newly developed PIM fellowship currently has institutional and philanthropic support, the sustainability of this training program is uncertain. Given that it is a completely new fellowship program, accreditation by the ACGME is likely years away. Currently, a two-year pilot by the hospital and Pediatrics Department is currently funding the fellow salary, program director effort, and coordinator time; philanthropy is funding the educational programming for the fellow.

Lastly, the concept of an integrative approach is, at times, a difficult philosophical mindset for patients and families. Behavior, lifestyle, and diet changes are frequently more challenging to implement than taking medications. These changes also take time. Referring providers and patients may be looking for a "quick fix", which may not be feasible. While evidence on integrative modalities is emerging in pediatrics, colleagues often remain skeptical and have reservations on the value of integrative therapies.

4.4. Future Directions

The PIM program at Stanford hopes to increase clinical services, education efforts, and research productivity. Clinically, a pilot inpatient integrative medicine consultation service is planned for Spring 2019. Discussions are underway to integrate mind–body and acupuncture treatment modalities to perioperative and postoperative treatment protocols. The program also needs to formally survey patients and families on patient satisfaction of its current programs.

On a national level, the faculty aims to collaborate with national organizations such as the American Academy of Pediatrics and other pediatric subspecialty organizations to have a broader reach for educational efforts. Several faculties have participated in discussions about developing an integrative medicine core competency requirement for all pediatric residents. Additionally, our program leadership advocates for other academic centers to establish pediatric integrative medicine clinical training fellowships.

Continued research is needed to establish evidenced-based safety and efficacy data for integrative therapies in pediatrics. Specific ongoing projects at our center include examining acupuncture for patients undergoing craniotomy, mind–body interventions for pediatric inflammatory bowel disease, and utilizing virtual reality for procedural pain and anxiety. Our program would be open to collaborating with other centers to develop the recently proposed multi-center PIM research network [139]. Continued growth in these areas will require ongoing institutional support for faculty time, resource allocation, and financial support.

5. Conclusions

Evidence of safety and efficacy of pediatric integrative treatment modalities within pediatric subspecialties continues to grow. The establishment of a pediatric integrative medicine program within an academic setting is feasible. It requires sufficient institutional support, funding, and adequately trained physician faculty and staff. Important contributors to our program's success include medical education to drive provider and trainee education, an emphasis on patient safety and evidence-based medicine, and an incredible team of enthusiastic physician leaders.

Author Contributions: Conceptualization, A.Y., J.M. and B.G.; writing—original draft preparation, G.R., J.A. and A.Y.; writing—review and editing, G.R., J.A., A.Y., J.M., D.G. and B.G.; supervision, A.Y., B.G., D.G. and J.M.

Acknowledgments: The authors would like to thank Kenneth Cox, Christy Sandborg, Daniel Murphy, and Mary Leonard for Stanford institutional leadership support. We acknowledge Leland Lei for assistance with pulling financial details for integrative clinics. We thank Ellen Gomes for technical editing, language editing, and proofreading. We would also like to thank Sudha K.V., the Weil Foundation, the Samuel Lawrence Foundation, and the Tracie Lawlor Foundation for philanthropic support.

References

1. Misra, S.M.; Guffey, D.; Roth, I.; Giardino, A.P. Complementary and Alternative Medicine Use in Uninsured Children in Texas. *Clin. Pediatr. (Phila.)* **2017**, *56*, 866–869. [CrossRef] [PubMed]
2. Kemper, K.J.; Vohra, S.; Walls, R. The Use of Complementary and Alternative Medicine in Pediatrics. *Pediatrics* **2008**, *122*, 1374–1386. [CrossRef] [PubMed]
3. McClafferty, H.; Vohra, S.; Bailey, M.; Brown, M.; Esparham, A.; Gerstbacher, D.; Golianu, B.; Niemi, A.-K.; Sibinga, E.; Weydert, J.; et al. Pediatric Integrative Medicine. *Pediatrics* **2017**, *140*, e20171961. [CrossRef]
4. Complementary, Alternative, or Integrative Health: What's In a Name? Available online: https://nccih.nih.gov/health/integrative-health (accessed on 20 July 2018).
5. Black, L.I.; Clarke, T.C.; Barnes, P.M.; Stussman, B.J.; Nahin, R.L. Use of Complementary Health Approaches Among Children Aged 4–17 Years in the United States: National Health Interview Survey, 2007–2012. *Natl. Health Stat. Rep.* **2015**, 1–19.
6. Clarke, T.C.; Black, L.I.; Stussman, B.J.; Barnes, P.M.; Nahin, R.L. Trends in the use of complementary health approaches among adults: United States, 2002–2012. *Natl. Health Stat. Rep.* **2015**, 1–16.
7. McCann, L.J.; Newell, S.J. Survey of paediatric complementary and alternative medicine use in health and chronic illness. *Arch. Dis. Child.* **2006**, *91*, 173–174. [CrossRef] [PubMed]
8. Eisenberg, D.M.; Davis, R.B.; Ettner, S.L.; Appel, S.; Wilkey, S.; Rompay, M.V.; Kessler, R.C. Trends in Alternative Medicine Use in the United States, 1990-1997: Results of a Follow-up National Survey. *JAMA* **1998**, *280*, 1569–1575. [CrossRef]
9. Taw, M.B. Integrative medicine, or not integrative medicine: That is the question. *J. Integr. Med.* **2015**, *13*, 350–352. [CrossRef]
10. Herman, P.M.; Poindexter, B.L.; Witt, C.M.; Eisenberg, D.M. Are complementary therapies and integrative care cost-effective? A systematic review of economic evaluations. *BMJ Open* **2012**, *2*, e001046. [CrossRef]
11. Ali, A.; Katz, D.L. Disease Prevention and Health Promotion: How Integrative Medicine Fits. *Am. J. Prev. Med.* **2015**, *49*, S230–S240. [CrossRef]
12. Vohra, S.; Schlegelmilch, M.; Jou, H.; Hartfield, D.; Mayan, M.; Ohinmaa, A.; Wilson, B.; Spavor, M.; Grundy, P. Comparative effectiveness of pediatric integrative medicine as an adjunct to usual care for pediatric inpatients of a North American tertiary care centre: A study protocol for a pragmatic cluster controlled trial. *Contemp. Clin. Trials Commun.* **2017**, *5*, 12–18. [CrossRef] [PubMed]
13. Cooney, G., Dwan, K.; Mead, G. Exercise for Depression. *JAMA* **2014**, *311*, 2432–2433. [CrossRef] [PubMed]
14. Ornish, D.; Scherwitz, L.W.; Billings, J.H.; Gould, K.L.; Merritt, T.A.; Sparler, S.; Armstrong, W.T.; Ports, T.A.; Kirkeeide, R.L.; Hogeboom, C.; et al. Intensive Lifestyle Changes for Reversal of Coronary Heart Disease. *JAMA* **1998**, *280*, 2001–2007. [CrossRef] [PubMed]
15. Knowler, W.C.; Barrett-Connor, E.; Fowler, S.E.; Hamman, R.F.; Lachin, J.M.; Walker, E.A.; Nathan, D.M. Reduction in the Incidence of Type 2 Diabetes with Lifestyle Intervention or Metformin. *N. Engl. J. Med.* **2002**, *346*, 393–403.
16. Loef, M.; Walach, H. The combined effects of healthy lifestyle behaviors on all cause mortality: A systematic review and meta-analysis. *Prev. Med.* **2012**, *55*, 163–170. [CrossRef] [PubMed]

17. Ornish, D.; Lin, J.; Chan, J.M.; Epel, E.; Kemp, C.; Weidner, G.; Marlin, R.; Frenda, S.J.; Magbanua, M.J.M.; Daubenmier, J.; et al. Effect of comprehensive lifestyle changes on telomerase activity and telomere length in men with biopsy-proven low-risk prostate cancer: 5-year follow-up of a descriptive pilot study. *Lancet Oncol.* **2013**, *14*, 1112–1120. [CrossRef]
18. Ornish, D.; Magbanua, M.J.M.; Weidner, G.; Weinberg, V.; Kemp, C.; Green, C.; Mattie, M.D.; Marlin, R.; Simko, J.; Shinohara, K.; et al. Changes in prostate gene expression in men undergoing an intensive nutrition and lifestyle intervention. *Proc. Natl. Acad. Sci. USA* **2008**, *105*, 8369–8374. [CrossRef]
19. He, Z.-Y.; Shi, C.-B.; Wen, H.; Li, F.-L.; Wang, B.-L.; Wang, J. Upregulation of p53 Expression in Patients with Colorectal Cancer by Administration of Curcumin. *Cancer Investig.* **2011**, *29*, 208–213. [CrossRef]
20. Supic, G.; Jagodic, M.; Magic, Z. Epigenetics: A New Link Between Nutrition and Cancer. *Nutr. Cancer* **2013**, *65*, 781–792. [CrossRef]
21. Patel, V.H. Nutrition and prostate cancer: An overview. *Expert Rev. Anticancer Ther.* **2014**, *14*, 1295–1304. [CrossRef]
22. Riccio, P.; Rossano, R. Nutrition Facts in Multiple Sclerosis. *ASN Neuro* **2015**, *7*, 1759091414568185. [CrossRef] [PubMed]
23. Gustafson, D.R.; Clare Morris, M.; Scarmeas, N.; Shah, R.C.; Sijben, J.; Yaffe, K.; Zhu, X. New Perspectives on Alzheimer's Disease and Nutrition. *J. Alzheimer's Dis.* **2015**, *46*, 1111–1127. [CrossRef] [PubMed]
24. Kawicka, A.; Regulska-Ilow, B. How nutritional status, diet and dietary supplements can affect autism. A review. *Roczniki Państwowego Zakładu Higieny* **2013**, *64*, 1–12. [PubMed]
25. Eilat-Adar, S.; Sinai, T.; Yosefy, C.; Henkin, Y. Nutritional Recommendations for Cardiovascular Disease Prevention. *Nutrients* **2013**, *5*, 3646–3683. [CrossRef] [PubMed]
26. Rodriguez-Leyva, D.; Weighell, W.; Edel, A.L.; LaVallee, R.; Dibrov, E.; Pinneker, R.; Maddaford, T.G.; Ramjiawan, B.; Aliani, M.; Guzman, R.; et al. Potent Antihypertensive Action of Dietary Flaxseed in Hypertensive PatientsNovelty and Significance. *Hypertension* **2013**, *62*, 1081–1089. [CrossRef] [PubMed]
27. Chen, T.; Yan, F.; Qian, J.; Guo, M.; Zhang, H.; Tang, X.; Chen, F.; Stoner, G.D.; Wang, X. Randomized Phase II Trial of Lyophilized Strawberries in Patients with Dysplastic Precancerous Lesions of the Esophagus. *Cancer Prev. Res.* **2012**, *5*, 41–50. [CrossRef] [PubMed]
28. Zeidan, F.; Martucci, K.T.; Kraft, R.A.; Gordon, N.S.; McHaffie, J.G.; Coghill, R.C. Brain Mechanisms Supporting the Modulation of Pain by Mindfulness Meditation. *J. Neurosci.* **2011**, *31*, 5540–5548. [CrossRef]
29. Jacob, J.A. As Opioid Prescribing Guidelines Tighten, Mindfulness Meditation Holds Promise for Pain Relief. *JAMA* **2016**, *315*, 2385–2387. [CrossRef]
30. Cherkin, D.C.; Sherman, K.J.; Balderson, B.H.; Cook, A.J.; Anderson, M.L.; Hawkes, R.J.; Hansen, K.E.; Turner, J.A. Effect of Mindfulness-Based Stress Reduction vs Cognitive Behavioral Therapy or Usual Care on Back Pain and Functional Limitations in Adults With Chronic Low Back Pain: A Randomized Clinical Trial. *JAMA* **2016**, *315*, 1240–1249. [CrossRef]
31. Nidich, S.I.; Rainforth, M.V.; Haaga, D.A.F.; Hagelin, J.; Salerno, J.W.; Travis, F.; Tanner, M.; Gaylord-King, C.; Grosswald, S.; Schneider, R.H. A Randomized Controlled Trial on Effects of the Transcendental Meditation Program on Blood Pressure, Psychological Distress, and Coping in Young Adults. *Am. J. Hypertens.* **2009**, *22*, 1326–1331. [CrossRef]
32. Davidson, R.J.; Kabat-Zinn, J.; Schumacher, J.; Rosenkranz, M.; Muller, D.; Santorelli, S.F.; Urbanowski, F.; Harrington, A.; Bonus, K.; Sheridan, J.F. Alterations in Brain and Immune Function Produced by Mindfulness Meditation. *Psychosom. Med.* **2003**, *65*, 564. [CrossRef] [PubMed]
33. Cotton, S.; Luberto, C.M.; Sears, R.W.; Strawn, J.R.; Stahl, L.; Wasson, R.S.; Blom, T.J.; Delbello, M.P. Mindfulness-based cognitive therapy for youth with anxiety disorders at risk for bipolar disorder: A pilot trial. *Early Interv. Psychiatry* **2016**, *10*, 426–434. [CrossRef] [PubMed]
34. Spigelblatt, L.; Laîné-Ammara, G.; Pless, I.B.; Guyver, A. The Use of Alternative Medicine by Children. *Pediatrics* **1994**, *94*, 811–814. [PubMed]
35. Sawni-Sikand, A.; Schubiner, H.; Thomas, R.L. Use of Complementary/Alternative Therapies Among Children in Primary Care Pediatrics. *Ambul. Pediatr.* **2002**, *2*, 99–103. [CrossRef]
36. Sibinga, E.M.S.; Ottolini, M.C.; Duggan, A.K.; Wilson, M.H. Parent-Pediatrician Communication about Complementary and Alternative Medicine Use for Children. *Clin. Pediatr. (Phila.)* **2004**, *43*, 367–373. [CrossRef] [PubMed]

37. Pappas, S.; Perlman, A. Complementary and alternative medicine: The importance of doctor-patient communication. *Med. Clin. N. Am.* **2002**, *86*, 1–10. [CrossRef]
38. Eisenberg, D.M. Advising Patients Who Seek Alternative Medical Therapies. *Ann. Intern. Med.* **1997**, *127*, 61. [CrossRef]
39. Perlman, A.I.; Eisenberg, D.M.; Panush, R.S. Talking with Patients about Alternative and Complementary Medicine. *Rheum. Dis. Clin. N. Am.* **1999**, *25*, 815–822. [CrossRef]
40. Sugarman, J.; Burk, L. Physicians' Ethical Obligations Regarding Alternative Medicine. *JAMA* **1998**, *280*, 1623–1625. [CrossRef]
41. Kemper, K.J.; O'Connor, K.G. Pediatricians' Recommendations for Complementary and Alternative Medical (CAM) Therapies. *Ambul. Pediatr.* **2004**, *4*, 482–487. [CrossRef]
42. Sawni, A.; Thomas, R. Pediatricians' attitudes, experience and referral patterns regarding complementary/ alternative medicine: A national survey. *BMC Complement. Altern. Med.* **2007**, *7*, 18. [CrossRef] [PubMed]
43. Winslow, L.C.; Shapiro, H. Physicians Want Education About Complementary and Alternative Medicine to Enhance Communication With Their Patients. *Arch. Intern. Med.* **2002**, *162*, 1176–1181. [CrossRef]
44. Vohra, S.; Surette, S.; Mittra, D.; Rosen, L.D.; Gardiner, P.; Kemper, K.J. Pediatric integrative medicine: Pediatrics' newest subspecialty? *BMC Pediatr.* **2012**, *12*, 123. [CrossRef]
45. Institute of Medicine (US) Committee on the Use of Complementary and Alternative Medicine by the American Public. *Complementary and Alternative Medicine in the United States*; The National Academies Collection: Reports funded by National Institutes of Health; National Academies Press (US): Washington, DC, USA, 2005; ISBN 978-0-309-09270-8.
46. McClafferty, H.; Dodds, S.; Brooks, A.J.; Brenner, M.G.; Brown, M.L.; Frazer, P.; Mark, J.D.; Weydert, J.A.; Wilcox, G.M.G.; Lebensohn, P.; et al. Pediatric Integrative Medicine in Residency (PIMR): Description of a New Online Educational Curriculum. *Children* **2015**, *2*, 98–107. [CrossRef] [PubMed]
47. Frank, E.; Breyan, J.; Elon, L. Physician disclosure of healthy personal behaviors improves credibility and ability to motivate. *Arch. Fam. Med.* **2000**, *9*, 287–290. [CrossRef] [PubMed]
48. McClafferty, H.; Brown, O.W.; Section on Integrative Medicine, Committee on Practice and Ambulatory Medicine. Physician Health and Wellness. *Pediatrics* **2014**, *134*, 830–835. [CrossRef] [PubMed]
49. Dewa, C.S.; Loong, D.; Bonato, S.; Thanh, N.X.; Jacobs, P. How does burnout affect physician productivity? A systematic literature review. *BMC Health Serv. Res.* **2014**, *14*, 325. [CrossRef]
50. Tawfik, D.S.; Profit, J.; Morgenthaler, T.I.; Satele, D.V.; Sinsky, C.A.; Dyrbye, L.N.; Tutty, M.A.; West, C.P.; Shanafelt, T.D. Physician Burnout, Well-being, and Work Unit Safety Grades in Relationship to Reported Medical Errors. *Mayo Clin. Proc.* **2018**, *93*, 1571–1580. [CrossRef]
51. Howe, A.; Smajdor, A.; Stöckl, A. Towards an understanding of resilience and its relevance to medical training. *Med. Educ.* **2012**, *46*, 349–356. [CrossRef]
52. Frank, E.; Rothenberg, R.; Lewis, C.; Belodoff, B.F. Correlates of physicians' prevention-related practices. Findings from the Women Physicians' Health Study. *Arch. Fam. Med.* **2000**, *9*, 359–367. [CrossRef]
53. Howe, M.; Leidel, A.; Krishnan, S.M.; Weber, A.; Rubenfire, M.; Jackson, E.A. Patient-Related Diet and Exercise Counseling: Do Providers' Own Lifestyle Habits Matter? *Prev. Cardiol.* **2010**, *13*, 180–185. [CrossRef] [PubMed]
54. Nguyen, C.T. Integrative Medicine as a Bridge to Physician Wellness. *Otolaryngol.-Head Neck Surg.* **2018**, *158*, 987–988. [CrossRef] [PubMed]
55. Vlieger, A.M.; Blink, M.; Tromp, E.; Benninga, M.A. Use of Complementary and Alternative Medicine by Pediatric Patients With Functional and Organic Gastrointestinal Diseases: Results From a Multicenter Survey. *Pediatrics* **2008**, *122*, e446–e451. [CrossRef] [PubMed]
56. Serpico, M.; Boyle, B.; Kemper, K.J.; Kim, S. Complementary and Alternative Medicine Use in Children with Inflammatory Bowel Diseases: A Single Center Survey. *J. Pediatr. Gastroenterol. Nutr.* **2016**, *63*, 651–657. [CrossRef] [PubMed]
57. Surette, S.; Vohra, S. Complementary, Holistic, and Integrative Medicine: Utilization Surveys of the Pediatric Literature. *Pediatr. Rev.* **2014**, *35*, 114–128. [CrossRef] [PubMed]
58. Misra, S.M. Integrative Therapies and Pediatric Inflammatory Bowel Disease: The Current Evidence. *Children* **2014**, *1*, 149–165. [CrossRef]

59. Miele, E.; Pascarella, F.; Giannetti, E.; Quaglietta, L.; Baldassano, R.N.; Staiano, A. Effect of a Probiotic Preparation (VSL#3) on Induction and Maintenance of Remission in Children With Ulcerative Colitis. *Am. J. Gastroenterol.* **2009**, *104*, 437–443.
60. Hanai, H.; Iida, T.; Takeuchi, K.; Watanabe, F.; Maruyama, Y.; Andoh, A.; Tsujikawa, T.; Fujiyama, Y.; Mitsuyama, K.; Sata, M.; et al. Curcumin Maintenance Therapy for Ulcerative Colitis: Randomized, Multicenter, Double-Blind, Placebo-Controlled Trial. *Clin. Gastroenterol. Hepatol.* **2006**, *4*, 1502–1506. [CrossRef]
61. Suskind, D.L.; Wahbeh, G.; Burpee, T.; Cohen, M.; Christie, D.; Weber, W. Tolerability of Curcumin in Pediatric Inflammatory Bowel Disease: A Forced-Dose Titration Study. *J. Pediatr. Gastroenterol. Nutr.* **2013**, *56*, 277. [CrossRef]
62. Ji, J.; Lu, Y.; Liu, H.; Feng, H.; Zhang, F.; Wu, L.; Cui, Y.; Wu, H. Acupuncture and Moxibustion for Inflammatory Bowel Diseases: A Systematic Review and Meta-Analysis of Randomized Controlled Trials. *J. Evid.-Based Complement. Altern. Med.* **2013**, *2013*, 158352. [CrossRef]
63. Timmer, A.; Preiss, J.C.; Motschall, E.; Rücker, G.; Jantschek, G.; Moser, G. Psychological interventions for treatment of inflammatory bowel disease. *Cochrane Database Syst. Rev.* **2011**. [CrossRef] [PubMed]
64. Cotton, S.; Roberts, Y.H.; Tsevat, J.; Britto, M.T.; Succop, P.; McGrady, M.E.; Yi, M.S. Mind-Body Complementary Alternative Medicine Use and Quality of Life in Adolescents with Inflammatory Bowel Disease. *Inflamm. Bowel Dis.* **2010**, *16*, 501–506. [CrossRef] [PubMed]
65. Mahler, T. Education and Hypnosis for Treatment of Functional Gastrointestinal Disorders (FGIDs) in Pediatrics. *Am. J. Clin. Hypn.* **2015**, *58*, 115–128. [CrossRef] [PubMed]
66. Mayer, E.A.; Tillisch, K. The brain-gut axis in abdominal pain syndromes. *Annu. Rev. Med.* **2011**, *62*, 381–396. [CrossRef] [PubMed]
67. Rutten, J.M.T.M.; Reitsma, J.B.; Vlieger, A.M.; Benninga, M.A. Gut-directed hypnotherapy for functional abdominal pain or irritable bowel syndrome in children: A systematic review. *Arch. Dis. Child.* **2013**, *98*, 252–257. [CrossRef] [PubMed]
68. Kline, R.M.; Kline, J.J.; Di Palma, J.; Barbero, G.J. Enteric-coated, pH-dependent peppermint oil capsules for the treatment of irritable bowel syndrome in children. *J. Pediatr.* **2001**, *138*, 125–128. [CrossRef] [PubMed]
69. Lin, Y.-C.; Lee, A.C.C.; Kemper, K.J.; Berde, C.B. Use of Complementary and Alternative Medicine in Pediatric Pain Management Service: A Survey. *Pain Med.* **2005**, *6*, 452–458. [CrossRef] [PubMed]
70. Young, L.; Kemper, K.J. Integrative care for pediatric patients with pain. *J. Altern. Complement. Med.* **2013**, *19*, 627–632. [CrossRef]
71. Palermo, T.M. Impact of recurrent and chronic pain on child and family daily functioning: A critical review of the literature. *J. Dev. Behav. Pediatr.* **2000**, *21*, 58–69. [CrossRef]
72. von Stülpnagel, C.; Reilich, P.; Straube, A.; Schäfer, J.; Blaschek, A.; Lee, S.-H.; Müller-Felber, W.; Henschel, V.; Mansmann, U.; Heinen, F. Myofascial trigger points in children with tension-type headache: A new diagnostic and therapeutic option. *J. Child Neurol.* **2009**, *24*, 406–409. [CrossRef]
73. Calvo-Muñoz, I.; Gómez-Conesa, A.; Sánchez-Meca, J. Physical therapy treatments for low back pain in children and adolescents: A meta-analysis. *BMC Musculoskelet. Disord.* **2013**, *14*, 55. [CrossRef] [PubMed]
74. Lee, B.H.; Scharff, L.; Sethna, N.F.; McCarthy, C.F.; Scott-Sutherland, J.; Shea, A.M.; Sullivan, P.; Meier, P.; Zurakowski, D.; Masek, B.J.; et al. Physical therapy and cognitive-behavioral treatment for complex regional pain syndromes. *J. Pediatr.* **2002**, *141*, 135–140. [CrossRef] [PubMed]
75. Cotton, S.; Luberto, C.M.; Bogenschutz, L.H.; Pelley, T.J.; Dusek, J. Integrative Care Therapies and Pain in Hospitalized Children and Adolescents: A Retrospective Database Review. *J. Altern. Complement. Med.* **2013**, *20*, 98–102. [CrossRef] [PubMed]
76. Lin, Y.-C.; Wan, L.; Jamison, R.N. Using Integrative Medicine in Pain Management: An Evaluation of Current Evidence. *Anesth. Analg.* **2017**, *125*, 2081.
77. Tsao, G.J.; Messner, A.H.; Seybold, J.; Sayyid, Z.N.; Cheng, A.G.; Golianu, B. Intraoperative acupuncture for posttonsillectomy pain: A randomized, double-blind, placebo-controlled trial. *Laryngoscope* **2015**, *125*, 1972–1978. [CrossRef] [PubMed]
78. Montgomery, G.H.; DuHamel, K.N.; Redd, W.H. A meta-analysis of hypnotically induced analgesia: How effective is hypnosis? *Int. J. Clin. Exp. Hypn.* **2000**, *48*, 138–153. [CrossRef] [PubMed]
79. Golianu, B.; Seybold, J.; D'Souza, G. Acupuncture as an Anesthetic Adjuvant for Pediatric Orthopedic Patients: A Pilot Study and Protocol Description. *Med. Acupunct.* **2015**, *27*, 475–480. [CrossRef]

80. Won, A.S.; Bailey, J.; Bailenson, J.; Tataru, C.; Yoon, I.A.; Golianu, B. Immersive Virtual Reality for Pediatric Pain. *Children* **2017**, *4*, 52. [CrossRef]
81. Yuan, J.C.; Rodriguez, S.; Caruso, T.J.; Tsui, J.H. Provider-controlled virtual reality experience may adjust for cognitive load during vascular access in pediatric patients. *Can. J. Anaesth.* **2017**, *64*, 1275–1276. [CrossRef]
82. Soo, I.; Mah, J.K.; Barlow, K.; Hamiwka, L.; Wirrell, E. Use of complementary and alternative medical therapies in a pediatric neurology clinic. *Can. J. Neurol. Sci.* **2005**, *32*, 524–528. [CrossRef]
83. Treat, L.; Liesinger, J.; Ziegenfuss, J.Y.; Humeniuk, K.; Prasad, K.; Tilburt, J.C. Patterns of Complementary and Alternative Medicine Use in Children with Common Neurological Conditions. *Glob. Adv. Health Med.* **2014**, *3*, 18–24. [CrossRef] [PubMed]
84. Kenney, D.; Jenkins, S.; Youssef, P.; Kotagal, S. Patient Use of Complementary and Alternative Medicines in an Outpatient Pediatric Neurology Clinic. *Pediatr. Neurol.* **2016**, *58*, 48–52.e7. [CrossRef] [PubMed]
85. Galicia-Connolly, E.; Adams, D.; Bateman, J.; Dagenais, S.; Clifford, T.; Baydala, L.; King, W.J.; Vohra, S. CAM Use in Pediatric Neurology: An Exploration of Concurrent Use with Conventional Medicine. *PLoS ONE* **2014**, *9*, e94078. [CrossRef] [PubMed]
86. Perrin, J.M.; Coury, D.L.; Hyman, S.L.; Cole, L.; Reynolds, A.M.; Clemons, T. Complementary and Alternative Medicine Use in a Large Pediatric Autism Sample. *Pediatrics* **2012**, *130*, S77–S82. [CrossRef] [PubMed]
87. Condò, M.; Posar, A.; Arbizzani, A.; Parmeggiani, A. Riboflavin prophylaxis in pediatric and adolescent migraine. *J. Headache Pain* **2009**, *10*, 361–365. [CrossRef] [PubMed]
88. Wang, F.; Van Den Eeden, S.K.; Ackerson, L.M.; Salk, S.E.; Reince, R.H.; Elin, R.J. Oral magnesium oxide prophylaxis of frequent migrainous headache in children: A randomized, double-blind, placebo-controlled trial. *Headache* **2003**, *43*, 601–610. [CrossRef] [PubMed]
89. Guidetti, V.; Dosi, C.; Bruni, O. The relationship between sleep and headache in children: Implications for treatment. *Cephalalgia* **2014**, *34*, 767–776. [CrossRef]
90. Legarda, S.B.; McMahon, D.; Othmer, S.; Othmer, S. Clinical Neurofeedback: Case Studies, Proposed Mechanism, and Implications for Pediatric Neurology Practice. *J. Child Neurol.* **2011**, *26*, 1045–1051. [CrossRef]
91. Tan, G.; Thornby, J.; Hammond, D.C.; Strehl, U.; Canady, B.; Arnemann, K.; Kaiser, D.A. Meta-Analysis of EEG Biofeedback in Treating Epilepsy. *Clin. Eeg. Neurosci.* **2009**, *40*, 173–179. [CrossRef]
92. Kanitz, J.L.; Camus, M.E.M.; Seifert, G. Keeping the balance—An overview of mind–body therapies in pediatric oncology. *Complement. Ther. Med.* **2013**, *21*, S20–S25. [CrossRef]
93. Laengler, A.; Spix, C.; Seifert, G.; Gottschling, S.; Graf, N.; Kaatsch, P. Complementary and alternative treatment methods in children with cancer: A population-based retrospective survey on the prevalence of use in Germany. *Eur. J. Cancer* **2008**, *44*, 2233–2240. [CrossRef] [PubMed]
94. Bishop, F.L.; Prescott, P.; Chan, Y.K.; Saville, J.; von Elm, E.; Lewith, G.T. Prevalence of Complementary Medicine Use in Pediatric Cancer: A Systematic Review. *Pediatrics* **2010**, *125*, 768–776. [CrossRef] [PubMed]
95. Jacobs, S.S. Integrative Therapy Use for Management of Side Effects and Toxicities Experienced by Pediatric Oncology Patients. *Children* **2014**, *1*, 424–440. [CrossRef] [PubMed]
96. Campbell, T.C. Cancer Prevention and Treatment by Wholistic Nutrition. *J. Nat. Sci.* **2017**, *3*.
97. Campbell, T.C. Nutrition and Cancer: An Historical Perspective—The Past, Present, and Future of Nutrition and Cancer. Part 2. Misunderstanding and Ignoring Nutrition. *Nutr. Cancer* **2017**, *69*, 962–968. [CrossRef] [PubMed]
98. Harvie, M.; Howell, A.; Evans, D.G. Can diet and lifestyle prevent breast cancer: What is the evidence? *Am. Soc. Clin. Oncol. Educ. Book* **2015**, e66–73. [CrossRef]
99. Lee, J.; Jeon, J.Y.; Meyerhardt, J.A. Diet and Lifestyle in Survivors of Colorectal Cancer. *Hematol. Oncol. Clin. N. Am.* **2015**, *29*, 1–27. [CrossRef] [PubMed]
100. Correa, P. Human Gastric Carcinogenesis: A Multistep and Multifactorial Process—First American Cancer Society Award Lecture on Cancer Epidemiology and Prevention. *Cancer Res.* **1992**, *52*, 6735–6740.
101. Vance, T.M.; Su, J.; Fontham, E.T.H.; Koo, S.I.; Chun, O.K. Dietary Antioxidants and Prostate Cancer: A Review. *Nutr. Cancer* **2013**, *65*, 793–801. [CrossRef]
102. Anand, P.; Kunnumakara, A.B.; Sundaram, C.; Harikumar, K.B.; Tharakan, S.T.; Lai, O.S.; Sung, B.; Aggarwal, B.B. Cancer is a Preventable Disease that Requires Major Lifestyle Changes. *Pharm. Res.* **2008**, *25*, 2097–2116. [CrossRef]

103. Chatzi, L.; Apostolaki, G.; Bibakis, I.; Skypala, I.; Bibaki-Liakou, V.; Tzanakis, N.; Kogevinas, M.; Cullinan, P. Protective effect of fruits, vegetables and the Mediterranean diet on asthma and allergies among children in Crete. *Thorax* **2007**, *62*, 677–683. [CrossRef] [PubMed]
104. Lozinsky, A.C.; Meyer, R.; Koker, C.D.; Dziubak, R.; Godwin, H.; Reeve, K.; Ortega, G.D.; Shah, N. Time to symptom improvement using elimination diets in non-IgE-mediated gastrointestinal food allergies. *Pediatr. Allergy Immunol.* **2015**, *26*, 403–408. [CrossRef] [PubMed]
105. Castro-Rodriguez, J.A.; Ramirez-Hernandez, M.; Padilla, O.; Pacheco-Gonzalez, R.M.; Pérez-Fernández, V.; Garcia-Marcos, L. Effect of foods and Mediterranean diet during pregnancy and first years of life on wheezing, rhinitis and dermatitis in preschoolers. *Allergol. Immunopathol. (Madrid)* **2016**, *44*, 400–409. [CrossRef] [PubMed]
106. Cramer, H.; Posadzki, P.; Dobos, G.; Langhorst, J. Yoga for asthma: A systematic review and meta-analysis. *Ann. Allergy Asthma Immunol.* **2014**, *112*, 503–510.e5.
107. Sankar, J.; Das, R.R. Asthma—A Disease of How We Breathe: Role of Breathing Exercises and Pranayam. *Indian J. Pediatr.* **2018**, *85*, 905–910. [CrossRef] [PubMed]
108. Burgess, J.; Ekanayake, B.; Lowe, A.; Dunt, D.; Thien, F.; Dharmage, S.C. Systematic review of the effectiveness of breathing retraining in asthma management. *Expert Rev. Respir. Med.* **2011**, *5*, 789–807. [CrossRef] [PubMed]
109. Mark, J.D. Pediatric Asthma. *Nutr. Clin. Pract.* **2009**, *24*, 578–588. [CrossRef]
110. Misra, S.M. The Current Evidence of Integrative Approaches to Pediatric Asthma. *Curr. Probl. Pediatr. Adolesc. Health Care* **2016**, *46*, 190–194. [CrossRef]
111. Guardamagna, O.; Abello, F.; Cagliero, P.; Lughetti, L. Impact of nutrition since early life on cardiovascular prevention. *Ital. J. Pediatr.* **2012**, *38*, 73. [CrossRef]
112. Kaikkonen, J.E.; Mikkilä, V.; Raitakari, O.T. Role of Childhood Food Patterns on Adult Cardiovascular Disease Risk. *Curr. Atheroscler. Rep.* **2014**, *16*, 443. [CrossRef]
113. Kavey, R.-E.W.; Allada, V.; Daniels, S.R.; Hayman, L.L.; McCrindle, B.W.; Newburger, J.W.; Parekh, R.S.; Steinberger, J. Cardiovascular Risk Reduction in High-Risk Pediatric Patients*: A Scientific Statement From the American Heart Association Expert Panel on Population and Prevention Science; the Councils on Cardiovascular Disease in the Young, Epidemiology and Prevention, Nutrition, Physical Activity and Metabolism, High Blood Pressure Research, Cardiovascular Nursing, and the Kidney in Heart Disease; and the Interdisciplinary Working Group on Quality of Care and Outcomes Research Endorsed by the American Academy of Pediatrics. *J. Cardiovasc. Nurs.* **2007**, *22*, 218–253. [PubMed]
114. Guarneri, M.; Mercado, N.; Suhar, C. Integrative Approaches for Cardiovascular Disease. *Nutr. Clin. Pract.* **2009**, *24*, 701–708. [CrossRef] [PubMed]
115. Boisvert, J.A.; Harrell, W.A. Integrative Treatment of Pediatric Obesity: Psychological and Spiritual Considerations. *Integr. Med. (Encinitas)* **2015**, *14*, 40–47. [PubMed]
116. Sibinga, E.M.S.; Webb, L.; Ghazarian, S.R.; Ellen, J.M. School-Based Mindfulness Instruction: An RCT. *Pediatrics* **2016**, *137*, e20152532. [CrossRef] [PubMed]
117. Nesvold, A.; Fagerland, M.W.; Davanger, S.; Ellingsen, Ø.; Solberg, E.E.; Holen, A.; Sevre, K.; Atar, D. Increased heart rate variability during nondirective meditation. *Eur. J. Prev. Cardiol.* **2012**, *19*, 773–780. [CrossRef] [PubMed]
118. Nijjar, P.S.; Puppala, V.K.; Dickinson, O.; Duval, S.; Duprez, D.; Kreitzer, M.J.; Benditt, D.G. Modulation of the autonomic nervous system assessed through heart rate variability by a mindfulness based stress reduction program. *Int. J. Cardiol.* **2014**, *177*, 557–559. [CrossRef] [PubMed]
119. Olex, S.; Newberg, A.; Figueredo, V.M. Meditation: Should a cardiologist care? *Int. J. Cardiol.* **2013**, *168*, 1805–1810. [CrossRef]
120. Painovich, J.; Longhurst, J. Integrating acupuncture into the cardiology clinic: Can it play a role? *Sheng Li Xue Bao* **2015**, *67*, 19–31.
121. McClafferty, H.; Brooks, A.J.; Chen, M.-K.; Brenner, M.; Brown, M.; Esparham, A.; Gerstbacher, D.; Golianu, B.; Mark, J.; Weydert, J.; et al. Pediatric Integrative Medicine in Residency Program: Relationship between Lifestyle Behaviors and Burnout and Wellbeing Measures in First-Year Residents. *Children* **2018**, *5*, 54. [CrossRef]
122. Won, A.S.; Tataru, C.A.; Cojocaru, C.M.; Krane, E.J.; Bailenson, J.N.; Niswonger, S.; Golianu, B. Two Virtual Reality Pilot Studies for the Treatment of Pediatric CRPS. *Pain Med.* **2015**, *16*, 1644–1647. [CrossRef]

123. Arruda, J.M.; Bogetz, A.L.; Vellanki, S.; Wren, A.; Yeh, A.M. Yoga as adjunct therapy for adolescents with inflammatory bowel disease: A pilot clinical trial. *Complement. Ther. Med.* **2018**, *41*, 99–104. [CrossRef] [PubMed]
124. Bodner, K.; D'Amico, S.; Luo, M.; Sommers, E.; Goldstein, L.; Neri, C.; Gardiner, P. A cross-sectional review of the prevalence of integrative medicine in pediatric pain clinics across the United States. *Complement. Ther. Med.* **2018**, *38*, 79–84. [CrossRef] [PubMed]
125. Kemper, K.J. Integrative medicine is becoming mainstream: Research on multimodal interventions needs to catch up. *Complement. Ther. Med.* **2018**, *39*, A1. [CrossRef] [PubMed]
126. Mark, J.D.; Chung, Y. Complementary and alternative medicine in pulmonology. *Curr. Opin. Pediatr.* **2015**, *27*, 334–340. [CrossRef]
127. Mark, J.D. Integrative medicine and asthma. *Pediatr. Clin. N. Am.* **2007**, *54*, 1007–1023. [CrossRef]
128. Coates, A.C.; Mark, J.D. Nutrition in Cystic Fibrosis. In *Nutrition in Pediatric Pulmonary Disease*; Dumont, R., Chung, Y., Eds.; Nutrition and Health; Springer: New York, NY, USA, 2014; pp. 81–97, ISBN 978-1-4614-8474-5.
129. Mark, J.D. Chapter 29—Asthma. In *Integrative Medicine (Fourth Edition)*; Rakel, D., Ed.; Elsevier: Amsterdam, The Netherlands, 2018; pp. 288–299.e2, ISBN 978-0-323-35868-2.
130. Yeh, A.M.; Wren, A.; Golianu, B. Mind-Body Interventions for Pediatric Inflammatory Bowel Disease. *Children* **2017**, *4*, 22. [CrossRef] [PubMed]
131. Kanak, M.; Park, K.T.; Yeh, A.M. Acupuncture and Integrative Medicine for Pediatric Gastroesophageal Reflux and Functional Dyspepsia. *Med. Acupunct.* **2015**, *27*, 467–474. [CrossRef]
132. Karamian, A.S.; Yeh, A.M.; Wusthoff, C. Integrative Medicine in Child Neurology: What do providers think and what do they need to learn? In Proceedings of the Annual Meeting of American Academy of Neurology, Los Angeles, CA, USA, 21 April 2018.
133. Staveski, S.L.; Boulanger, K.; Erman, L.; Lin, L.; Almgren, C.; Journel, C.; Roth, S.J.; Golianu, B. The Impact of Massage and Reading on Children's Pain and Anxiety After Cardiovascular Surgery: A Pilot Study. *Pediatr. Crit. Care Med.* **2018**, *19*, 725–732. [CrossRef]
134. Golianu, B.; Krane, E.; Seybold, J.; Almgren, C.; Anand, K.J.S. Non-pharmacological techniques for pain management in neonates. *Semin. Perinatol.* **2007**, *31*, 318–322. [CrossRef]
135. Sparrow, K.; Golianu, B. Does Acupuncture Reduce Stress Over Time? A Clinical Heart Rate Variability Study in Hypertensive Patients. *Med. Acupunct.* **2014**, *26*, 286–294. [CrossRef]
136. Mitchell, A.J.; Hall, R.W.; Golianu, B.; Yates, C.; Williams, D.K.; Chang, J.; Anand, K.J.S. Does noninvasive electrical stimulation of acupuncture points reduce heelstick pain in neonates? *Acta Paediatr.* **2016**, *105*, 1434–1439. [CrossRef] [PubMed]
137. NS-CSHCN Compare All Years: How Many Children/Youth Have Special Health Care Needs? Nationwide. Available online: http://childhealthdata.org/browse/survey/results?q=1792&r=1&t=1&ta=116 (accessed on 27 November 2018).
138. Eckert, M.; Amarell, C.; Anheyer, D.; Cramer, H.; Dobos, G. Integrative Pediatrics: Successful Implementation of Integrative Medicine in a German Hospital Setting-Concept and Realization. *Children* **2018**, *5*, 122. [CrossRef] [PubMed]
139. Esparham, A.; Misra, S.; Sibinga, E.; Culbert, T.; Kemper, K.; McClafferty, H.; Vohra, S.; Rosen, L. Pediatric Integrative Medicine: Vision for the Future. *Children* **2018**, *5*, 111. [CrossRef] [PubMed]
140. Bell, I.R.; Caspi, O.; Schwartz, G.E.R.; Grant, K.L.; Gaudet, T.W.; Rychener, D.; Maizes, V.; Weil, A. Integrative medicine and systemic outcomes research: Issues in the emergence of a new model for primary health care. *Arch. Intern. Med.* **2002**, *162*, 133–140. [CrossRef] [PubMed]

12

A Review of Non-Pharmacological Treatments for Pain Management in Newborn Infants

Avneet K. Mangat [1,2], Ju-Lee Oei [3], Kerry Chen [4], Im Quah-Smith [5] and Georg M. Schmölzer [2,6,*]

1 Faculty of Science, University of Alberta, Edmonton, AB T6G 2R3, Canada; amangat@ualberta.ca
2 Centre for the Studies of Asphyxia and Resuscitation, Neonatal Research Unit, Royal Alexandra Hospital, Edmonton, AB T6G 2R3, Canada
3 School of Women's and Children's Health, University of New South Wales, Kensington, NSW 2031, Australia; j.oei@unsw.edu.au
4 Faculty of Medicine, University of New South Wales, Kensington, NSW 2033, Australia; kerry.chen@unsw.edu.au
5 School of Women's and Children's Health University of New South Wales, Kensington, NSW 2033, Australia; quahsmith@gmail.com
6 Department of Pediatrics, University of Alberta, Edmonton, AB T6G 2R3, Canada
* Correspondence: georg.schmoelzer@me.com

Abstract: Pain is a major problem in sick newborn infants, especially for those needing intensive care. Pharmacological pain relief is the most commonly used, but might be ineffective and has side effects, including long-term neurodevelopmental sequelae. The effectiveness and safety of alternative analgesic methods are ambiguous. The objective was to review the effectiveness and safety of non-pharmacological methods of pain relief in newborn infants and to identify those that are the most effective. PubMed and Google Scholar were searched using the terms: "infant", "premature", "pain", "acupuncture", "skin-to-skin contact", "sucrose", "massage", "musical therapy" and 'breastfeeding'. We included 24 studies assessing different methods of non-pharmacological analgesic techniques. Most resulted in some degree of analgesia but many were ineffective and some were even detrimental. Sucrose, for example, was often ineffective but was more effective than music therapy, massage, breast milk (for extremely premature infants) or non-invasive electrical stimulation acupuncture. There were also conflicting results for acupuncture, skin-to-skin care and musical therapy. Most non-pharmacological methods of analgesia provide a modicum of relief for preterm infants, but none are completely effective and there is no clearly superior method. Study is also required to assess potential long-term consequences of any of these methods.

Keywords: infant; premature; pain; acupuncture; skin-to-skin contact; sucrose; massage; musical therapy; breastfeeding

---

1. Introduction

Newborn infants admitted to an Neonatal Intensive Care Unit (NICU) undergo an average of 134 painful procedures within the first two weeks [1,2]. Even more concerning, some infants might experience more than 3000 painful procedures during the entire course of their NICU stay [3]. These procedures are often necessary to ensure best care, such as heel pricks for blood sampling or endotracheal suctioning. Some of these procedures are also performed repeatedly on the same infant and have been shown to cause adverse physiological consequences, such as hypoxemia, bradycardia and hypertension [1].

Apart from acute discomfort, there is now growing evidence, that painful (and particularly, repetitive) procedures may have adverse consequences on long-term neurological development. Animal models demonstrate that painful events in early life can increase the number of glucocorticoid receptors in the hippocampus, which may affect future stress response [4]. Pain may not even need to be chronic or repetitive to elicit adverse future outcomes. For example, infants have increased stress behavior during routine immunizations at 4–6 months if circumcision was conducted at birth without analgesia [5]. This highlights the lifelong implications of pain management during this critical period in life [1,6].

Pharmacological methods are the most frequently used means to ameliorate or prevent pain in infants. However, many analgesics have adverse effects. For example, opioids can have troublesome adverse effects including somnolence, and respiratory depression making it unsuitable for use in spontaneously breathing, opioid-naïve patients [7].

Adjuvants to pharmacological analgesia are therefore needed. Non-pharmacological analgesic methods include acupuncture, non-nutritive sucking (NNS), breastfeeding (BF), sucrose/glucose solution, skin-to-skin care (SSC), swaddling, therapeutic massage, musical therapy (MT) and facilitated tucking (Table 1). These methods utilize environmental, behavioral, and pharmacological approaches by activating a "gate control mechanism" that prevents the pain sensation from traveling to the central nervous system [8]. While evidence exists for non-pharmacological analgesic methods, the strategies are not used universally. We therefore aimed to summarize the current evidence about the efficacy, safety, and feasibility of non-pharmacological interventions for pain management in newborn infants to determine if they could be considered an alternative to other methods of analgesia, including medications.

Table 1. Non-pharmacological treatments for pain relief.

Environmental Control
Skin-to-skin care Swaddling Facilitated tucking Therapeutic touch/massage Musical therapy
Feeding Methods
Non-nutritive sucking Breastfeeding
Other Interventions
Acupuncture Sucrose/glucose solutions

2. Methods

PubMed and Google Scholar were systematically searched include the following search-terms "infants", "pain", "acupuncture", "skin-to-skin contact", "sucrose", "massage", "musical therapy" and "breastfeeding" between 1965 and 2018 (Appendix A). List of references of identified articles were manually searched. Articles were included if they described non-pharmacological techniques in preterm or term infants and excluded if they compared pharmacological and non-pharmacological intervention or there was no behavioral measurement of pain (e.g., PIPP (Premature Infant Pain Profile), or NIPS (Neonatal Infant Pain Scale)). Only human studies were included and no language restrictions were applied.

3. Results

A total of 26 studies describing acupuncture (n = 3), skin to skin care (n = 3), non-nutritive sucking (n = 1), swaddling (n = 3), sucrose/glucose solution (n = 3), massage (n = 4), musical therapy (n = 5), breastfeeding (n = 3) and facilitated tucking (n = 1) were identified (Table 2). A total of 10 studies were done in preterm infants, 12 studies were in term infants and four studies were done in preterm and term infants. It was not possible to make a distinction between preterm and term infants since many studies did not separate their samples by gestation.

Table 2. Randomized controlled trials for non-pharmacological methods of pain relief in infants.

First Author, Year	Population	Intervention	Other Intervention	Primary Outcome		p-Value
				Intervention	Control	
Shabani, 2016 [9]	Preterm (n = 20)	MT	N/A	Facial pain expressions M (SD): MT: 0.4 (0.1)	Control: 2.1 (0.4)	0.001
Seo, 2016 [10]	Term (n = 56)	SSC	N/A	PIPP M ± SD: SSC: 4.1 ± 2.3	Control: 6.3 ± 3.5	0.01
Freire, 2008 [11]	Preterm (n = 95)	SSC	Glucose	HR M ± SD: SSC: 5.1 ± 3.9 bpm Glucose: 9.9 ± 6.1 bpm	Control: 10.8 ± 6.5 bpm	SSC vs. glucose: 0.0001 SSC vs. control: 0.0001
Olsson, 2016 [12]	Preterm (n = 10)	SSC	N/A	PIPP M: 5.7	Control: 5.0	>0.05 (NS)
Efendi, 2018 [13]	Preterm (n = 30)	Pacifier and swaddling	N/A	Increase in pain score: Swaddle: 5.9 ± 2.2 to 6.1 ± 2.0	Control: 5.4 ± 1.8 to 7.7 ± 2.7	Swaddling: NS Control: 0.003
Erkut, 2017 [14]	Term (n = 74)	Swaddle	N/A	NIPS M ± SD: Swaddle: 1.6 ± 0.8	Control: 3.3 ± 1.5	0.01
Ho, 2016 [15]	Preterm (n = 54)	Swaddle	N/A	PIPP M ± SD: Swaddle: 7.0 ± 2.7	Control: 14.7 ± 2.9	<0.001
Axelin, 2006 [16]	Preterm (n = 20)	FT	N/A	NIPS Median (IQR): FT: 3 (2–6)	Control: 5 (2–7)	<0.001
Arikan, 2008 [17]	Preterm/term (n = 175)	Massage	Sucrose herbal tea, hydrolyzed formula	Crying time after procedure M ± SD: Massage: 4.4 ± 1.8 s Sucrose: 3.9 ± 1.5 s Tea: 3.2 ± 1.2 s Formula: 2.7 ± 1.1 s	Control: 5.3 ± 1.76 s	Comparing before and after procedure: $p < 0.001$ for all but control ($p > 0.05$)
Chik, 2017 [18]	Preterm/term (n = 80)	Massage	N/A	PIPP M (SD): Massage: 6 (3.3)	Control: 12 (4.3)	<0.001
Jain, 2006 [19]	Preterm (n = 23)	Massage	N/A	NIPS M (SD): Massage: 1.5 (0.9)	Control: 3.5 (1.6)	<0.001
Zhu, 2015 [20]	Term (n = 250)	MT	BF	NIPS M (SD): MT: not significant MT + BF: not significant BF: 3.1 (1.9)	Control: 6.4 (0.2)	BF vs. control: <0.001
Shah, 2017 [21]	Preterm/term (n = 35)	MT	Sucrose	PIPP median (IQR): MT: 6 (3–11) MT + sucrose: 3 (0–4)	Sucrose: 5 (3–10)	MT vs. sucrose: >0.05 MT + sucrose vs. sucrose: <0.001 MT + sucrose vs. MT: <0.001

Table 2. *Cont.*

First Author, Year	Population	Intervention	Other Intervention	Primary Outcome		p-Value
				Intervention	Control	
Zurita-Cruz, 2017 [22]	Term ($n = 144$)	BF	MS	Crying time Median (IQR): BF: 19 (0–136) MS: 41.5 (0–184)	Control: 41 (0–161)	BF vs. control: 0.007 Control vs. MS: >0.05
Erkul, 2017 [23]	Term ($n = 100$)	BF	N/A	NIPS M ± SD: BF: 1.9 ± 2.2	Control: 6.8 ± 0.7	<0.05
Simonse, 2012 [24]		BF	Bottle fed, sucrose	PIPP M (95%CI): BF: 7.0 (5.3–8.7) Bottle fed: 5.4 (3.7–7.1)	Sucrose: 5.3 (3.6–6.9)	BF vs. bottle fed: >0.05 BF vs. sucrose: >0.05
Baudesson, 2017 [25]	Preterm ($n = 33$)	MO	N/A	PIPP M (SD): MO: 7.3 (3.0)	Control: 10 (3.5)	0.03
Mitchell, 2016 [26]	Term ($n = 162$)	NESAP	Sucrose	PIPP M ± SD: NESAP: 5.0 ± 4.0 Sucrose: 4.0 ± 1.8 NESAP + sucrose: 3.6 ± 1.2	Control: 4.9 ± 4.0	<0.01
Chen, 2017 [27]	Preterm/term ($n = 30$)	MA	N/A	PIPP M ± SD: MA: 5.9 ± 3.7	Control: 8.3 ± 4.7	0.04
Abbasoglu, 2015 [28]	Preterm ($n = 32$)	Acupressure	N/A	PIPP M ± SD: Acupressure: 9.1 ± 2.0	Control: 9.6 ± 1.7	0.5
Lima, 2017 [29]	Term ($n = 78$)	NNS	Glucose	NIPS M ± SD: NNS: 33.9 ± 17.6	Glucose: 10.9 ± 11.3	<0.001
Gouin, 2018 [30]	Term ($n = 245$)	Sucrose	N/A	NIPS M ± SD: Sucrose: 2.3 ± 0.5	Control: 1.6 ± 0.5	0.6
Collados-Gómez, 2018 [31]	Preterm ($n = 66$)	Sucrose	EBM	PIPP Median (IQR): Sucrose: 6 (4–8)	EBM: 7 (4–9)	0.28

M: mean, SD: standard deviation, IQR: interquartile range, NS: not significant, HR: heart rate, SSC: skin-to-skin care, FT: facilitated tuck, MT: musical therapy, BF: breast feeding, MO: milk odor, NS: non-significant, NNS: non-nutritive sucking, NESAP: non-invasive electrical stimulation at acupuncture points, N/A: not/applicable, MS: milk substitute, EBM: expressed breastmilk, PIPP: Premature Infant Pain Profile, NIPS: Neonatal Infant Pain Scale, bpm: beats per minute.

3.1. Environmental Control

Creating a more comforting environment with SSC, swaddling, therapeutic touch/massage, music therapy and comfort positioning for the infant can produce analgesic effects. Cholecystokinin, a neuropeptide associated with analgesia, is released when the infant is exposed to familiar smell of the mother [32]. Therefore, providing an infant with SSC with the mother can have an analgesic effect [32]. Swaddling, the practice of wrapping infants in blankets and can help simulate the environment of the womb which may translate to analgesia [33,34]. Massage can potentially saturate the senses and decrease the pain signals that are sent to the central nervous system [35]. Music uses distraction to activate the infant's attention and thus distracts them from the pain and decreases their sensation of pain [9]. Holding the infant in a flexed position, which is known as facilitated tucking, can also have analgesic effects due to saturation of senses similar to massage therapy [35].

3.1.1. Skin-to-Skin Care

Overall, most studies reported decreased pain responses during SSC compared to placebo methods. Seo et al. reported 35% less pain and an 88% decrease in crying duration with SSC compared to controls during heel pricks [10]. Similarly, Freire et al. compared SSC with oral glucose solution or placebo for pain relief of 95 preterm infants during heel prick. The infants randomized to SSC had significantly lower heart rates (mean $\pm$ standard deviation (SD), 5 ± 4 vs. control 11 ± 7 vs. oral glucose 10 ± 6 beats per minute (bpm); $p = 0.0001$) and oxygen saturation variation (1.5 ± 1.7 vs. control 2.6 ± 1.5 vs. oral glucose $1.9 \pm 1.5\%$; $p = 0.0012$) than those given glucose or to controls [11]. Olsson et al. reported similar pain scores between SSC and placebo during venepuncture of 10 preterm infants [12]. In summary, SSC might reduce pain in preterm and term infants.

3.1.2. Swaddling

Efendi et al. randomized 30 preterm infants to either swaddling and pacifier or control during painful procedures and demonstrated a significantly lower heart rate and pain scores in infants receiving swaddling and a pacifier [13]. As the study combined NNS and swaddling, it is therefore impossible to differentiate which of these methods might have provided pain relief. Other studies have reported that swaddling alone decreases pain during heel prick [14,15]. Erkut et al. reported a 50% pain reduction, a 30% decrease in duration of crying time, and a significantly increased oxygen saturation (mean $\pm$ SD, 97 ± 2 vs. control: $95 \pm 2\%$, $p = 0.006$) in the swaddled group after a heel prick procedure in 74 term infants [14]. Ho et al. randomized 54 premature infants to swaddling or control and reported lower pain scores (7 ± 3 vs. control: 145 ± 3, $p < 0.001$), lower heart rate (162 ± 10 vs. control: 182 ± 17 bpm, $p < 0.001$), and higher oxygen saturation (96 ± 4 vs. control $87 \pm 7\%$, $p < 0.001$) after heel prick [15]. These studies suggest that swaddling alone or combining with a pacifier has the potential to decrease pain in preterm and term infants.

3.1.3. Facilitated Tucking

Axelin et al. randomized 20 preterm infants to either control or facilitated tucking (flexed position by their parents) [16]. Overall, facilitated tucking reduced pain by 40% ($p < 0.001$) and crying time was significantly shorter 5 s vs. 17 s, $p = 0.024$ when compared to no tucking [16].

3.1.4. Therapeutic Touch/Massage

Two observational studies reported that massage therapy significantly reduced mean crying time (4.4 ± 1.8 vs. control: 5.3 ± 1.7 h/day, $p < 0.001$) in infants with infant colic [17] and decreased NIPS scores (3.9 vs. control: 4.8, $p = 0.002$) in term infants [34]. Two randomized trials reported that an upper limb massage significantly decreased pain responses during venipuncture in preterm and term infants [18,19]. Chik et al. randomized 80 infants and found significantly lower pain scores between the massage and control group (-6.0, $p < 0.001$) [18]. Similarly, Jain et al. found a 60% decrease in pain and a significant decrease in heart rate (mean ± SD: 149 ± 14 vs. control: 159 ± 13 bpm, $p = 0.03$) after venipuncture of 23 infants [19]. These studies suggest that a gentle massage prior a heel prick is safe and can decrease pain.

3.1.5. Musical Therapy

Using MT, a case study with five infants in a cardiac intensive care unit showed a decreased average heart rate in 4/5 infants in 66% of the sessions [36]. In addition, respiratory rate and blood pressure were also decreased, while oxygen saturation increased in some of the infants [36]. Furthermore, Olischar et al. reported more mature sleep-wake cycles in newborn infants > 32 weeks' gestation exposed to music when compared to controls suggesting a calming effect on quiet sleep [37]. These data suggest that MT has a stabilizing effect on physiological parameters and sleep, which could be translate to a decreased pain response. However, currently available evidence has conflicting results.

Shabani et al. randomized 20 preterm infants to MT or control during venous blood sampling and reported a significant decrease in heart rate (mean ± SD: 148 ± 4 vs. control 163 ± 4 bpm, $p = 0.005$) and an 80% decrease in the infants' mean facial pain expressions with MT [9]. Zhu et al. randomized 250 term infants to either MT, MT + BF, BF, or control and observed that the BF group had a 50% decrease in pain and a 70% decrease in duration of crying time [20]. In addition, no difference between BF or BF + MT was observed, suggesting that MT was ineffective for pain relief [20]. Shah et al. randomized 35 infants to MT, sucrose, or MT + sucrose using a cross-over design [21]. Overall, median interquartile range pain scores were significantly lower in the MT + sucrose group (3, 0–4) compared to MT (6, 3–11) or sucrose (5, 3–10) alone [21]. In addition, pain scores were similar between the MT and sucrose groups [21]. These data suggest that a combination of MT + sucrose provides improved pain relief compared to sucrose or music alone.

3.2. Feeding Methods

Breastfeeding and NNS are believed to support analgesia through the release of cholecystokinin (neuropeptide) [32,38]. With BF, cholecystokinin is believed to be released due to familiar odors of the mother [32]. Non-nutritive sucking has been associated with the activation of sensory nerves that can lead to the release of cholecystokinin which can then interact with opioids and produce analgesia [1].

3.2.1. Breastfeeding

Zurita-Cruz et al. randomized 144 infants to either BF, milk substitute, or no analgesia (control group) during vaccination and reported that infants who received BF had reduced pain and 50% reduction in median crying time compared with milk substitute or controls [22]. There were no significant differences in any of the parameters between the milk substitute and control groups suggesting that milk substitute was ineffective at decreasing pain [22]. Similarly, Erkul et al. randomized 100 infants to either BF or control prior vaccination and observed lower pain scores (mean ± SD: 1.9 ± 2.2 vs. 6.8 ± 0.7, $p < 0.05$), lower duration of crying (mean ± SD: 20.5 ± 16.2 vs. 45.1 ± 14.5 s, $p = 0.005$), lower heart rate (mean ± SD: 164 ± 17 vs. 172 ± 15 bpm, $p < 0.05$), and higher mean oxygen saturation (mean ± SD: 98 ± 3 vs. 94 ± 7%, $p < 0.05$) [23]. One may assume that there is a difference between the analgesic effects of BF compared to oral administering breast milk, due to BF having the additive analgesic effects from other factors such as parental presence and SSC. However, a randomized controlled trial of 71 preterm neonates reported a surprising distinction between BF and bottle feeding [24]. Bottle feeding significantly decreased the mean COMFORTneo pain score compared to breast feeding (BF: 19.0 vs. bottle-fed: 16.3, $p = 0.03$) [24]. The study also compared the analgesic effects of breast milk to sucrose and found no significant differences in PIPP scores eluding that both were just as effective [24]. It is also noteworthy that, in premature infants, even the smell of breast milk had a 50% reduction in pain scores during venipuncture and a decrease in percent of duration of crying (0.17 ± 0.6 vs. 9.7 ± 17.3 s, $p = 0.04$) after venipuncture [25]. These results are important in situations where breast feeding is not feasible in the NICU (e.g., mother not present) since the smell of breast milk has the potential to decrease pain.

3.2.2. Non-Nutritive Sucking

A case-control study compared infants who sucked on an adult's little finger ($n = 20$) with BF ($n = 20$) and without any analgesia ($n = 23$, control group) during venipuncture [39]. Overall outcomes with BF and NNS were similar (35 vs. 24%, $p > 0.05$) suggesting a similar efficacy in analgesia [39]. While NNS has some effect on pain relief further studies are needed to examine different approaches of NNS (e.g., use of finger or pacifier) or combination with glucose.

3.3. Other Interventions

3.3.1. Acupuncture

Body acupuncture and pain management is well known with the spinal pain pathways being recruited for attenuation of pain signaling in needle acupuncture. Manual acupuncture activates different afferent fibers (Aβ, Aδ, and C) and these signals ascend mainly through the spinal ventrolateral funiculus to the brain [26]. Many brain nuclei compose the network involved in processing acupuncture analgesia such as locus coeruleus and arcuate nucleus [26]. However, more recent research reveals the bigger impact of acupuncture on the individual. Now considered a complex sensory stimulation, acupuncture effects also include autonomic re-regulation and regulatory changes in functional connectivity centrally—mitigating the effects of physical and emotional trauma in the individual [40,41]. The non-invasive approach (no needling modalities of acupuncture such as low-level laser and magnet application), is more autonomically driven to gain direct access to central pain control centers [40]. Neuroimaging studies have confirmed the re-regulatory capacity of acupuncture centrally [42].

Several studies examined the effects of non-invasive acupuncture on neonatal pain [27,28,43]. Chen et al. randomized 30 term infants to either auricular non-invasive magnetic acupuncture or placebo to decrease infant pain during heel pricks [27]. The study reported a 30% reduction in pain in infants receiving magnetic acupuncture [27]. Abbasoglu et al. reported a 45% reduction in mean duration of crying with acupressure compared to control infants during heel pricks in 32 preterm infants, but no significant differences in pain score between groups [28]. Differences in these studies could have been due to the use of varying techniques (e.g., acupuncture or acupressure) or different acupuncture points. Future studies should distinguish between the optimal points and duration of treatment (e.g., duration of placement of acupuncture) and to elucidate the long-term implications of different methods of acupuncture.

3.3.2. Sucrose/Glucose Solutions

Oral sucrose solution is most commonly used as non-pharmacological interventions for pain management in newborn infants. Sucrose may exert its analgesic effects through endogenous opioid pathways or via an increase in dopamine and acetylcholine [1,44]. However, the evidence for pain relief is conflicting. Lima et al. reported a 40% reduction in pain scores and a 70% reduction in crying time with oral glucose compared to NNS in 78 healthy newborns during immunization [29]. Gouin et al. randomized 1–3 months old children undergoing a venipuncture to either sucrose or placebo and found similar pain scores (mean $\pm$ SD: sucrose 2.3 ± 0.5 vs. placebo 1.6 ± 0.5, $p = 0.6$), heart rate variability (mean $\pm$ SD: sucrose 33 ± 6 vs. placebo 24 ± 5 bpm, $p = 0.44$), and crying time (mean $\pm$ SD: sucrose 63 ± 3 vs. placebo 49 ± 5 sec, $p = 0.17$) for both groups [30]. Similarly, a randomized trial with 66 preterm infants > 28 weeks gestation administered expressed breast milk or oral sucrose for pain management during venipuncture [31]. Overall, similar pain scores with 7 (range 4–9) with expressed breast milk and 6 (range 4–8) with sucrose were observed [31]. These studies suggest that oral sucrose might not be effective in all infants and that expressed breast milk has similar analgesic effects. Furthermore, the analgesia effect of sucrose might be ineffective in infants' experience opioid withdrawal [45]. However, a recent study reported similar pain scores for opioid exposed and non-exposed infants suggesting that oral sucrose might be effective in both exposed and non-exposed infants [46].

There may, however, be negative effects of oral sucrose. Asmerom et al. randomized 131 premature infants undergoing a heel lance procedure to either control, placebo with NNS, or sucrose [47]. Although, a 22% decrease in median pain scores was observed with sucrose compared to control, increased markers of oxidative stress and increased use of adenosine triphosphate could indicate cellular injury in infants receiving sucrose. Furthermore, infants receiving sucrose had a significant increase in the heart rate from (mean $\pm$ SD): 155 $\pm$ 14 to 171 $\pm$ 155 bpm compared to infants the control (154 $\pm$ 13 to 155 $\pm$ 14 bpm) and placebo groups (156 $\pm$ 14 to 165 $\pm$ 15 bpm, $p < 0.001$) [47].

However, there might be also some positive long-term effects of sucrose on spatial learning and memory [48]. Rat models showed that chronic pain impaired short-term memory, but sucrose prevented such impairment and increased endorphin levels [48]. Sucrose also prevented a decrease levels of brain derived neurotropic factor, which occurs during chronic pain [48]. This conflicting evidence suggests that further studies are needed to examine long-term effects (e.g., long-term neurodevelopmental outcomes or obesity) of oral sucrose.

4. Discussion

Non-pharmacological techniques have the potential to provide pain relief for preterm and term infants. Most studies included in this review demonstrated an improvement in behavioral pain responses including facial expressions, duration of crying or latency to first cry, and physiological parameters (e.g., heart rate, oxygen saturation). This indicates that non-pharmacological techniques are beneficial and were successful at reducing pain. However, this finding was not reproducible in sucrose vs. placebo, breastmilk vs. sucrose, and breast feeding vs. musical therapy studies [20,30,31]. These contradictory results raise questions about the potential mechanism of these interventions. Further research is needed to determine the best non-pharmacological intervention, duration of the intervention, and dose response for optimal pain relief in newborn infants.

While sucrose is now considered the gold standard in non-pharmacological pain relief, the current evidence remains contradictory. Although, several studies identified a clear benefit of sucrose compared to other techniques (e.g., music, massage or NNS) [16,20,26,29], other studies reported lower pain score with alternative techniques including magnetic acupuncture or SSC [11,27]. The mechanism of sucrose has also been controversial. Many believe that sucrose decreases pain through opioid mechanisms but methadone-exposed newborn infants do not appear to be susceptible to the effects of sucrose, probably because of opioid-receptor blockade by methadone [45]. However, Marceau et al. reported that opioid exposed neonates had decreased pain responses with the use of sucrose which suggests additional other mechanisms for sucrose's analgesic effects [46]. There is also conflicting evidence regarding any long-term effects of sucrose. Rat models reported that sucrose increased endorphins and brain-derived neurotrophic factor, which up-regulates neurogenesis and restores memory functions [48–50]. Interestingly, an increase in oxidative stress markers, which might lead to cellular damage was also reported after sucrose administration [47]. This raises questions as to whether sucrose can be should be the gold standard for non-pharmacological pain relief and studies examining long-term effects are needed.

The main limitation of the studies included in this review was the differences in the way pain was assessed. In preterm infants, heart rate or oxygen saturation variations may also have been due to physiological immaturity, entirely unrelated to the painful procedure or to the intervention. There is no standardized approach to the measurement of pain and each study used different scores e.g., Premature Infant Pain Profile score, Neonatal Infant Pain Scale score, Douleur Aiguë du Nouveau-né scale (a French scale of neonatal pain) [24], Face, Legs, Activity, Cry and Consolability Pain Scale [30], which makes it impossible to compare studies in a meta-analysis.

There are also limitations to the effectiveness of the non-pharmacological methods depending on many factors. Studies suggest that gestational age might influence the response to non-pharmacological treatments. Studies comparing sucrose with breast milk reported similar pain scores in infants >28 weeks' gestation [23], while infants <28 weeks' gestation had significantly lower pain scores after oral sucrose but not after breast milk [31]. Skin-to-skin care, swaddling and facilitated tucking is limited to times when the infant's position is not crucial and is not suitable for emergency procedures or for procedures dependent on position (e.g., lumbar puncture). Breastfeeding also may not always be available (e.g., in NICU or mother not present). If the infant is very ill, a lot of the interventions may not be possible.

One of the major advantages to using these non-pharmacological methods is their high safety profile. Most importantly, all these interventions have a very favorable benefit to risk ratio, even if the benefits are modest—the risk is extremely low. Supervision and support from staff helps with safety concerns for SSC, swaddling, massage therapy, facilitated tucking and BF such as improper technique, holding or positioning [51]. When using laser acupuncture, the infant and acupuncturists must wear protective ear-gear as well as cover any reflective surface to prevent the laser from hitting one's eye. Yates et al. assessed the safety of non-invasive electrical stimulation at acupuncture points (NESAP) by observing skin reactions, vital signs and PIPP scores [52]. There were no significant changes found in these measures and no adverse events occurred, which concludes that NESAP is safe [52]. Some of the main challenges in implementation is reluctance from staff or parents, due to disbelief or the invasiveness of the procedure (e.g., use of needle acupuncture in infants).

The major benefit of non-pharmacological treatments includes (i) ease of use, (ii) apparent safety, (iii) feasibility, and (iv) ease of learning, which would allow universal implementation of any of these interventions. However, acupuncture using needle or laser would require training and experience about the specific acupuncture points, and lasers might not be readily available. The long-term effects of any non-pharmacological intervention have not been studied and is a major knowledge gap, that needs to be addressed.

5. Conclusions

Newborn infants in an NICU undergo many painful but necessary procedures during hospitalizations. The implications of the pain associated with these procedures and the types of pain relief given to the infants have considerable implication for both short- and long-term outcomes. The evidence for non-pharmacological analgesia is sparse and needs further study. While most appear to be safe and relatively effective, their effects on the long-term outcomes of the infants is unknown, especially when coupled with pharmacological analgesia.

Author Contributions: Conception and design: G.M.S., J.-L.O., I.Q.-S., A.K.M.; Collection and assembly of data: G.M.S., J.-L.O., I.Q.-S., A.K.M.; Analysis and interpretation of the data: G.M.S., J.-L.O., I.Q.-S., A.K.M., K.C.; Drafting of the article: G.M.S., J.-L.O., I.Q.-S., A.K.M., K.C.; Critical revision of the article for important intellectual content: G.M.S., J.-L.O., I.Q.-S., A.K.M., K.C.; Final approval of the article: G.M.S., J.-L.O., I.Q.-S., A.K.M., K.C.

Appendix A

Search of PubMed—last performed 4 June 2018

#1 infant (n = 1,119,189)

#2 infants (n = 1,159,867)

#3 preterm (n = 62,246)

#4 premature (n = 170,785)
#5 pain (n = 733,273)
#6 relief (n = 84,761)
#6 acupuncture (n = 28,139)
#7 skin-to-skin care (n = 47,999)
#8 non-nutritive sucking (n = 367)
#9 sucrose (n = 74,579)
#10 massage (n = 13,982)
#11 music (n = 22,562)
#12 breastfeeding (n = 49,518)
#13 non-pharmacological (n = 6513)
Search of Google Scholar—last performed 4 June 2018
#1 infant (n = 3,220,000)
#2 infants (n = 2,080,000)
#3 preterm (n = 1,010,000)
#4 premature (n = 2,840,000)
#5 pain (n = 3,770,000)
#6 relief (n = 2,390,000)
#6 acupuncture (n = 592,000)
#7 skin-to-skin care (n = 3,820,000)
#8 non-nutritive sucking (n = 21,900)
#9 sucrose (n = 2,640,000)
#10 massage (n = 773,000)
#11 music (n = 3,770,000)
#12 breastfeeding (n = 649,000)
#13 non-pharmacological (n = 2,540,000)

References

1. Cignacco, E.; Hamers, J.P.; Stoffel, L.; Lingen, R.A.; Gessler, P.; McDougall, J.; Nelle, M. The efficacy of non-pharmacological interventions in the management of procedural pain in preterm and term neonates. *Eur. J. Pain* **2007**, *11*, 139–152. [CrossRef] [PubMed]
2. Saad, H.H.; Bours, G.J.J.W.; Stevens, B.; Hamers, J.P.H. Assessment of pain in the neonate. *Semin. Perinatol.* **1998**, *22*, 402–416. [CrossRef]
3. Barker, D.P.; Rutter, N. Exposure to invasive procedures in neonatal intensive care unit admissions. *Arch. Dis. Child.-Fetal Neonatal Ed.* **1995**, *72*, 47–48. [CrossRef]
4. Meaney, M.J.; Aitken, D.H. The effects of early postnatal handling on hippocampal glucocorticoid receptor concentrations: Temporal parameters. *Brain Res.* **1985**, *354*, 301–304. [CrossRef]
5. Taddio, A.; Katz, J.; Ilersich, A.L.; Koren, G. Effect of neonatal circumcision on pain response during subsequent routine vaccination. *Lancet* **1997**, *349*, 599–603. [CrossRef]
6. American and Canadian Academy of Pediatrics. Prevention and management of pain and stress in the neonate. *Pediatrics* **2000**, *15*, 454–461.
7. Taddio, A. Opioid analgesia for infants in the neonatal intensive care unit. *Clin. Perinatol.* **2002**, *29*, 493–509. [CrossRef]
8. Melzack, R.; Wall, P.D. Pain mechanism: A new theory. *Science* **1965**, *150*, 971–979. [CrossRef] [PubMed]
9. Shabani, F.; Nayeri, N.D.; Karimi, R.; Zarei, K.; Chehrazi, M. Effects of music therapy on pain responses induced by blood sampling in premature infants: A randomized cross-over trial. *Iran. J. Nurs. Midwifery Res.* **2016**, *21*, 391–396. [PubMed]
10. Seo, Y.S.; Lee, J.; Ahn, H.Y. Effects of Kangaroo Care on Neonatal Pain in South Korea. *J. Trop. Pediatr.* **2016**, *62*, 246–249. [CrossRef] [PubMed]
11. Freire, N.B.; Garcia, J.B.; Lamy, Z.C. Evaluation of analgesic effect of skin-to-skin contact compared to oral glucose in preterm neonates. *Pain* **2008**, *139*, 28–33. [CrossRef] [PubMed]
12. Olsson, E.; Ahlsén, G.; Eriksson, M. Skin-to-skin contact reduces near-infrared spectroscopy pain responses in premature infants during blood sampling. *Acta Paediatr.* **2016**, *105*, 376–380. [CrossRef] [PubMed]

13. Efendi, D.; Rustina, Y.; Gayatri, D. Pacifier and swaddling effective in impeding premature infant's pain score and heart rate. *Enferm. Clin.* **2018**, *1*, 46–50. [CrossRef]
14. Erkut, Z.; Yildiz, S. The Effect of Swaddling on Pain, Vital Signs, and Crying Duration during Heel Lance in Newborns. *Pain Manag. Nurs.* **2017**, *18*, 328–336. [CrossRef] [PubMed]
15. Ho, L.P.; Ho, S.S.; Leung, D.Y.; So, W.K.; Chan, C.W. A feasibility and efficacy randomized controlled trial of swaddling for controlling procedural pain in preterm infants. *J. Clin. Nurs.* **2016**, *25*, 472–482. [CrossRef] [PubMed]
16. Axelin, A.; Salanteräa, S.; Lehtonenb, L. Facilitated tucking by parents' in pain management of preterm infants—A randomized crossover trial. *Early Hum. Dev.* **2006**, *8*, 241–247. [CrossRef] [PubMed]
17. Arikan, D.; Alp, H.; Gözüm, S.; Orbak, Z.; Cifçi, E.K. Effectiveness of massage, sucrose solution, herbal tea or hydrolysed formula in the treatment of infantile colic. *J. Clin. Nurs.* **2008**, *17*, 1754–1761. [PubMed]
18. Chik, Y.M.; Ip, W.Y.; Choi, K.C. The Effect of Upper Limb Massage on Infants' Venipuncture Pain. *Pain Manag. Nurs.* **2017**, *18*, 50–57. [CrossRef] [PubMed]
19. Jain, S.; Kumar, P.; McMillan, D.D. Prior leg massage decreases pain responses to heel stick in preterm babies. *J. Paediatr. Child Health* **2006**, *42*, 505–508. [CrossRef] [PubMed]
20. Zhu, J.; Hong-Gu, H.; Zhou, X.; Wei, H.; Gao, Y.; Ye, B.; Liu, Z.; Chan, S.W. Pain relief effect of breast feeding and music therapy during heel lance for healthy-term neonates in China: A randomized controlled trial. *Midwifery* **2015**, *31*, 365–372. [CrossRef] [PubMed]
21. Shah, S.R.; Kadage, S.; Sinn, J. Trial of Music, Sucrose, and Combination Therapy for Pain Relief during Heel Prick Procedures in Neonates. *J. Pediatr.* **2017**, *190*, 153–158.e2. [CrossRef] [PubMed]
22. Zurita-Cruz, J.N.; Rivas-Ruiz, R.; Gordillo-Álvarez, V.; Villasis-Keever, M.Á. Breastfeeding for acute pain control on infants: A randomized controlled trial. *Nutr. Hosp.* **2017**, *34*, 301–307. [CrossRef] [PubMed]
23. Erkul, M.; Efe, E. Efficacy of Breastfeeding on Babies' Pain During Vaccinations. *Breastfeed. Med.* **2017**, *12*, 110–115. [CrossRef] [PubMed]
24. Simonse, E.; Mulder, P.G.; van Beek, R.H. Analgesic effect of breast milk versus sucrose for analgesia during heel lance in late preterm infants. *Pediatrics* **2012**, *129*, 657–663. [CrossRef] [PubMed]
25. Baudesson de Chanville, A.; Brevaut-Malaty, V.; Garbi, A.; Tosello, B.; Baumstarck, K.; Gire, C. Analgesic Effect of Maternal Human Milk Odor on Premature Neonates: A Randomized Controlled Trial. *J. Hum. Lact.* **2017**, *33*, 300–308. [CrossRef] [PubMed]
26. Zhao, Z. Neural mechanism underlying acupuncture analgesia. *Prog. Neurobiol.* **2008**, *85*, 355–375. [CrossRef] [PubMed]
27. Chen, K.L.; Lindrea, K.B.; Quah-Smith, I.; Schmölzer, G.M.; Daly, M.; Schindler, T.; Oei, J.L. Magnetic noninvasive acupuncture for infant comfort (MAGNIFIC)—A single-blinded randomised controlled pilot trial. *Acta Paediatr.* **2017**, *106*, 1780–1786. [CrossRef] [PubMed]
28. Abbasoğlu, A.; Cabıoğlu, M.T.; Tuğcu, A.U.; İnce, D.A.; Tekindal, M.A.; Ecevit, A.; Tarcan, A. Acupressure at BL60 and K3 Points Before Heel Lancing in Preterm Infants. *EXPLORE J. Sci. Heal.* **2015**, *11*, 363–366. [CrossRef] [PubMed]
29. Lima, A.; Santos, V.; Nunes, M.; Barreto, J.; Ribeiro, C.; Carvalho, J.; Ribeiro, M. Glucose solution is more effective in relieving pain in neonates than non-nutritive sucking: A randomized clinical trial. *Eur. J. Pain* **2017**, *21*, 159–165. [CrossRef] [PubMed]
30. Gouin, S.; Gaucher, N.; Lebel, D.; Desjardins, M.P. A Randomized Double-Blind Trial Comparing the Effect on Pain of an Oral Sucrose Solution vs. Placebo in Children 1 to 3 Months Old Undergoing Simple Venipuncture. *J. Emerg. Med.* **2018**, *54*, 33–39. [CrossRef] [PubMed]
31. Collados-Gómez, L.; Ferrera-Camacho, P.; Fernandez-Serran, E.; Camacho-Vicente, V.; Flores-Herrero, C.; García-Pozo, A.; Jiménez-García, R. Randomised crossover trial showed that using breast milk or sucrose provided the same analgesic effect in preterm infants of at least 28 weeks. *Acta Paediatr.* **2018**, *107*, 436–441. [CrossRef] [PubMed]
32. Hebb, A.L.; Poulin, J.F.; Roach, S.P.; Zacharko, R.M.; Drolet, G. Cholecystokinin and endogenous opioid peptides: Interactive influence on pain, cognition, and emotion. *Prog. Neuropsychopharmacol. Biol. Psychiatry* **2005**, *29*, 1225–1238. [CrossRef] [PubMed]
33. Huang, C.M.; Tung, W.S.; Kuo, L.L.; Chang, Y.J. Comparison of pain responses of premature infants to the heelstick between containment and swaddling. *J. Nurs. Res.* **2004**, *12*, 31–35. [CrossRef] [PubMed]

34. Esfahani, M.S.; Sheykhi, S.; Abdeyazdan, Z.; Jodakee, M.; Boroumandfar, K. A comparative study on vaccination pain in the methods of massage therapy and mothers' breastfeeding during injection of infants referring to Navabsafavi Health Care Center in Isfahan. *Iran. J. Nurs. Midwifery Res.* **2013**, *18*, 494–498. [PubMed]
35. Bellieni, C.V.; Buonocore, G.; Nenci, A.; Franci, N.; Cordelli, D.M.; Bagnoli, F. Sensorial saturation: An effective analgesic tool for heel-prick in preterm infants. *Neonatology* **2001**, *80*, 15–18. [CrossRef] [PubMed]
36. Yurkovich, J.; Burns, D.S.; Harrison, T. The Effect of Music Therapy Entrainment on Physiologic Measures of Infants in the Cardiac Intensive Care Unit: Single Case Withdrawal Pilot Study. *J. Music Ther.* **2018**, *55*, 62–82. [CrossRef] [PubMed]
37. Olischar, M.; Shoemark, H.; Holton, T.; Weninger, M.; Hunt, R.W. The influence of music on aEEG activity in neurologically healthy newborns ≥32 weeks' gestational age. *Acta Paediatr.* **2011**, *100*, 670–675. [CrossRef] [PubMed]
38. Porter, R.H.; Winberg, J. Unique salience of maternal breast odors for newborn infants. *Neurosci. Biobehav. Rev.* **1999**, *23*, 439–449. [CrossRef]
39. Lima, A.H.; Hermont, A.P.; Friche, A.A.L. Analgesia in newborns: A case-control study of the efficacy of nutritive and non-nutritive sucking stimuli. *CoDAS* **2013**, *25*, 365–368. [CrossRef] [PubMed]
40. Napadow, V.; Ahn, A.; Longhurst, J.; Lao, L.; Stener-Victorin, E.; Harris, R.; Langevin, H.M. The status and future of acupuncture mechanism research. *J. Altern. Complement. Med.* **2008**, *14*, 861–869. [CrossRef] [PubMed]
41. Quah-Smith, I.; Sachdev, P.S.; Wen, W.; Chen, X.; Williams, M.A. The Brain Effects of Laser Acupuncture in Healthy Individuals: An fMRI Investigation. *PLoS ONE* **2010**, *5*, e12619. [CrossRef] [PubMed]
42. Cho, Z.H.; Oleson, T.D.; Alimi, D.; Niemtzow, R.C. Acupuncture: The search for biologic evidence with functional magnetic resonance imaging and positron emission tomography techniques. *J. Altern. Complement. Med.* **2002**, *8*, 399–401. [CrossRef] [PubMed]
43. Mitchell, A.J.; Hall, R.W.; Golianu, B.; Yates, C.; Williams, D.K.; Chang, J.; Anand, K.J. Does noninvasive electrical stimulation of acupuncture points reduce heelstick pain in neonates? *Acta Paediatr.* **2016**, *105*, 1434–1439. [CrossRef] [PubMed]
44. Holsti, L.; Grunau, R.E. Considerations for using sucrose to reduce procedural pain in preterm infants. *Pediatrics* **2010**, *125*, 1042–1047. [CrossRef] [PubMed]
45. Blass, E.M.; Ciaramitaro, V. A new look at some old mechanisms in newborns: Taste and tactile determinants of state, affect and action. *Monogr. Soc. Child Dev.* **1994**, *59*, 1–81. [CrossRef]
46. Marceau, J.R.; Murray, H.; Nanan, R.K. Efficacy of oral sucrose in infants of methadone-maintained mothers. *Neonatology* **2010**, *97*, 67–70. [CrossRef] [PubMed]
47. Asmerom, Y.; Slater, L.; Boskovic, D.S.; Bahjri, K.; Holden, M.S.; Phillips, R.; Deming, D.; Ashwal, S.; Fayard, E.; Angeles, D.M. Oral sucrose for heel lance increases adenosine triphosphate use and oxidative stress in preterm neonates. *J. Pediatr.* **2013**, *163*, 29–35. [CrossRef] [PubMed]
48. Nuseir, K.Q.; Alzoubi, K.H.; Alabwaini, J.; Khabour, O.F.; Kassab, M.I. Sucrose-induced analgesia during early life modulates adulthood learning and memory formation. *Physiol. Behav.* **2015**, *145*, 84–90. [CrossRef] [PubMed]
49. Siuciak, J.A.; Wong, V.; Perasall, D.; Weigand, S.J.; Lindsay, R.M. BDNF produces analgesia in the formalin test and modifies neuropeptide levels in rat brain and spinal cord areas associated with nociception. *Eur. J. Neurosci.* **1995**, *7*, 663–670. [CrossRef] [PubMed]
50. Zhang, H.; Torregrossa, M.M.; Jutkiewica, E.M. Endogenous opioids upregulate brain-derived neurotrophic factor mRNA through delta- and micro-opioid receptors independent of antidepressant-like effects. *Eur. J. Neurosci.* **2006**, *23*, 984–994. [CrossRef] [PubMed]
51. Feldman-Winter, L.; Goldsmith, J.P. Safe Sleep and Skin-to-Skin Care in the Neonatal Period for Healthy Term Newborns. *Pediatrics* **2016**, *138*, e20161889. [CrossRef] [PubMed]
52. Yates, C.C.; Mitchell, A.J.; Lowe, L.M.; Lee, A.; Hall, R.W. Safety of Noninvasive Electrical Stimulation of Acupuncture Points During a Routine Neonatal Heel Stick. *Med. Acupunct.* **2013**, *25*, 285–290. [CrossRef] [PubMed]

13

Mind–Body Interventions for Pediatric Inflammatory Bowel Disease

Ann Ming Yeh [1,*], Anava Wren [1] and Brenda Golianu [2]

[1] Department of Pediatrics, Division of Pediatric Gastroenterology, Hepatology and Nutrition, Stanford University, Palo Alto, CA 94304, USA; awren2@stanford.edu
[2] Department of Anesthesia, Perioperative and Pain Medicine, Stanford University, Palo Alto, CA 94304, USA; bgolianu@stanford.edu
* Correspondence: annming@stanford.edu

Abstract: Pediatric inflammatory bowel disease is an autoimmune disease that causes chronic inflammation of the gastrointestinal mucosa. There is emerging evidence that the brain–gut connection affects inflammatory bowel disease (IBD) patients more than previously thought. This is evidenced by comorbid mood disorders, irritable bowel symptoms concurrent with quiescent IBD, and the potential of psychosocial stressors to trigger IBD flares. Mind–body interventions such as psychotherapy, relaxation, mindfulness, biofeedback, yoga, and clinical hypnosis offer an adjunct to standard medical treatment for IBD. We will review the current evidence base for these mind–body interventions in the treatment of pediatric IBD, illustrate a case study, and offer suggestions for future research for this promising field.

Keywords: mind-body; inflammatory bowel disease; pediatric; biofeedback; psychotherapy; hypnosis; yoga; relaxation

1. Introduction

Inflammatory bowel disease (IBD) is a chronic and relapsing inflammatory condition involving all or part of the gastrointestinal (GI) tract. The most common forms of IBD are Crohn's Disease (CD) and Ulcerative Colitis (UC), where CD may involve the entire GI tract and UC involves only the large intestine. The pathophysiology of IBD is thought to be multifactorial, involving a complex interplay between genetic predisposition, the gut microbiota, gut mucosal integrity, the immune system, and environmental triggers such as nutrition and psychosocial stressors [1,2]. Conventional treatments for pediatric IBD include anti-inflammatory pharmacologic therapies (5-aminosalicylic acid derivatives), corticosteroids, immunomodulators (6-mercaptopurine, methotrexate), and biologics [3]. Nutritional therapies such as enteral nutrition can also be effective for small bowel Crohn's disease [4–6].

Patients with IBD commonly seek integrative and complementary medicine treatment due to beliefs that medications are not effective, concern about medication side effects/risks, and interest in adjunct therapies to optimize disease management and help to improve symptoms and quality of life [7]. Integrative medicine is considered a healing-oriented medicine that reaffirms the importance of the relationship between practitioner and patient, focuses on the whole person, and utilizes empirically supported therapeutic approaches. According to the National Institute of Health, integrative medicine is an umbrella term that can include various modalities such as natural products (e.g., herbs and supplements), whole systems medicine (e.g., traditional Chinese medicine, Ayurveda), and mind–body interventions (e.g., relaxation, yoga, clinical hypnosis). The term integrative refers to the coordinated approach of utilizing conventional and complementary therapies together in an integrative way [8].

Over the past decade, mind–body interventions (MBI) have received increased attention. These interventions are categorized as those that 'employ a variety of techniques designed to facilitate the mind's capacity to affect bodily function and symptoms' [9]. Mind–body interventions are thought to be dynamic, and some definitions of MBI include manipulative modalities such as acupuncture, massage, and spinal manipulation. For the purposes of this review, however, we will focus on non-manipulative MBI, including psychotherapy, relaxation techniques, mindfulness-based therapies, biofeedback, yoga, and clinical hypnosis. Mind–body interventions are emerging as popular treatment modalities amongst IBD patients [10] and provide safe, inexpensive, non-pharmacologic ways to target the autonomic nervous system by decreasing the stress response and increasing the relaxation response.

The aim of this paper is to: (1) provide background information and a rationale for the use of mind–body interventions in pediatric IBD populations; (2) provide a brief overview of key mind–body interventions for pediatric IBD; (3) review the safety and efficacy of these mind–body interventions and highlight areas for future research; and (4) present a sample case demonstrating a multidisciplinary approach to mind–body IBD treatment.

Regarding the criteria for considering studies for this review, all controlled clinical trials, quasi-randomized trials, and non-randomized trials including pediatric patients with UC or CD and mind–body interventions were included. The search criteria were expanded to include adult patients with IBD or youth with irritable bowel syndrome (IBS) when no literature was available in pediatric IBD samples. Studies published between 1980 and 2017 were considered in this review. Pubmed was utilized as the primary search engine. The search strategies included terms related to pediatrics, IBD, IBS, mind–body interventions identified for this review, and common synonyms for the aforementioned terms.

2. Background

While the pathophysiology of IBD is thought to be due to interrelated factors, increasing evidence has shown the intimate connection between the brain and the gut and the effect of this bidirectional interaction on gut and psychological health [11]. It is noteworthy to highlight that IBD patients readily identify stress as a contributing factor to disease flares [12,13]. Numerous studies have noted a significant association between perceived stress, negative mood, and major life events and disease relapse, hospitalization, and abdominal surgery risk [12,14]. Prospective studies show that exposure to stressful events as well as perceived stress (i.e., the individual's view of a demand relative to their resources) may contribute to relapse risk [15–17]. One study found that pediatric patients with IBD who had low stress levels and used non-avoidant coping strategies had fewer relapses [15], suggesting the potential benefit of stress management interventions in this population.

The bidirectional brain-gut relationship is especially notable in youth who have IBD with associated IBS-type symptoms. Despite adequate control of their IBD, patients may continue to suffer from refractory IBS symptoms. At times, this situation may present a diagnostic and treatment challenge, as it may be difficult to distinguish between 'true' IBS symptoms versus a subclinical form of IBD. Children with IBD in clinical remission, as defined in the abbreviated-PCDAI (pediatric Crohn's disease activity index) or the PUCAI (pediatric ulcerative colitis activity index), have a 6.4% prevalence of IBS-type symptoms. In patients who have biochemical markers of quiescent or minimal disease, with a calprotectin of <250 μg/g, IBS symptom prevalence is 16.1% (95% confidence interval (CI): 7.6–25.8%; Crohn's disease: 16.7%; ulcerative colitis: 10.8% [18]. A meta-analysis of 1703 patients showed that patients with IBD had a higher prevalence of IBS symptoms, compared to non-IBD controls [19].

Patients in IBD remission may suffer from a variety of somatic complaints, including recurrent abdominal pain, urgency, diarrhea, constipation, bloating, gas, and cramping sensations. Symptoms of pain and discomfort may persist even after inflammation is adequately controlled due to visceral hyperalgesia, somatic-parietal abdominal pain, referred pain, strictures or adhesions, small intestinal bacterial overgrowth (SIBO), dysmotility, and central sensitization [20]. Factors that may increase central sensitization include disordered sleep, social stressors, and the presence of anxiety or depression [20]. IBD and IBS have overlapping and interacting mechanisms of illness. Subsets of IBS patients may have low grade inflammation, and some studies suggest that IBS and IBD exist on a similar disease continuum [21,22]. Furthermore, both IBD and IBS patients may have derangements in the gut microbiota that lead to disease [23–25].

A multidisciplinary approach to the management of IBD and IBS symptoms is essential to successful symptom improvement and disease treatment [26–28]. This approach includes thorough assessment and management by a pediatrician in consultation with a gastroenterology specialist to ensure adequate control of inflammation and gut physiological factors. Additional providers include a dietician to assess nutritional concerns; a pain specialist if pain is a presenting complaint; a physical or occupational therapist if there is significant deconditioning or loss of quality of life; and a clinical psychologist, pediatric pain psychologist, or other mental health therapist if there are psychosocial, adjustment, or symptom management concerns. An effective multidisciplinary team will work in tandem to guide appropriate interventions and disease modifying therapies for patients, optimize their physiologic and psychological wellbeing, and help to improve and sustain their ongoing quality of life [29].

IBD patients, specifically those with persistent IBS symptoms despite quiescent inflammation, may benefit from integrating mind–body interventions into multidisciplinary care. Research has demonstrated that mind–body interventions are commonly utilized by patients with IBS and IBD and may help to decrease anxiety and improve coping abilities [10]. Of note, up to 84% of pediatric patients with IBD already utilize some sort of integrative medicine therapy, according to a single-center survey at a tertiary care center [10]. Among these, 61% of patients used stress management and 35% utilized special exercises (e.g., yoga, swimming). In another survey of 67 adolescents with IBD, 40% used relaxation and 21% used guided imagery once a day to once a week for symptom management [30]. Younger adolescents were more likely to regularly use meditation, and adolescents with more severe disease were more willing to consider using relaxation as an adjunct therapy. Given the high utilization of mind–body interventions among pediatric IBD patients and the potential efficacy of MBI for this population, providers should be knowledgeable and open to discussing common mind–body interventions.

3. Mind–Body Interventions

3.1. Psychotherapy

Patients with IBD endorse elevated levels of emotional distress and poor quality of life compared to the general population [28,31]. Anxiety and depressive disorders have been documented to be higher among patients with IBD compared to non-IBD cohorts [31–33]. In pediatric IBD populations, high rates of anxiety and depression have been documented and there is an increased risk of developing depression compared to youth with other chronic illnesses and healthy controls [33–35]. Symptoms of anxiety and depression have been negatively associated with psychological well-being and disease-related outcomes in IBD populations, including lower quality of life, increased perceived stress, IBD relapse, inflammation, pain, poor medication adherence, and increased risk of surgery [28,33,36–39]. Unfortunately, psychiatric comorbidities are often under-diagnosed and undertreated across the lifespan. Recently, there has been growing support for multidisciplinary IBD treatment in order to treat the whole patient, including psychological interventions for youth and adults with IBD [28]. Psychological interventions have received increasing attention in the mind–body IBD literature [7], given the comorbidity between psychological conditions and IBD and the preliminary efficacy of such treatments on both psychological and physical outcomes.

Psychological interventions aimed at improving emotional distress and disease outcomes among IBD patients have generally focused on psychotherapy, stress management, hypnosis, and psychoeducation [40]. Over the past decade, numerous systematic reviews and meta-analyses have explored the effect of psychological interventions on children, adolescents, and adults with IBD. Overall, the findings have been mixed. A Cochrane review from 2011 [41] concluded that there was no evidence for psychological interventions in adults with IBD; however, the authors noted more empirical evidence for the use of psychotherapy among pediatric populations with IBD. Specifically, such interventions were found to improve depression and quality of life among youth [41]. More recent reviews have found psychological interventions to have some benefit on psychological outcomes and growing potential to reduce physical symptoms such as pain and fatigue, relapse rate, hospitalization, and medication adherence [40,42]. These mixed findings have been partially attributed to the limited body of research, comparing interventions with varying psychological content and methodological limitations.

Cognitive Behavioral Therapy

Cognitive behavioral therapy (CBT) is one type of psychological intervention that has demonstrated particular promise among pediatric populations with IBD. While there are many types of psychotherapy, CBT is the most common and has the greatest evidence base in pediatric IBD populations [35,43]. CBT is based on the premise that emotions, thoughts, and behaviors are interconnected and that psychological functioning can improve by working to understand and change maladaptive thoughts and behaviors. Significant literature supports the use of CBT among children with anxiety and mood disorders [44,45], and growing research has demonstrated the efficacy of CBT protocols among youth with chronic illnesses [46].

Szigethy and colleagues conducted some of the first studies exploring the effectiveness of CBT among youth with IBD [47]. They modified a manual-based CBT protocol to address the impact of physical illness on youth with depression. The intervention focused on physical illness narrative, social skills training, and family education. The protocol consists of nine individual modules focused on behavioral activation, cognitive restructuring, and problem-solving skills and three family sessions focused on psychoeducation and family problem-solving skills. An early pilot study demonstrated promising results among 11 adolescents (12–17 years). Specifically, there were significant reductions in child and parent-reported depression symptoms pre- to post-treatment ($p < 0.001$; 0.65–0.92 effect size), as well as significant improvements in global adjustment ($p < 0.01$) and physical functioning ($p < 0.05$) among youth [47]. Despite these positive results, there were several study limitations, including the small sample size and the lack of a control group and long-term follow-up, limiting assumptions of causality and generalizability.

Later larger randomized controlled groups by Szigethy et al. [48] demonstrated that, among 41 youth with IBD, the protocol could lead to clinically significant improvements in depression symptoms ($p < 0.01$; 1.01 effect size) and functioning ($p < 0.05$, 0.86 effect size), compared to treatment as usual. Of note, these benefits persisted one-year post-treatment. When the protocol was compared to supportive non-directive therapy (SNDT), the results showed that both interventions equally reduced depression symptoms (37.3% for CBT; 31.9% for SNDT) among 217 youth [43]. There were also significant improvements across groups on measures of global functioning, quality of life, and disease activity; however, the CBT intervention showed a significantly greater reduction in IBD activity compared to SNDT ($p = 0.04$). Disease activity was measured by the PCDAI and PUCAI disease activity scoring scales for CD and UC, respectively. Lastly, follow-up analyses on a smaller study sample of youth with CD ($N = 70$) showed that both CBT and SNDT were associated with decreased GI-related health care utilization, specifically GI-hospitalization frequency, inpatient days, ER visits, and endoscopies [49]. Overall, these results support CBT as a beneficial adjunct to the medical management of IBD among pediatric patients.

Recent research supports Szigethy and colleagues' findings over the past decade, demonstrating the benefits of CBT protocols for youth with IBD and emotional distress. Of note, Levy et al. [50] randomized 187 youth (8–17 years) to a brief three session CBT intervention or an education support condition and conducted follow-up assessments up to one year post-treatment. The findings demonstrated that the CBT intervention led to significantly more pre- to post-treatment improvement compared to the control group on measures of pain coping abilities ($p < 0.05$), IBD-related quality of life ($p < 0.05$), parent-reported solicitous behavior ($p < 0.05$), and missed days of school in the six months following treatment ($p < 0.05$). Children reported significant improvement in depression symptoms post-treatment with no significant between group differences ($p = 0.10$). Interestingly, exploratory sub-group analyses demonstrated that children in the CBT intervention with higher levels of flares pre-baseline had significantly fewer flares post-treatment compared to the control (16.7% versus 52.9%; $p < 0.05$). Future studies should further explore the possibility that brief CBT protocols can affect disease activity in a larger sample of youth with IBD using more rigorous methodology, such as PCDAI/PUCAI measures of disease activity, and the concurrent measurement of calprotectin and inflammatory cytokines. The strengths of this study include the large sample size, controlling for time and attention in the educational support condition, and developing a brief intervention to address the accessibility and adherence issues common to psychotherapy protocols.

Currently, a multicenter randomized controlled trial (RCT) is underway to investigate the efficacy of a CBT protocol in reducing symptoms of depression and anxiety and improving quality of life and disease course in youth with IBD [51]. Larger RCTs such as this are greatly needed in order to address past study limitations and further assess the feasibility, efficacy, and generalizability of CBT interventions for youth with IBD and co-occurring emotional distress.

Overall, there is promising preliminary evidence for the feasibility of CBT interventions in tertiary pediatric GI/IBD clinics and the efficacy of such protocols in improving psychological wellbeing and disease-related outcomes. Effective non-pharmacological treatments for emotional distress are especially important given the comorbidity between IBD and depression and anxiety and the potential for antidepressants to exacerbate GI symptoms and complicate medical regimens [47].

3.2. Relaxation and Stress Management

Given the relationship between stress, emotional distress, and negative IBD-related outcomes, researchers have explored the efficacy of relaxation and stress-management protocols for IBD patients. The goal of such interventions is to teach patients skills to relax and reduce daily stress in order to support improved psychological and physical wellbeing. The content of these interventions varies, as well as the format (individual versus group sessions), delivery (nurse, psychiatrist, psychologist), and duration (one session versus eight weekly sessions). Relaxation-based interventions usually focus on teaching patients a subset of relaxation strategies, such diaphragmatic breathing techniques, guided imagery (e.g., focus on imagination and distraction), progressive muscle relaxation (PMR) (e.g., focus on building and releasing muscle tension), and autogenic training (i.e., focus on physical manifestations of relaxation in the body like heaviness in the musculoskeletal system or warmth of the circulatory system) [41]. Stress management protocols tend to include psychoeducation (e.g., related to IBD and treatment; stress and relaxation response) and a variety of relaxation and coping skills (e.g., problem solving, communication, identifying and modifying negative thoughts). Exercise and diet support are also integrated into some stress management treatments [40,41].

The majority of research investigating the use of relaxation and stress management interventions in IBD populations has been conducted in adult samples. Randomized controlled trials investigating the efficacy of PMR and guided imagery-based relaxation protocols have shown significant improvements in psychological functioning, quality of life, and pain variables among adults with IBD [52,53]. Stress management interventions have shown mixed efficacy. Some RCTs have demonstrated that stress management protocols can improve psychological functioning [54–56] and disease-related outcomes [55,57,58], while other studies show no significant changes in IBD outcomes across conditions [59].

Research exploring more integrative CBT interventions (CBT with greater emphasis on relaxation-based coping skills) has shown promise in pediatric patients with IBD. McCormick and colleagues [60] developed a one-day CBT intervention for adolescents and parents focused on disease-related coping skills, pain management, relaxation, communication, and limit setting

($N = 24$ parent–child dyads). Treatment was followed by six weeks of web-based skill review that focused on weekly homework, coping skills, and group chat sessions related to treatment modules. Separate adolescent and parent sites were created. Following the integrative CBT treatment, there were significant improvements in child and parent-reports of somatic symptoms ($p < 0.01$) and adaptive coping ($p < 0.05$). While there were no significant differences between the CBT and wait-list control condition, no changes in the above symptoms were found for the control group. Despite preliminary support for the intervention among adolescents with IBD and their parents, there was a lack of random assignment to groups, limiting conclusions about intervention efficacy. Overall, it appears that no studies to date have explored the efficacy of relaxation or stress management interventions in pediatric IBD populations.

Future research exploring the feasibility and efficacy of relaxation-focused interventions among pediatric samples is needed. Brief relaxation protocols could be particularly helpful in pediatric GI clinics, as they could be easily delivered by a variety of providers and integrated into multidisciplinary care.

3.3. *Mindfulness*

Over the past decade, mindfulness-based interventions have received increasing attention in mind–body research and are emerging as a point of interest among researchers exploring psychotherapeutic interventions for patients with IBD. Mindfulness-based stress reduction (MBSR) and mindfulness-based cognitive therapy (MBCT) are typically the most common mindfulness treatments in clinical and research settings. Across these protocols, the primary treatment aim is to teach patients mindfulness, which is the ability to be aware of the present moment and one's thoughts, emotions, and body sensations in a purposeful, non-judgmental manner [61,62]. Mindfulness is usually practiced via a series of breathing, meditation, and movement exercises, all of which support non-judgmental and compassionate awareness. Bringing one's focus and attention to the present can buffer one from ruminating on negative cognitions (e.g., catastrophizing about IBD flares) or bothersome physical sensations (e.g., abdominal pain).

To date, it appears that mindfulness-based interventions for patients with IBD have been exclusively conducted in adult samples. One of the first randomized controlled studies investigated the feasibility and efficacy of an eight week mindfulness-based stress reduction (MBSR) group among 55 patients with ulcerative colitis compared to an attention control condition with mind–body psychoeducation [63]. MBSR was developed by John Kabat-Zinn and consists of eight weekly 2.5 h sessions, weekly homework, and a seven hour weekend session, all focused on promoting mindfulness in daily life. Results demonstrated that the MBSR intervention was highly feasible and acceptable among IBD patients; however, the protocol did not impact psychological or disease outcomes compared to the control condition. Interestingly, among patients who flared during the study, those randomized to the MBSR condition reported significantly higher quality of life compared to the control condition ($p = 0.001$). Additionally, post-hoc analyses demonstrated that MBSR may be effective in reducing flares among patients with heightened states of stress, supporting the approach of tailoring treatments to patient characteristics as is routinely done with pharmacotherapy [63].

A more recent controlled trial [64] provided preliminary support for the feasibility, acceptability, and efficacy of an eight week modified MBSR protocol for adults with IBD ($N = 60$). Post-treatment, there were significant improvements in anxiety ($p < 0.05$), depression ($p < 0.05$), quality of life ($p < 0.01$), and mindfulness ($p < 0.01$), compared to a treatment as usual control condition. Of note, significant reductions in depression and improvements in mindfulness were present six months following the intervention ($p < 0.001$). The corresponding effect sizes ranged from medium ($d = 0.56$) to large ($d = 1.27$), providing support for clinically meaningful outcomes. However, additional randomized controlled trials are needed to further support these findings.

Schoultz and colleagues [65] have also explored the efficacy of a MBCT intervention among 44 adults with IBD. MBCT was developed by Zindel Segal and colleagues and is largely based on

MBSR [66]. It is an eight-week group treatment that integrates mindfulness and cognitive therapy techniques to support stress management and self-care. Schoultz et al. [65] found that MBCT led to significant improvements in depression ($p < 0.05$), trait anxiety ($p < 0.05$), and dispositional mindfulness ($p < 0.05$) among patients with IBD, compared to a wait-list control condition. These findings persisted at a six-month follow-up assessment. No changes were noted on disease activity and IBD quality of life. Thomas and colleagues also developed a form of psychotherapy, entitled multi-convergent therapy (MCT), that combines mindfulness with cognitive and behavioral techniques [67]. A randomized controlled pilot study assessed the efficacy of MCT among 66 adults with IBD. The results demonstrated significant pre- to post-treatment improvements in the MCT condition, compared to the control on quality of life among IBD patients with IBS-type symptoms (determined by Rome III criteria at baseline) ($p = 0.021$) [68]. These findings offer further support to the notion that mindfulness protocols could be effective for sub-groups of IBD patients.

While, to our knowledge, there is no published research investigating the use of mindfulness-based interventions among youth with IBD, preliminary support for mindfulness protocols in adult IBD populations and youth with IBS [69] suggest that this could be a promising line of future research. Going forward, investigators should explore the feasibility and efficacy of age appropriate mindfulness treatments among children and adolescents with IBD, particularly in patients with heighted states of stress, concurrent psychological diagnoses, or IBS-IBD symptoms. This research should also address some of the methodological limitations highlighted in the adult literature. Specifically, future studies should include a bigger sample size and multiple control groups and include attention and wait list control, assess treatment adherence and engagement, and collect psychological, physiological, and disease activity-related outcomes.

3.4. *Biofeedback*

Biofeedback is a process in which the electronic monitoring of normally automatic bodily functions (e.g., heart rate, blood pressure, skin temperature) is used to train a patient to acquire voluntary control of that function. The autonomic nervous system is the primary target of biofeedback, particularly the sympathetic nervous system, or the body's 'fight or flight' system. The autonomic nervous system received its name because it was once believed that this system operated without our control. However, research has shown that a person can, in fact, control this part of the nervous system when provided with appropriate feedback of its functioning [70]. In pediatric gastroenterology, mind–body research suggests that biofeedback may be helpful in treating symptoms of IBS and functional abdominal pain (FAP) such as dyspepsia, bloating, and cramping [71,72].

Heart Rate Variability Biofeedback

Heart rate variability biofeedback (HRVB) is a type of biofeedback that can directly improve autonomic dysfunction and restore vagal tone [70]. Heart rate variability (HRV) is the change in time intervals between adjacent heartbeats. HRV can be measured non-invasively as a physiologic marker of autonomic nervous system function. Optimal HRV reflects a self-regulatory capacity, specifically a person's adaptability and resilience to respond to and recover from stressful stimuli [73]. HRV varies from person to person depending on age, gender, health, and fitness. Lower HRV, or less variability in heart rate in various positions and activities, suggests higher persistent sympathetic tone and less resilience to stressful triggers [73]. Analysis of HRV involves power spectral analysis filtering techniques to separate the heart rate waveform into frequency ranges [74,75]. The high frequency (HF) band reflects parasympathetic activity, whereas the low frequency (LF) band reflects sympathetic activity [76]. The LF/HF ratio is used by some researchers to assess the balance between sympathetic and parasympathetic activity [74,77]. Non-invasive instruments that connect to an earlobe, finger, or to the chest via electrocardiogram leads measure HRV. The user then engages in breathing and relaxation exercises to visualize how this may affect their HRV directly on the screen [73]. HRVB is a novel modality and research on its efficacy and utilization is still emerging.

A study by Sowder et al. [72] investigated the effect of HRVB in children with FAP. Children participated in six sessions of HRVB aimed at normalizing autonomic balance. At baseline, children with FAP in this study had greater autonomic dysregulation than children without FAP, as indicated by a higher LF/HF ratio ($t_{(28)} = 2.95$; $p = 0.006$). After the treatment sessions, the FAP group was able to significantly reduce their symptoms which correlated with significant increases in their autonomic balance, as evidenced by a decrease in the LF/HF ratio($t_{(19)} = 2.57$, $p = 0.019$). Another prospective open-label study by Stern et al. looked at 27 children with either IBS or FAP who underwent HRVB to treat their presenting symptoms for an average of eight 30-min sessions. They concluded that almost 70% of IBS patients and 63% of FAP patients achieved full remission (defined as having no symptoms for at least two full weeks) [71]. Qualitative data from this study showed that patients with both IBS and FAP expressed satisfaction with the intervention and their clinical outcomes and felt validated in the 'reality' of their symptoms.

Although no studies to date have looked at HRVB in IBD patients, a study by Jelenova et al. found that adolescents with mild IBD had less adaptability to stress compared to healthy controls [78]. The HRV of the IBD patients showed significantly lower levels of spectral activity in low frequency bands of HRV at both supine and standing positions ($p < 0.005$ and $p < 0.01$ respectively). This study was limited by the small sample size (25 IBD patients, 35 controls) and the fact that HRV was measured over five min, which may not be as accurate as 24 h measurements. Larger studies investigating normal values of HRV within healthy adolescent populations as compared to IBD populations would help to identify clinically significant HRV abnormalities within a pediatric IBD population. Although the effect of biofeedback on pediatric IBD has not yet been explored in depth, this modality offers a non-invasive way to decrease physiologic reactivity to stress, which may lead to IBD flares, decreased pain threshold, and IBS-IBD symptoms. Further research in this area is clearly warranted.

3.5. Yoga

Yoga is a mind–body technique arising from ancient India that combines physical postures, breath control, and meditation to promote health and relaxation. Yoga is believed to have mood-enhancing properties that inhibit physiologic stress and inflammation [79,80]. A systematic review of 25 randomized controlled trials provides evidence that yoga improves regulation of the sympathetic nervous system and hypothalamic–pituitary–adrenal system, as evidenced by multiple physiologic parameters including blood pressure, heart rate, cortisol, and cytokine expression [81]. Yoga also increases personal empowerment, which is the ability to develop the confidence and strength to set realistic goals and fulfill one's potential [82]. Personal empowerment is a measure vital to one's wellness and emotional health, and increased empowerment leads to improved patient activation. Of note, patient activation towards medical care can improve health outcomes, reduce medical system costs, and improve the patient's overall healthcare experience [83,84]. Yoga is a low cost, high reward form of self-care that has the potential to fill a known health care gap by decreasing stress, promoting wellness, and reducing disease burden.

Yoga protocols have been shown to be a feasible and safe adjunctive therapy for adolescents and young adults with IBS [85]. Nearly half of the participants in a brief yoga intervention for adolescents with IBS reported a significant reduction in pain and global symptom improvement, and young adults in the yoga group were significantly more likely to endorse symptom improvement compared to wait-list controls ($\chi^2 = 11.13$, $p = 0.03$) [85]. Another randomized trial of yoga for adolescents with IBS found significantly improved gastrointestinal symptoms ($p < 0.01$), lower levels of functional disability ($p = 0.073$), less use of emotion-focused avoidance ($p = 0.09$), and less anxiety ($p = 0.09$) compared to wait-list controls [86]. A systematic review of six randomized controlled trials studying yoga as a treatment for IBS in adults found significant improvements in quality of life, global improvement, and physical functioning [87]. However, the review was limited by the small overall sample size (total of 273 patients), heterogeneity of control groups, and unclear risk of bias in observed studies (no allocation concealment or adequate random sequence generation described). Despite these studies' positive findings, there are no studies to date evaluating yoga as a potentially effective adjunct therapy for youth with IBD. Given the overlapping and interacting mechanisms between IBD and IBS, these preliminary yoga studies for IBS may also apply to the IBD population. Thus, there is a clear need for studies to investigate the potential benefits of yoga as a mind–body therapy in children and adolescents with IBD.

3.6. Clinical Hypnosis

Clinical hypnosis is a common MBI and refers to the specific ability to focus one's attention narrowly and deepen one's concentration, while simultaneously diminishing awareness of external stimuli. In this state of awareness, it is thought that the individual may be able to modulate some physiological processes not ordinarily under conscious control [88]. In the treatment of abdominal pain, most hypnosis or hypnotherapy studies have focused on the management of symptoms related to IBS, while a few have examined the action of hypnosis on IBD [89]. The strongest evidence for the efficacy of hypnotherapy in IBD is its association with reduced IBD related inflammation and improved quality of life. Mixed results have been obtained regarding its effects on psychological and pain outcomes [90]. The mechanism of action of hypnotherapy is believed to be via the 'brain–gut axis', through the modulation of vagal visceral afferent signals via the pontomedullary nuclei, limbic regions including the amygdala, hippocampus, and insula, and vagal efferent signaling via pathways of descending modulation. These pathways may be dysregulated by cognitive and environmental demands, leading to the overriding of local reflex functions that occur during sleep or in the context of digestion [11].

Hypnotherapy normally begins with an introduction by the practitioner, development of rapport, and receipt of permission to perform the hypnosis exercise. Following, a hypnosis induction is performed, with the aim of allowing the individual to enter an altered consciousness or trance state (e.g., similar to a narrow state of focused attention). This state is readily achieved by children, who naturally are able to enter a state of focus and attention during play or while engaging their imagination. Once in the hypnotic state, gentle suggestions are made for enhancing one's ability to regulate or normalize gastro-intestinal function, including the minimization of pain, nausea, vomiting or other symptomatology. Various metaphors can be employed to facilitate this process; for example, the gut may be likened to a smoothly flowing river, whose flow can be guided by the patient's gentle encouragement. The placing of the patient's hands over the abdomen, or taking specific medicines, can be seen as a way to engender calm and protection against pain, bloating, discomfort, or abnormal bowel habits. Subsequently, patients are encouraged to utilize the technique to calm their symptoms at other times during their daily life. Hypnotherapy has been demonstrated to be safe and effective for use in youth; however, it should only be employed by appropriately trained individuals [91].

In a randomized controlled study of 54 adult patients with ulcerative colitis, clinical remission was prolonged in 26 patients by a mean of 78 days compared to 29 attention controls. The intervention consisted of a seven-session standardized treatment protocol. Patients were also provided with an audio recording to practice outside of sessions five days per week during the study. The control intervention consisted of non-directive discussion about Ulcerative Colitis and the 'mind–body connection'. In addition, analysis of the group maintaining remission at one year showed a significantly higher remission rate among those in the hypnosis condition (68%) compared to control patients (40%) [92]. While mechanisms of action are unknown, stress management and increased self-efficacy have been posited as possible mediators.

In another study, 15 adult patients with severe or very severe IBD on corticosteroids, but not responding to medication, received 12 sessions of 'gut-focused hypnotherapy' and were followed up for a mean duration of 5.4 years. Sixty percent of patients were able to entirely stop corticosteroids and did not require them at follow-up [93]. In a similar study, 15 patients with severe IBD underwent 12 sessions of gut directed hypnosis, which focused on tactile stimuli as well as visualization. In 14 out of the 15 patients, disease severity was reduced from severe to either mild or moderate following treatment, and quality of life was improved from 'very poor' and 'poor' to 'good' and 'excellent' [94]. Of note, one session of 'gut-directed hypnotherapy' has been shown to reduce systemic and rectal mucosal inflammatory responses. Serum interleukin-6 concentration was reduced by 53%, circulating natural killer cell numbers were reduced by 18%, rectal mucosal release of substance P was reduced by 81%, histamine was reduced by 35%, and interleukin-13 was reduced by 53% [95].

In the pediatric population, hypnotherapy was successfully utilized in a case series for six children with IBD. The children received between four and 12 sessions over three months, and treatment resulted in improved symptoms and decreased inflammatory markers, though the exact values are not provided in the report [96]. In a randomized controlled study of 53 pediatric patients (aged eight to 18) with IBS and functional abdominal pain, patients underwent six sessions of hypnotherapy (HT) over a three-month period. The control intervention was standard medical care, with six sessions of supportive therapy. Pain intensity decreased in the HT group from 13.5 to 1.3 and in the control group from 14.1 to 8 ($p < 0.001$). Pain frequency reporting also decreased in the HT group from 13.1 to 1.1 and in the control group from 14.4 to 9.3 ($p = 0.007$). The three-month pain remission rate was 59% in the HT group compared to 12% in the standard care group ($p < 0.001$). Interestingly, there continued to be post-treatment improvement and remission rates at one year (85% and 25% respectively; $p < 0.001$) [97].

While no larger studies have investigated how some of these effects might be mediated in children with IBD, an interesting study in adults with IBS showed that gut-directed hypnotherapy had a normalizing effect on the aberrant central processing of visceral signals. Forty-four female adult patients were randomized to hypnosis or educational therapy. They received seven weekly one hour long sessions of hypnotherapy, including CD recordings for home use. Rectal distention was performed while the patient underwent functional magnetic resonance imaging of the brain to assess the central nervous system response to the distention stimulus. Both groups showed reduction in blood oxygen level dependent signals, including anterior insula, albeit by different centrally acting mechanisms [98]. The normalization of autonomic nervous system functions may also play a role in symptom management, as gut directed hypnotherapy has been shown to reduce heart and respiratory rates independently of emotional content [99]. Hypnotherapy is a promising therapy that may support symptom management in inflammatory bowel disease and potentially decrease the inflammatory response itself. More studies are needed to explore the feasibility, efficacy, and dose-response relationship of hypnotherapy interventions among pediatric patients suffering from IBD.

4. Sample Case

A 14-year-old female with a diagnosis of ileocolonic Crohn's disease for one year presented for a second opinion for IBD evaluation and management. The important findings on initial endoscopy were chronic ileitis of the terminal ileum, moderately active chronic colitis of the ascending colon, and colonic mucosa with rare branching crypt. Magnetic resonance enterography demonstrated a segment of borderline mild circumferential thickening of the small bowel in the ileum. Previous laboratories showed an elevated C-reactive protein (17 mg/L) and erythrocyte sedimentation rate (42 mm/h), fecal calprotectin (839 mcg/g), and low vitamin D (12 ng/mL). Her weight was 48 kg (24%), and her BMI was 21.28 kg/m^2 (50%). She was initially started on sulfasalazine, folic acid, and prednisone taper with the plan to transition to 6-mercaptopurine. However, she was only currently compliant with iron supplementation due to concerns about medication side effects.

The patient's presenting symptoms included watery diarrhea two times daily without hematochezia, frequent abdominal pain limiting her activity, and fatigue requiring a three hour nap every afternoon. She described significant stress related to Crohn's and school and became tearful when discussing her disease and desire to be normal. She also endorsed medical-related anxiety, needle phobia, and increasing frustration about her recurrent abdominal pain. During the evaluation, disease management options were discussed, including biologics, re-induction with steroids, use of immunomodulators, and enteral therapy. The patient was also referred for psychotherapy with a pediatric pain psychologist.

Psychological evaluation suggested significant academic and social anxiety related to IBD. Specifically, the patient endorsed difficulties concentrating in class due to symptoms, embarrassment about bathroom needs at school, body image concerns around peers, pain catastrophizing when out with friends, and anxiety around upcoming required blood draws. Weekly psychotherapy was initiated, and treatment goals included teaching her anxiety and pain management strategies, increasing daily functioning, and supporting her adjustment to life with a chronic illness.

Treatment initially focused on validating her past experiences, supporting increased trust with medical professionals, and empowering her to be more engaged in her health care. The mind–body modalities used in treatment included: (1) biofeedback for stress and pain management (e.g., HRV via emWave—a commonly used biofeedback program by HeartMath LLC, Boulder Creek, CA, USA); (2) hypnosis for needle phobia and pain management (e.g., comfort and relaxation dials in her 'control center', the brain); (3) mindfulness for stress and anxiety management; (4) CBT for needle phobia (e.g., graded exposures to feared stimulus like needles and blood draw); (5) and CBT for general anxiety and pain management (e.g., increasing awareness of negative pain-related thoughts, cognitive restructuring, behavioral activation to increase daily functioning).

During the first month of treatment, each session began with biofeedback and/or hypnosis exercises, such as playing the Garden Game on emWave (HeartMath LLC, Boulder Creek, CA, USA) or utilizing her relaxation dial to release worries and tension. CBT techniques were incorporated into the last 30 min of the session, focusing on graded needle exposures. For example, she practiced looking at pictures of blood draws and preparing her arm for a blood draw, with rubbing alcohol and tourniquet placement, and applying relaxation-based coping skills. Daily homework included practicing mind–body skills using biofeedback applications such as Bellybio [100] and Breathe2Relax [101], listening to a hypnosis recording about her comfort dial, and creating a weekly behavioral activation log. Treatment focused on a top-down and bottom-up approach to anxiety and pain management. After four weekly sessions working with these mind–body interventions, the patient was able to have her blood drawn with minimal difficulty. She also endorsed less anxiety at school and spent more time out of the house with friends.

At the patient's follow-up gastroenterology visit, she agreed to restart disease modifying medications. Of note, her calprotectin values subsequently normalized to 70 mcg/g, and her anemia and inflammatory markers also improved. The patient continued psychotherapy for 12 weeks. This multidisciplinary approach allowed for shared decision making in a case where the patient and family had at first demonstrated medical noncompliance due to medical-related anxiety. This case highlights the benefit of integrating mind–body interventions into IBD treatment.

When considering this case, and the biopsychosocial challenges associated with IBD, it is also important to highlight that ongoing psychotherapy is often recommended by multidisciplinary IBD teams to support mood, IBD symptom management, and health promotion (e.g., medication adherence, transitioning care). As studies have demonstrated, psychotherapy can have long-term positive effects on psychological and IBD-related outcomes. While most empirical evidence supports CBT for youth with IBD, acceptance and mindfulness-based treatment strategies should be considered when working with patients on adjustment and identity concerns related to IBD. Continued research in this area is warranted.

5. Conclusions

Mind–body interventions may be an effective non-invasive adjunctive therapy to standard medical care in pediatric IBD populations. Research shows that psychotherapy, specifically cognitive behavioral therapy, may be helpful in improving depression, functioning, and quality of life in youth with IBD. Relaxation and mindfulness-based interventions appear to improve psychological functioning among adult IBD populations, with particular benefit for subpopulations of patients experiencing heightened states of stress and concurrent IBS symptoms. Heart rate variability biofeedback and yoga may offer a way to help patients decrease pain and IBS-IBD symptoms, as well as improve anxiety and elevated persistent sympathetic tone. Preliminary data also suggests that clinical hypnosis and other mind–body interventions may have the potential to affect IBD activity (e.g., reduced inflammatory response). Further research needs to be conducted in pediatric samples in order to further validate the feasibility, efficacy, and cost effectiveness of these mind–body interventions in pediatric IBD. Manipulative therapies, such as acupuncture and massage, and dietary therapies may also improve overall well-being in IBD patients and be an area worthy of further investigation.

Mind–body interventions can be implemented in the clinical setting by various providers, including GI physicians, nurse practitioners, and physician assistants. Mental health providers such as social workers, pediatric pain psychologists, or clinical psychologists can also be trained in mind–body interventions. For the time being, insurance may not cover specific mind–body treatments. However, providers often can bill for services through evaluation and management codes based on time (for medical providers) or health and behavior codes based on time (for mental health providers). As evidence emerges on the efficacy of mind–body interventions to improve IBD outcomes, hopefully insurance companies will deem these interventions as medically necessary and gradually incorporate them into part of mainstream care.

We encourage pediatric IBD providers to reflect on the importance of the brain–gut connection with patients and families, assess their interest in mind–body interventions, and engage in multidisciplinary treatment with mind–body treatments when appropriate and supported by empirical evidence. This integrative treatment approach has the promise to improve patients' disease activity and overall well-being.

Acknowledgments: We thank Jenna Arruda for assistance with literature search and writing, and Srisindu Vellanki for assistance with literature search.

Author Contributions: A.W., A.M.Y., and B.G wrote the manuscript and commented on the manuscript at all stages.

References

1. Cho, J.H. The genetics and immunopathogenesis of inflammatory bowel disease. *Nat. Rev. Immunol.* **2008**, *8*, 458–466. [CrossRef] [PubMed]
2. Mackner, L.M.; Greenley, R.N.; Szigethy, E.; Herzer, M.; Deer, K.; Hommel, K.A. Psychosocial issues in pediatric inflammatory bowel disease: Report of the North American Society for Pediatric Gastroenterology, Hepatology, and Nutrition. *J. Pediatr. Gastroenterol. Nutr.* **2013**, *56*, 449–458. [CrossRef] [PubMed]
3. Wilson, D.C.; Thomas, A.G.; Croft, N.M.; Newby, E.; Akobeng, A.K.; Sawczenko, A.; Fell, J.M.E.; Murphy, M.S.; Beattie, R.M.; Sandhu, B.K.; et al. Systematic review of the evidence base for the medical treatment of paediatric inflammatory bowel disease. *J. Pediatr. Gastroenterol. Nutr.* **2010**, *50* (Suppl. 1), S14–S34. [CrossRef] [PubMed]
4. Zachos, M.; Tondeur, M.; Griffiths, A.M. Enteral nutritional therapy for induction of remission in Crohn's disease. *Cochrane Database Syst. Rev.* **2007**. [CrossRef]
5. Day, A.S.; Whitten, K.E.; Lemberg, D.A.; Clarkson, C.; Vitug-Sales, M.; Jackson, R.; Bohane, T.D. Exclusive enteral feeding as primary therapy for Crohn's disease in Australian children and adolescents: A feasible and effective approach. *J. Gastroenterol. Hepatol.* **2006**, *21*, 1609–1614. [CrossRef] [PubMed]
6. Heuschkel, R.B.; Menache, C.C.; Megerian, J.T.; Baird, A.E. Enteral nutrition and corticosteroids in the treatment of acute Crohn's disease in children. *J. Pediatr. Gastroenterol. Nutr.* **2000**, *31*, 8–15. [CrossRef] [PubMed]
7. Cheifetz, A.S.; Gianotti, R.; Luber, R.; Gibson, P.R. Complementary and Alternative Medicines Used by Patients with Inflammatory Bowel Diseases. *Gastroenterology* **2017**, *152*, 415–429.e15. [CrossRef] [PubMed]
8. Complementary, Alternative, or Integrative Health: What's in a Name? Available online: https://nccih.nih.gov/health/integrative-health (accessed on 10 February 2017).
9. Mind and Body Practices. Available online: https://nccih.nih.gov/health/mindbody (accessed on 15 February 2017).

10. Serpico, M.; Boyle, B.; Kemper, K.J.; Kim, S. Complementary and Alternative Medicine Use in Children with Inflammatory Bowel Diseases: A Single Center Survey. *J. Pediatr. Gastroenterol. Nutr.* **2016**, *63*, 651–657. [CrossRef] [PubMed]
11. Mayer, E.A.; Tillisch, K. The brain–gut axis in abdominal pain syndromes. *Annu. Rev. Med.* **2011**, *62*, 381–396. [CrossRef] [PubMed]
12. Maunder, R.G.; Levenstein, S. The role of stress in the development and clinical course of inflammatory bowel disease: Epidemiological evidence. *Curr. Mol. Med.* **2008**, *8*, 247–252. [CrossRef] [PubMed]
13. Levenstein, S.; Prantera, C.; Varvo, V.; Scribano, M.L.; Berto, E.; Andreoli, A.; Luzi, C. Psychological stress and disease activity in ulcerative colitis: A multidimensional cross-sectional study. *Am. J. Gastroenterol.* **1994**, *89*, 1219–1225. [PubMed]
14. Bonaz, B.L.; Bernstein, C.N. Brain–gut interactions in inflammatory bowel disease. *Gastroenterology* **2013**, *144*, 36–49. [CrossRef] [PubMed]
15. Bitton, A.; Dobkin, P.L.; Edwardes, M.D.; Sewitch, M.J.; Meddings, J.B.; Rawal, S.; Cohen, A.; Vermeire, S.; Dufresne, L.; Franchimont, D.; et al. Predicting relapse in Crohn's disease: A biopsychosocial model. *Gut* **2008**, *57*, 1386–1392. [CrossRef] [PubMed]
16. Duffy, L.C.; Zielezny, M.A.; Marshall, J.R.; Weiser, M.M.; Phillips, J.F.; Byers, T.E.; Calkins, B.M.; Graham, S.; Ogra, P.L. Lag time between stress events and risk of recurrent episodes of inflammatory bowel disease. *Epidemiology* **1991**, *2*, 141–145. [CrossRef] [PubMed]
17. Collins, S.M. Stress and the Gastrointestinal Tract IV. Modulation of intestinal inflammation by stress: Basic mechanisms and clinical relevance. *Am. J. Physiol. Gastrointest. Liver Physiol.* **2001**, *280*, G315–G318. [PubMed]
18. Diederen, K.; Hoekman, D.R.; Hummel, T.Z.; de Meij, T.G.; Koot, B.G.P.; Tabbers, M.M.; Vlieger, A.M.; Kindermann, A.; Benninga, M.A. The prevalence of irritable bowel syndrome-type symptoms in paediatric inflammatory bowel disease, and the relationship with biochemical markers of disease activity. *Aliment. Pharmacol. Ther.* **2016**, *44*, 181–188. [CrossRef] [PubMed]
19. Halpin, S.J.; Ford, A.C. Prevalence of symptoms meeting criteria for irritable bowel syndrome in inflammatory bowel disease: Systematic review and meta-analysis. *Am. J. Gastroenterol.* **2012**, *107*, 1474–1482. [CrossRef] [PubMed]
20. Srinath, A.; Young, E.; Szigethy, E. Pain management in patients with inflammatory bowel disease: Translational approaches from bench to bedside. *Inflamm. Bowel Dis.* **2014**, *20*, 2433–2449. [CrossRef] [PubMed]
21. Bercik, P.; Verdu, E.F.; Collins, S.M. Is irritable bowel syndrome a low-grade inflammatory bowel disease? *Gastroenterol. Clin. N. Am.* **2005**, *34*, 235–245. [CrossRef] [PubMed]
22. Abdul Rani, R.; Raja Ali, R.A.; Lee, Y.Y. Irritable bowel syndrome and inflammatory bowel disease overlap syndrome: Pieces of the puzzle are falling into place. *Intest. Res.* **2016**, *14*, 297–304. [CrossRef] [PubMed]
23. Chung, C.-S.; Chang, P.-F.; Liao, C.-H.; Lee, T.-H.; Chen, Y.; Lee, Y.-C.; Wu, M.-S.; Wang, H.-P.; Ni, Y.-H. Differences of microbiota in small bowel and faeces between irritable bowel syndrome patients and healthy subjects. *Scand. J. Gastroenterol.* **2016**, *51*, 410–419. [CrossRef] [PubMed]
24. Shankar, V.; Reo, N.V.; Paliy, O. Simultaneous fecal microbial and metabolite profiling enables accurate classification of pediatric irritable bowel syndrome. *Microbiome* **2015**, *3*, 73. [CrossRef] [PubMed]
25. Putignani, L.; Del Chierico, F.; Vernocchi, P.; Cicala, M.; Cucchiara, S.; Dallapiccola, B.; Dysbiotrack Study Group. Gut Microbiota Dysbiosis as Risk and Premorbid Factors of IBD and IBS Along the Childhood–Adulthood Transition. *Inflamm. Bowel Dis.* **2016**, *22*, 487–504. [CrossRef] [PubMed]
26. Ricci, C.; Lanzarotto, F.; Lanzini, A. The multidisciplinary team for management of inflammatory bowel diseases. *Dig. Liver Dis.* **2008**, *40*, S285–S288. [CrossRef]
27. Goodhand, J.; Hedin, C.R.; Croft, N.M.; Lindsay, J.O. Adolescents with IBD: The importance of structured transition care. *J. Crohns Colitis* **2011**, *5*, 509–519. [CrossRef] [PubMed]
28. Regueiro, M.; Greer, J.B.; Szigethy, E. Etiology and Treatment of Pain and Psychosocial Issues in Patients with Inflammatory Bowel Diseases. *Gastroenterology* **2017**, *152*, 430–439.e4. [CrossRef] [PubMed]
29. Day, A.S.; Ledder, O.; Leach, S.T.; Lemberg, D.A. Crohn's and colitis in children and adolescents. *World J. Gastroenterol.* **2012**, *18*, 5862–5869. [CrossRef] [PubMed]

30. Cotton, S.; Humenay Roberts, Y.; Tsevat, J.; Britto, M.T.; Succop, P.; McGrady, M.E.; Yi, M.S. Mind–body complementary alternative medicine use and quality of life in adolescents with inflammatory bowel disease. *Inflamm. Bowel Dis.* **2010**, *16*, 501–506. [CrossRef] [PubMed]
31. Fuller-Thomson, E.; Sulman, J. Depression and inflammatory bowel disease: Findings from two nationally representative Canadian surveys. *Inflamm. Bowel Dis.* **2006**, *12*, 697–707. [CrossRef] [PubMed]
32. Kappelman, M.D.; Long, M.D.; Martin, C.; DeWalt, D.A.; Kinneer, P.M.; Chen, W.; Lewis, J.D.; Sandler, R.S. Evaluation of the patient-reported outcomes measurement information system in a large cohort of patients with inflammatory bowel diseases. *Clin. Gastroenterol. Hepatol.* **2014**, *12*, 1315–1323.e2. [CrossRef] [PubMed]
33. Mikocka-Walus, A.; Knowles, S.R.; Keefer, L.; Graff, L. Controversies Revisited: A Systematic Review of the Comorbidity of Depression and Anxiety with Inflammatory Bowel Diseases. *Inflamm. Bowel Dis.* **2016**, *22*, 752–762. [CrossRef] [PubMed]
34. Greenley, R.N.; Hommel, K.A.; Nebel, J.; Raboin, T.; Li, S.-H.; Simpson, P.; Mackner, L. A meta-analytic review of the psychosocial adjustment of youth with inflammatory bowel disease. *J. Pediatr. Psychol.* **2010**, *35*, 857–869. [CrossRef] [PubMed]
35. Keethy, D.; Mrakotsky, C.; Szigethy, E. Pediatric inflammatory bowel disease and depression: Treatment implications. *Curr. Opin. Pediatr.* **2014**, *26*, 561–567. [CrossRef] [PubMed]
36. Graff, L.A.; Walker, J.R.; Bernstein, C.N. Depression and anxiety in inflammatory bowel disease: A review of comorbidity and management. *Inflamm. Bowel Dis.* **2009**, *15*, 1105–1118. [CrossRef] [PubMed]
37. Gray, W.N.; Denson, L.A.; Baldassano, R.N.; Hommel, K.A. Treatment adherence in adolescents with inflammatory bowel disease: The collective impact of barriers to adherence and anxiety/depressive symptoms. *J. Pediatr. Psychol.* **2012**, *37*, 282–291. [CrossRef] [PubMed]
38. Goodhand, J.R.; Wahed, M.; Mawdsley, J.E.; Farmer, A.D.; Aziz, Q.; Rampton, D.S. Mood disorders in inflammatory bowel disease: Relation to diagnosis, disease activity, perceived stress, and other factors. *Inflamm. Bowel Dis.* **2012**, *18*, 2301–2309. [CrossRef] [PubMed]
39. Mittermaier, C.; Dejaco, C.; Waldhoer, T.; Oefferlbauer-Ernst, A.; Miehsler, W.; Beier, M.; Tillinger, W.; Gangl, A.; Moser, G. Impact of depressive mood on relapse in patients with inflammatory bowel disease: A prospective 18-month follow-up study. *Psychosom. Med.* **2004**, *66*, 79–84. [CrossRef] [PubMed]
40. Knowles, S.R.; Monshat, K.; Castle, D.J. The efficacy and methodological challenges of psychotherapy for adults with inflammatory bowel disease: A review. *Inflamm. Bowel Dis.* **2013**, *19*, 2704–2715. [CrossRef] [PubMed]
41. Timmer, A.; Preiss, J.C.; Motschall, E.; Rücker, G.; Jantschek, G.; Moser, G. Psychological interventions for treatment of inflammatory bowel disease. *Cochrane Database Syst. Rev.* **2011**. [CrossRef]
42. McCombie, A.; Gearry, R.; Andrews, J.; Mulder, R.; Mikocka-Walus, A. Does Computerized Cognitive Behavioral Therapy Help People with Inflammatory Bowel Disease? A Randomized Controlled Trial. *Inflamm. Bowel Dis.* **2016**, *22*, 171–181. [CrossRef] [PubMed]
43. Szigethy, E.; Bujoreanu, S.I.; Youk, A.O.; Weisz, J.; Benhayon, D.; Fairclough, D.; Ducharme, P.; Gonzalez-Heydrich, J.; Keljo, D.; Srinath, A.; et al. Randomized efficacy trial of two psychotherapies for depression in youth with inflammatory bowel disease. *J. Am. Acad. Child Adolesc. Psychiatry* **2014**, *53*, 726–735. [CrossRef] [PubMed]
44. Kendall, P.C.; Flannery-Schroeder, E.; Panichelli-Mindel, S.M.; Southam-Gerow, M.; Henin, A.; Warman, M. Therapy for youths with anxiety disorders: A second randomized clinical trial. *J. Consult. Clin. Psychol.* **1997**, *65*, 366–380. [CrossRef] [PubMed]
45. March, J.; Silva, S.; Petrycki, S.; Curry, J.; Wells, K.; Fairbank, J.; Burns, B.; Domino, M.; McNulty, S.; Vitiello, B.; et al. Fluoxetine, cognitive-behavioral therapy, and their combination for adolescents with depression: Treatment for Adolescents With Depression Study (TADS) randomized controlled trial. *JAMA* **2004**, *292*, 807–820. [PubMed]
46. Thompson, R.D.; Delaney, P.; Flores, I.; Szigethy, E. Cognitive-behavioral therapy for children with comorbid physical illness. *Child Adolesc. Psychiatr. Clin. N. Am.* **2011**, *20*, 329–348. [CrossRef] [PubMed]
47. Szigethy, E.; Whitton, S.W.; Levy-Warren, A.; DeMaso, D.R.; Weisz, J.; Beardslee, W.R. Cognitive-behavioral therapy for depression in adolescents with inflammatory bowel disease: A pilot study. *J. Am. Acad. Child Adolesc. Psychiatry* **2004**, *43*, 1469–1477. [CrossRef] [PubMed]

48. Szigethy, E.; Kenney, E.; Carpenter, J.; Hardy, D.M.; Fairclough, D.; Bousvaros, A.; Keljo, D.; Weisz, J.; Beardslee, W.R.; Noll, R.; et al. Cognitive-behavioral therapy for adolescents with inflammatory bowel disease and subsyndromal depression. *J. Am. Acad. Child Adolesc. Psychiatry* **2007**, *46*, 1290–1298. [CrossRef] [PubMed]
49. Keerthy, D.; Youk, A.; Srinath, A.I.; Malas, N.; Bujoreanu, S.; Bousvaros, A.; Keljo, D.; DeMaso, D.R.; Szigethy, E.M. Effect of Psychotherapy on Health Care Utilization in Children With Inflammatory Bowel Disease and Depression. *J. Pediatr. Gastroenterol. Nutr.* **2016**, *63*, 658–664. [CrossRef] [PubMed]
50. Levy, R.L.; van Tilburg, M.A.L.; Langer, S.L.; Romano, J.M.; Walker, L.S.; Mancl, L.A.; Murphy, T.B.; Claar, R.L.; Feld, S.I.; Christie, D.L.; et al. Effects of a Cognitive Behavioral Therapy Intervention Trial to Improve Disease Outcomes in Children with Inflammatory Bowel Disease. *Inflamm. Bowel Dis.* **2016**, *22*, 2134–2148. [CrossRef] [PubMed]
51. Van den Brink, G.; Stapersma, L.; El Marroun, H.; Henrichs, J.; Szigethy, E.M.; Utens, E.M.; Escher, J.C. Effectiveness of disease-specific cognitive-behavioural therapy on depression, anxiety, quality of life and the clinical course of disease in adolescents with inflammatory bowel disease: Study protocol of a multicentre randomised controlled trial (HAPPY-IBD). *BMJ Open Gastroenterol.* **2016**, *3*, e000071. [PubMed]
52. Shaw, L.; Ehrlich, A. Relaxation training as a treatment for chronic pain caused by ulcerative colitis. *Pain* **1987**, *29*, 287–293. [CrossRef]
53. Mizrahi, M.C.; Reicher-Atir, R.; Levy, S.; Haramati, S.; Wengrower, D.; Israeli, E.; Goldin, E. Effects of guided imagery with relaxation training on anxiety and quality of life among patients with inflammatory bowel disease. *Psychol. Health* **2012**, *27*, 1463–1479. [CrossRef] [PubMed]
54. Langhorst, J.; Mueller, T.; Luedtke, R.; Franken, U.; Paul, A.; Michalsen, A.; Schedlowski, M.; Dobos, G.J.; Elsenbruch, S. Effects of a comprehensive lifestyle modification program on quality-of-life in patients with ulcerative colitis: A twelve-month follow-up. *Scand. J. Gastroenterol.* **2007**, *42*, 734–745. [CrossRef] [PubMed]
55. Gerbarg, P.L.; Jacob, V.E.; Stevens, L.; Bosworth, B.P.; Chabouni, F.; DeFilippis, E.M.; Warren, R.; Trivellas, M.; Patel, P.V.; Webb, C.D.; et al. The Effect of Breathing, Movement, and Meditation on Psychological and Physical Symptoms and Inflammatory Biomarkers in Inflammatory Bowel Disease: A Randomized Controlled Trial. *Inflamm. Bowel Dis.* **2015**, *21*, 2886–2896. [CrossRef] [PubMed]
56. Smith, G.D.; Watson, R.; Roger, D.; McRorie, E.; Hurst, N.; Luman, W.; Palmer, K.R. Impact of a nurse-led counselling service on quality of life in patients with inflammatory bowel disease. *J. Adv. Nurs.* **2002**, *38*, 152–160. [CrossRef] [PubMed]
57. Milne, B.; Joachim, G.; Niedhardt, J. A stress management programme for inflammatory bowel disease patients. *J. Adv. Nurs.* **1986**, *11*, 561–567. [CrossRef] [PubMed]
58. García-Vega, E.; Fernandez-Rodriguez, C. A stress management programme for Crohn's disease. *Behav. Res. Ther.* **2004**, *42*, 367–383. [CrossRef]
59. Larsson, K.; Sundberg Hjelm, M.; Karlbom, U.; Nordin, K.; Anderberg, U.M.; Lööf, L. A group-based patient education programme for high-anxiety patients with Crohn disease or ulcerative colitis. *Scand. J. Gastroenterol.* **2003**, *38*, 763–769. [PubMed]
60. McCormick, M.; Reed-Knight, B.; Lewis, J.D.; Gold, B.D.; Blount, R.L. Coping skills for reducing pain and somatic symptoms in adolescents with IBD. *Inflamm. Bowel Dis.* **2010**, *16*, 2148–2157. [CrossRef] [PubMed]
61. Kabat-Zinn, J. *Wherever You Go, There You Are*; Hyperion: New York, NY, USA, 1994.
62. Baer, R.A. Mindfulness Training as a Clinical Intervention: A Conceptual and Empirical Review. *Clin. Psychol. Sci. Pract.* **2003**, *10*, 125–143. [CrossRef]
63. Jedel, S.; Hoffman, A.; Merriman, P.; Swanson, B.; Voigt, R.; Rajan, K.B.; Shaikh, M.; Li, H.; Keshavarzian, A. A randomized controlled trial of mindfulness-based stress reduction to prevent flare-up in patients with inactive ulcerative colitis. *Digestion* **2014**, *89*, 142–155. [PubMed]
64. Neilson, K.; Ftanou, M.; Monshat, K.; Salzberg, M.; Bell, S.; Kamm, M.A.; Connell, W.; Knowles, S.R.; Sevar, K.; Mancuso, S.G.; et al. A Controlled Study of a Group Mindfulness Intervention for Individuals Living With Inflammatory Bowel Disease. *Inflamm. Bowel Dis.* **2016**, *22*, 694–701. [CrossRef] [PubMed]
65. Schoultz, M.; Atherton, I.; Watson, A. Mindfulness-based cognitive therapy for inflammatory bowel disease patients: Findings from an exploratory pilot randomised controlled trial. *Trials* **2015**, *16*, 379. [CrossRef] [PubMed]
66. Segal, Z.; Williams, J.; Teasdale, J. *Mindfulness-Based Cognitive Therapy for Depression: A New Approach to Preventing Relapse*; The Guilford Press: New York, NY, USA, 2002.

67. Thomas, M.; Sadlier, M.; Smith, A. The effect of Multi Convergent Therapy on the psychopathology, mood and performance of Chronic Fatigue Syndrome patients: A preliminary study. *Couns. Psychother. Res.* **2006**, *6*, 91–99. [CrossRef]
68. Berrill, J.W.; Sadlier, M.; Hood, K.; Green, J.T. Mindfulness-based therapy for inflammatory bowel disease patients with functional abdominal symptoms or high perceived stress levels. *J. Crohns Colitis* **2014**, *8*, 945–955. [CrossRef] [PubMed]
69. Ali, A.; Weiss, T.R.; Dutton, A.; McKee, D.; Jones, K.D.; Kashikar-Zuck, S.; Silverman, W.K.; Shapiro, E.D. Mindfulness-Based Stress Reduction for Adolescents with Functional Somatic Syndromes: A Pilot Cohort Study. *J. Pediatr.* **2017**, *183*, 184–190. [CrossRef] [PubMed]
70. Lehrer, P.M.; Gevirtz, R. Heart rate variability biofeedback: How and why does it work? *Front. Psychol.* **2014**, *5*, 756. [CrossRef] [PubMed]
71. Stern, M.J.; Guiles, R.A.F.; Gevirtz, R. HRV biofeedback for pediatric irritable bowel syndrome and functional abdominal pain: A clinical replication series. *Appl. Psychophysiol. Biofeedback* **2014**, *39*, 287–291. [CrossRef] [PubMed]
72. Sowder, E.; Gevirtz, R.; Shapiro, W.; Ebert, C. Restoration of vagal tone: A possible mechanism for functional abdominal pain. *Appl. Psychophysiol. Biofeedback* **2010**, *35*, 199–206. [CrossRef] [PubMed]
73. Shaffer, F.; McCraty, R.; Zerr, C.L. A healthy heart is not a metronome: An integrative review of the heart's anatomy and heart rate variability. *Front. Psychol.* **2014**, *5*, 1040. [CrossRef] [PubMed]
74. Pagani, M.; Lombardi, F.; Guzzetti, S.; Rimoldi, O.; Furlan, R.; Pizzinelli, P.; Sandrone, G.; Malfatto, G.; Dell'Orto, S.; Piccaluga, E. Power spectral analysis of heart rate and arterial pressure variabilities as a marker of sympatho-vagal interaction in man and conscious dog. *Circ. Res.* **1986**, *59*, 178–193. [CrossRef] [PubMed]
75. Axelrod, S.; Lishner, M.; Oz, O.; Bernheim, J.; Ravid, M. Spectral Analysis of Fluctuations in Heart Rate: An Objective Evaluation of Autonomic Nervous Control in Chronic Renal Failure. *Nephron* **2004**, *45*, 202–206. [CrossRef]
76. Eckberg, D.L. Human sinus arrhythmia as an index of vagal cardiac outflow. *J. Appl. Physiol.* **1983**, *54*, 961–966. [PubMed]
77. Pal, G.K.; Adithan, C.; Ananthanarayanan, P.H.; Pal, P.; Nanda, N.; Durgadevi, T.; Lalitha, V.; Syamsunder, A.N.; Dutta, T.K. Sympathovagal Imbalance Contributes to Prehypertension Status and Cardiovascular Risks Attributed by Insulin Resistance, Inflammation, Dyslipidemia and Oxidative Stress in First Degree Relatives of Type 2 Diabetics. *PLoS ONE* **2013**, *8*, e78072. [CrossRef] [PubMed]
78. Jelenova, D.; Ociskova, M.; Prasko, J.; Hunkova, M.; Karaskova, E.; Kolarova, J.; Vydra, D.; Mihal, V. Heart rate variability in children with inflammatory bowel diseases. *Neuro Endocrinol. Lett.* **2015**, *36*, 72–79. [PubMed]
79. Twal, W.O.; Wahlquist, A.E.; Balasubramanian, S. Yogic breathing when compared to attention control reduces the levels of pro-inflammatory biomarkers in saliva: A pilot randomized controlled trial. *BMC Complement. Altern. Med.* **2016**, *16*, 294. [CrossRef] [PubMed]
80. Sharma, P.; Poojary, G.; Vélez, D.M.A.; Dwivedi, S.N.; Deepak, K.K. Effect of Yoga-Based Intervention in Patients with Inflammatory Bowel Disease. *Int. J. Yoga Ther.* **2015**, *25*, 101–112. [CrossRef] [PubMed]
81. Pascoe, M.C.; Bauer, I.E. A systematic review of randomised control trials on the effects of yoga on stress measures and mood. *J. Psychiatr. Res.* **2015**, *68*, 270–282. [CrossRef] [PubMed]
82. Hibbard, J.H.; Stockard, J.; Mahoney, E.R.; Tusler, M. Development of the Patient Activation Measure (PAM): Conceptualizing and Measuring Activation in Patients and Consumers. *Health Serv. Res.* **2004**, *39*, 1005–1026. [CrossRef] [PubMed]
83. Greene, J.; Hibbard, J.H. Why does patient activation matter? An examination of the relationships between patient activation and health-related outcomes. *J. Gen. Intern. Med.* **2012**, *27*, 520–526. [CrossRef] [PubMed]
84. Shah, S.L.; Siegel, C.A. Increasing Patient Activation Could Improve Outcomes for Patients with Inflammatory Bowel Disease. *Inflamm. Bowel Dis.* **2015**, *21*, 2975–2978. [CrossRef] [PubMed]
85. Evans, S.; Lung, K.C.; Seidman, L.C.; Sternlieb, B.; Zeltzer, L.K.; Tsao, J.C.I. Iyengar Yoga for Adolescents and Young Adults With Irritable Bowel Syndrome. *J. Pediatr. Gastroenterol. Nutr.* **2014**, *59*, 244–253. [CrossRef] [PubMed]
86. Kuttner, L.; Chambers, C.T.; Hardial, J.; Israel, D.M.; Jacobson, K.; Evans, K. A randomized trial of yoga for adolescents with irritable bowel syndrome. *Pain Res. Manag.* **2006**, *11*, 217–223. [CrossRef] [PubMed]

87. Schumann, D.; Anheyer, D.; Lauche, R.; Dobos, G.; Langhorst, J.; Cramer, H. Effect of Yoga in the Therapy of Irritable Bowel Syndrome: A Systematic Review. *Clin. Gastroenterol. Hepatol.* **2016**, *14*, 1720–1731. [CrossRef] [PubMed]
88. Sugarman, L.I. Hypnosis: Teaching children self-regulation. *Pediatr. Rev.* **1996**, *17*, 5–11. [CrossRef] [PubMed]
89. Ballou, S.; Keefer, L. Psychological Interventions for Irritable Bowel Syndrome and Inflammatory Bowel Diseases. *Clin. Transl. Gastroenterol.* **2017**, *8*, e214. [CrossRef] [PubMed]
90. Szigethy, E. Hypnotherapy for Inflammatory Bowel Disease Across the Lifespan. *Am. J. Clin. Hypn.* **2015**, *58*, 81–99. [CrossRef] [PubMed]
91. Section on Integrative Medicine. Mind–bodyTherapies in Children and Youth. *Pediatrics* **2016**, *138*, e20161896.
92. Keefer, L.; Taft, T.H.; Kiebles, J.L.; Martinovich, Z.; Barrett, T.A.; Palsson, O.S. Gut-directed hypnotherapy significantly augments clinical remission in quiescent ulcerative colitis. *Aliment. Pharmacol. Ther.* **2013**, *38*, 761–771. [CrossRef] [PubMed]
93. Keefer, L.; Keshavarzian, A. Feasibility and acceptability of gut-directed hypnosis on inflammatory bowel disease: A brief communication. *Int. J. Clin. Exp. Hypn.* **2007**, *55*, 457–466. [CrossRef] [PubMed]
94. Miller, V.; Whorwell, P.J. Treatment of inflammatory bowel disease: A role for hypnotherapy? *Int. J. Clin. Exp. Hypn.* **2008**, *56*, 306–317. [CrossRef] [PubMed]
95. Mawdsley, J.E.; Jenkins, D.G.; Macey, M.G.; Langmead, L.; Rampton, D.S. The effect of hypnosis on systemic and rectal mucosal measures of inflammation in ulcerative colitis. *Am. J. Gastroenterol.* **2008**, *103*, 1460–1469. [CrossRef]
96. Shaoul, R.; Sukhotnik, I.; Mogilner, J. Hypnosis as an adjuvant treatment for children with inflammatory bowel disease. *J. Dev. Behav. Pediatr.* **2009**, *30*, 268. [CrossRef] [PubMed]
97. Vlieger, A.M.; Menko-Frankenhuis, C.; Wolfkamp, S.C.S.; Tromp, E.; Benninga, M.A. Hypnotherapy for children with functional abdominal pain or irritable bowel syndrome: A randomized controlled trial. *Gastroenterology* **2007**, *133*, 1430–1436. [CrossRef] [PubMed]
98. Lowén, M.B.O.; Mayer, E.A.; Sjöberg, M.; Tillisch, K.; Naliboff, B.; Labus, J.; Lundberg, P.; Ström, M.; Engström, M.; Walter, S.A. Effect of hypnotherapy and educational intervention on brain response to visceral stimulus in the irritable bowel syndrome. *Aliment. Pharmacol. Ther.* **2013**, *37*, 1184–1197. [CrossRef] [PubMed]
99. Yapko, M. *Trancework: An Introduction to the Practice of Clinical Hypnosis*, 4th ed.; Routledge: New York, NY, USA, 2012.
100. *Bellybio Interactive Breathing*, version 1.1.3; RelaxLine, 2010.
101. *Breathe2Relax*, version 1.7; The National Center for Telehealth and Technology: Joint Base Lewis-McChord, WA, USA, 2016.

14

Pediatric Headache Clinic Model: Implementation of Integrative Therapies in Practice

Anna Esparham *, Anne Herbert, Emily Pierzchalski, Catherine Tran, Jennifer Dilts, Madeline Boorigie, Tammie Wingert, Mark Connelly and Jennifer Bickel

Children's Mercy Hospital, University of Missouri-Kansas City School of Medicine, Division of Child Neurology, 2401 Gillham Rd., Kansas City, MO 64108, USA; ajherbert@cmh.edu (A.H.); ecpierzchalski@cmh.edu (E.P.); ctq44@mail.umkc.edu (C.T.); jjdilts@cmh.edu (J.D.); meboorigie@cmh.edu (M.B.); twingert@cmh.edu (T.W.); mconnelly1@cmh.edu (M.C.); jlbickel@cmh.edu (J.B.)

* Correspondence: aeesparham@cmh.edu

Abstract: The demand for integrative medicine has risen in recent years as research has demonstrated the efficacy of such treatments. The public has also become more conscientious of the potential limitations of conventional treatment alone. Because primary headache syndromes are often the culmination of genetics, lifestyle, stress, trauma, and environmental factors, they are best treated with therapies that are equally multifaceted. The Children's Mercy Hospital, Kansas City, Missouri Headache Clinic has successfully incorporated integrative therapies including nutraceuticals, acupuncture, aromatherapy, biofeedback, relaxation training, hypnosis, psychology services, and lifestyle recommendations for headache management. This paper provides a detailed review of the implementation of integrative therapies for headache treatment and discusses examples through case studies. It can serve as a model for other specialty settings intending to incorporate all evidenced-based practices, whether complementary or conventional.

Keywords: headache; migraine; integrative medicine; complementary therapies; pediatric; mind-body; clinic model; multidisciplinary; implementation

---

1. Introduction

Headaches are one of the most common disorders in childhood, with 60–75% of children reporting that they have had a significant headache by the age of 15 [1,2]. Headache disorders in children are truly a biopsychosocial phenomenon, best addressed with a holistic approach utilizing multidisciplinary therapeutic strategies [3,4]. Integrative medicine aims to make use of all evidence-based therapies, whether complementary or conventional, especially when treating chronic conditions [5,6]. Integrative medicine fosters optimal team dynamics, supports interdisciplinary providers and their staff, encourages healthy communication and mutual respect, and ultimately results in better care for patients [5]. As certain integrative therapies have been proven effective for certain conditions, healthcare providers may benefit from an understanding of the "how-to" of practical implementation of these integrative therapies into their practice [3,4].

Several studies have demonstrated that integrative therapies such as acupuncture, biofeedback, relaxation and stress coping skills, nutraceuticals/supplements, and aromatherapy are efficacious for headaches [7–14]. The use of complementary and integrative therapies in children with headaches may be as high as 76% in some populations [15]. Non-pharmacologic therapies implemented in practice with conventional medicine may prevent medication overuse and chronification of headaches. Because medical prophylaxis alone may often be insufficient, integrative approaches optimize clinical outcomes and provide patients with the best treatment experience [3,16]. Integrative therapies also increase patient self-care and empowerment by taking steps toward better health [17].

Much of the literature on integrative and complementary treatment modalities focuses on the public's use of such therapies as well as their efficacy and safety. There is a paucity of literature on the various ways in which integrative therapies can be implemented in clinical practice. We describe how integrative therapies have been incorporated into a pediatric headache clinic in a Midwest academic medical center, Children's Mercy Hospital and Clinics, Kansas City, Missouri (CMH). In this descriptive article, we outline integrative therapies and the evidence to support their use. Utilizing case studies, we describe how integrative therapies have been successfully incorporated into an academic headache practice. The case studies were deemed exempt by the CMH institutional review board.

2. Integrative Approaches and Their Implementation in Practice

2.1. Nutraceuticals/Dietary Supplements

Magnesium, riboflavin, and coenzyme Q10 are dietary supplements that are more commonly used for migraine headaches, based on the American Academy of Neurology and American Headache Society (AHS/AAN) guidelines [7]. Magnesium is involved in over 300 enzymatic reactions and participates in neuronal homeostasis through antagonizing the *N*-methyl-D-aspartate (NMDA) receptor, blocking calcium channels, and decreasing neurogenic inflammation [18]. Riboflavin plays a role in membrane stability, energy-related cellular function, and mediation of oxidative stress. Coenzyme Q10 (CoQ10) is involved in healthy mitochondrial function and acts as an antioxidant [19]. Butterbur exhibits anti-inflammatory effects by inhibiting leukotriene synthesis and regulating calcium channels [20]. Magnesium and riboflavin are considered by the AHS and AAN as Level B evidence: Probably effective for migraine prevention [7]. CoQ10 is considered Level C: Possibly effective for migraine prevention [7]. The American Academy of Neurology withdrew butterbur from their 2012 migraine prevention guidelines due to the associated risk of hepatotoxicity, as butterbur may contain petazolides [21]. The dietary supplement industry does not regulate the removal of petazolides, so caution is required.

In the CMH pediatric headache clinic, providers typically initiate a preventive supplement and/or medication for patients having four or more headaches per month. Preventive supplements or medications are each trialed one at a time for three months in order to determine therapeutic effect with the goal of decreasing headache severity and frequency. Potential risks, benefits, and side effects of supplements and medications are discussed with patients and their families to determine which preventive option is the best fit.

2.2. Acupuncture

Acupuncture's mechanisms of action include activating the endorphin-enkephalin system, inhibiting pain pathways in the spinal cord and midbrain through neurotransmitter release, and cell-to-cell signaling through connective tissue manipulation [22–25]. Acupuncture has demonstrated efficacy for prevention of both episodic migraines and episodic tension-type headaches [8,9]. A 2016 Cochrane review demonstrated that acupuncture may be more effective at reducing migraine frequency compared to prophylactic drug treatment (Standard Mean Deviation (SMD) −0.25; 95% Confidence Interval (CI) −0.39–−0.10: 3 trials, 739 participants), but not at long-term follow-up [8]. Migraine frequency decreased by 50% in 41% of participants receiving acupuncture versus 17% of those not receiving acupuncture (Risk Ratio (RR) 2.40; 95% CI 2.08–2.76; 4 studies; 2519 participants) [8].

One large trial of 1265 participants in a Cochrane review, comparing acupuncture to routine care in the treatment of tension type headaches, showed a 50% reduction of headache frequency in 48% of acupuncture recipients versus 19% of those with routine treatment (RR 2.52; 95% CI 2.11–3.02; number needed to treat 3; 95% CI 3–5) [9]. A second trial of 207 participants, comparing acupuncture to routine care found 45% versus 4% improvement, respectively; (RR 11.36; 95% CI 3.69–34.98; number needed to treat 2; 95% CI 1–9) [9].

Acupuncture began to be utilized for our headache patients in 2015. Dr. Jennifer Bickel, MD, a neurologist and medical acupuncturist, developed the acupuncture program, which now includes three medical acupuncturists, all trained via a 300 h medical acupuncture course. According to a market data report by the CMH de-identified information database approved by CMH, the majority of patients treated with acupuncture included older adolescents, predominantly female, and of white race. One hundred and thirty patients received acupuncture between October 2015 and November 2017. The average number of acupuncture visits per patient was 4.1. The number of new and total acupuncture visits increased in relation to the addition of medical acupuncturists. Patients with refractory headaches were more likely to receive acupuncture, compared to patients with less frequent headaches. A significant proportion of acupuncture patients had also tried more aggressive treatments, such as OnabotulinumtoxinA injections (16%) and valproic acid (10%), suggesting that the patients receiving acupuncture had complex and intractable headaches.

CMH marketed the acupuncture program by developing a page on their website that launched in April 2017. The acupuncture page has received nearly 200 views and is currently ranked second in Google searches for the keyword phrase "acupuncture for headaches in children". The acupuncture clinic has expanded to include referrals from other CMH providers, predominantly from general neurology, pain management, rehabilitation, gastroenterology, and physical therapy. Acupuncture training privileges for acute pain protocols have also recently been approved by the CMH credentialing committee. The acupuncture training program will target physicians in the acute care setting (i.e., emergency department, urgent care) teaching two acute pain protocols.

2.3. *Aromatherapy*

Aromatherapy refers to the medicinal or therapeutic use of essential oils derived from plant sources [26]. Lavender essential oil has been commonly used for its anxiolytic and mood stabilizing properties. It has been evaluated for migraines in a placebo-controlled clinical trial. Inhaling lavender essential oil for 15 min reduced headache severity on the Visual Analogue Scale (VAS) from 3.6 ± 2.8 to 1.6 ± 1.6 and was statistically significant compared to the control group [10].

Aromatherapy started in the CMH Headache Clinic as a nurse-driven project, utilized as an adjunctive therapy with acupuncture. CMH provided training to personnel on aromatherapy through an online module course. Acupuncture patients were offered a hospital-approved lavender essential oil patch and asked to evaluate their experience. The survey asked if "using the essential oil patch enhanced my acupuncture experience" on a Likert scale of 1 (not at all) to 5 (very much). Twelve respondents completed the survey with an average Likert scale score of 3.5. All respondents unanimously responded "yes" to "I would like to use essential oil patches in the future". On the basis of the positive responses, lavender essential oil patches continue to be utilized during acupuncture.

2.4. *Evidence-Based Behavioral and Self-Regulation Interventions*

The United States Headache Consortium Guidelines has recommended (grade A evidence) that relaxation, biofeedback, and cognitive behavioral therapies may be considered as options for the prevention of migraines [27].

2.4.1. Biofeedback

Biofeedback teaches self-regulation of autonomic functions related to stress and pain, including heart rate, respiratory rate, and skin temperature. A meta-analysis, including five studies with 137 participants, found that biofeedback reduced pediatric migraine frequency (Mean Difference (MD) −1.97 (95% CI, −2.72–−1.21); $p < 0.00001$), attack duration (MD −3.94 (95% CI, −5.57–−2.31); $p < 0.00001$), and headache intensity (MD, −1.77 (95% CI, −2.42–−1.11); $p < 0.00001$) compared with waiting-list control patients [11].

The CMH biofeedback clinic is staffed by a clinical pain psychologist and trained nursing staff. The biofeedback approach utilizes audio-visual technology to teach regulation of heart rate, respiratory rate, and skin temperature. Additionally, the pain psychologist utilizes cognitive behavioral therapy techniques, including acceptance and commitment therapy, to facilitate generalization and application of strategies in pain management. Patients who consistently practice self-regulation skills independently see the most success with this program.

2.4.2. Relaxation Training

Relaxation training includes deep/diaphragmatic breathing, progressive muscle relaxation, guided imagery, and mindfulness/meditation. Relaxation training, like biofeedback, increases patients' control over physiological responses to headache pain, reducing stress and anxiety, and decreasing sympathetic overdrive. While little data exists on relaxation in children, progressive muscle relaxation (PMR) was shown to decrease migraine frequency in adults by up to 41% after a six-week intervention [12]. In a meta-analysis, relaxation training in adult studies demonstrated an effect size of 0.55 (CI: 0.14–0.96), representing a moderate improvement in migraine headaches [28].

The CMH headache providers utilize a website, www.headachereliefguide.com, to teach relaxation strategies to patients and families. The website, developed by Dr. Jennifer Bickel, MD and Dr. Mark Connelly, PhD, contains a "relaxation section" with videos demonstrating relaxed breathing, PMR, and guided imagery. Additionally, CMH pain psychologists teach relaxation strategies during some headache clinic visits.

2.4.3. Hypnosis

Clinical hypnosis is a self-regulation strategy using self-directed suggestions to facilitate the mind-body connection, ultimately cultivating a sense of awareness and positive well-being [29]. A clinical hypnosis case series demonstrated a therapeutic benefit for adolescents with comorbid chronic daily headaches and anxiety [13]. Mind-body strategies, including clinical hypnosis, may regulate connections in the prefrontal structures of the adolescent brain, reducing the impact of stress-related conditions [30]. Mind-body therapies also balance dysregulation of the autonomic nervous system that may occur in migraines [31,32].

A headache-trained nurse practitioner at CMH received certification in clinical hypnosis at the National Pediatric Hypnosis Training Institute. This nurse practitioner offers clinical hypnosis during clinic visits to assist children and teens in self-guided relaxation, thus optimizing resilience.

2.4.4. Psychological Services

Depression and anxiety may contribute to functional impairment in children and adolescents with migraines [33]. A 2016 meta-analysis found that cognitive behavioral therapy demonstrated clinically significant improvement (50% or greater reduction of headache activity) after treatment and at follow-up three months later (Odds Ratio (OR) 9.11 (95% CI: 5.01–16.58, $p < 0.001$) and OR 9.18 (95% CI: 5.69–14.81, $p < 0.001$), respectively) [14]. A 2014 Cochrane review demonstrated that face-to-face psychological treatments reduced pain intensity in pediatric headache patients, with long-term benefits [34].

CMH Headache Clinic patients who are missing multiple days of school due to headache and/or have comorbid psychological concerns are referred to the CMH Comprehensive Headache Clinic. In this multidisciplinary clinic, patients and their families are treated by a headache physician, a clinical pain psychologist, and a headache social worker. Pain psychologists provide education in relaxation and self-regulation, pain coping strategies, and lifestyle modification. Additionally, acceptance and commitment therapy and other cognitive behavioral strategies are utilized. Pain psychologists frequently help patients and their families to find counseling services near their homes, facilitating ongoing psychological care. The headache social worker provides parental support and headache-specific school accommodations. This often includes a school letter and, when indicated, a 504 plan.

2.4.5. Lifestyle Strategies

Nutrition, sleep, water, caffeine, and physical activity all affect headaches. Skipping meals, not getting enough sleep, and decreased physical activity have been associated with recurrent headaches in the adolescent population [35]. Modifying sleep hygiene in children may play a significant role in improving headache symptoms [36]. Caffeine and food additives including monosodium glutamate, cocoa, aspartame, cheese, citrus, and nitrites are common triggers for headaches in children [37]. Caffeine abstinence has been associated with improved headache outcomes [38]. Increasing water intake may result in increased quality of life and decreased headache duration [39,40].

CMH Headache Clinic practitioners evaluate and discuss lifestyle factors at each clinic visit, often helping patients to identify a particular lifestyle factor on which to focus their improvement efforts for the next few months. Headache Clinic nurses provide additional patient education at the end of clinic visits, and written information is also provided. Additionally, patients and families are referred to www.headachereliefguide.com to review lifestyle recommendations. Lifestyle "check-ins" are done through telephone triage by nursing staff. Parents are encouraged to call a live nurse phone line regarding questions, concerns, and updates regarding their child. Nursing staff routinely ask about lifestyle behaviors and provide education, utilizing provider recommendations and the headache relief guide website. This empowers patients and families to take ownership of their own health outcomes.

3. Case Studies

All names have been changed to protect privacy.

3.1. Case Study: Claire

Claire is an 18 year-old female with diagnoses of migraine without aura, vestibular dysfunction, and ulcerative colitis. At age 14, she sought care with a neurologist at an outside facility. At that time, headaches occurred once a week. Claire's headaches worsened at the age of 15 after sustaining three mild traumatic brain injuries within a six-week time period. Screening labs and brain MRI were normal. Claire's headaches were refractory to multiple medications including nortriptyline, propranolol, topiramate, amitriptyline, CoQ10, zolmitriptan, hydrocodone-acetaminophen, and two OnabotulinumtoxinA treatments. She had not attended school for one year (due to headaches) prior to her first appointment at the CMH Headache Clinic.

Claire began treatment with a nurse practitioner at the CMH Headache Clinic at the age of 16. At her initial visit, she reported continuous occipital headaches associated with visual scotoma, dizziness, and nausea. Her nurse practitioner noted signs of vestibular dysfunction on exam and referred Claire to vestibular therapy, in addition to initiating preventive and abortive medications. The nurse practitioner counseled Claire on the importance of good headache hygiene, specifically focusing on increasing water intake and regulating sleep. Claire was receiving counseling for stress, which her nurse practitioner recommended continuing. Claire received occipital nerve blocks twice after that visit without headache improvement. She tried several preventives including tizanidine, cyproheptadine, atenolol, and lisinopril. She practiced vestibular exercises consistently and the dizziness partially improved.

Claire's nurse practitioner ordered the CMH comprehensive aggressive migraine protocol (CAMP) after nine additional months of intractable headaches despite multiple interventions. CAMP is a five-day outpatient dihydroergotamine (DHE) and magnesium infusion program. CAMP patients and their parents receive visits from a nurse practitioner, pain psychologist, and social worker. Massage, aromatherapy, hypnosis, Cefaly (an FDA-approved transcutaneous electrical nerve stimulation unit device to prevent and abort headaches), and acupuncture can also be provided during a CAMP session. Claire's headache decreased from 6 out of 10 to 1 out of 10 on the VAS by the end of the fourth day of CAMP.

Claire began monthly acupuncture sessions after CAMP. Acupuncture procedures varied at each monthly session and included electroacupuncture, scalp, auricular, neck and back, abdominal, and extremity acupoints. After each acupuncture session, she had two to three weeks of complete headache relief. She was able to wean off of preventive medication completely for several months but has since restarted daily amitriptyline and occasionally requires rizatriptan or a combination abortive treatment of ibuprofen, an antiemetic, and an antihistamine. She now attends college and is managing classes and a part time job successfully. She continues to receive monthly acupuncture for prevention of migraines and sees her nurse practitioner at regular intervals.

3.2. Case Study: Allison

Allison is an 18 year-old female with diagnoses of chronic daily headache, asthma, allergic rhinitis, and anxiety. She began treatment with a nurse practitioner at the CMH Headache Clinic at the age of 16, approximately three months after sustaining her third concussion. Her examination showed vestibular dysfunction but was otherwise normal. Allison's nurse practitioner ordered vestibular therapy, magnesium oxide daily for headache prevention, and an abortive cocktail of ibuprofen and diphenhydramine. Her abortive cocktail was limited to two to three times weekly. Lifestyle counseling on hydration, nutrition, sleep, and stress was given at the time of visit and www.headachereliefguide.com was used to teach relaxation strategies.

At her three-month follow-up visit, Allison had been compliant with her medication regimen, vestibular therapy, and lifestyle modifications. She continued to have daily headaches, but with decreased headache intensity. Additionally, she reported dizziness, fogginess, and increased anxiety. Her headache provider added a second preventive medication, amitriptyline daily, and encouraged her to initiate counseling. She was prescribed a new abortive cocktail of hydroxyzine, prochlorperazine, and ibuprofen. She was also referred for biofeedback therapy.

Allison started weekly biofeedback visits with a trained psychologist for a total of five weekly sessions. Biofeedback entailed utilizing four different sensors that measure physiologic correlates to stress or autonomic regulation: A surface electromyograph on the frontalis muscle of the forehead to measure muscle tension, a temperature sensor on pad of middle finger for thermoregulation and vascular reactivity, an electrodermal sensor on index and fourth fingers to measure skin conductance (i.e., sweat/moisture level), and a pneumograph strain gauge just below the rib cage to measure respiratory patterns. At the first visit, Allison exhibited sympathetic and vascular activation in response to stress. She was instructed to practice diaphragmatic breathing for three minutes, three times daily. At the second session, she was taught PMR. By the third session, her daily headaches had decreased to one headache per week. She completed a guided imagery exercise and was instructed to practice this in addition to diaphragmatic breathing and PMR at home. At her fourth session, she reported one headache per week, which responded well to abortive therapy. She was also taught autogenic relaxation during her fourth biofeedback session. At her fifth session, she continued to only report one headache weekly. At the end of biofeedback, she demonstrated improvement in all four biofeedback measures including reduced heart rate, reduced muscle tension on electromyography, increased skin temperature, and reduced respiratory rate. This is indicative of improvements in her ability to regulate stress or the autonomic nervous system. After biofeedback, she has continued practicing autogenic relaxation, guided imagery, PMR, and diaphragmatic breathing exercises at home.

Three months following biofeedback treatments, Allison returned for a follow-up Headache Clinic visit. Her exam, including vestibular function, was normal. Allison's headaches were still transformed from chronic daily headaches to episodic as she reported only one headache per week, alleviated by ibuprofen and sleep. She was advised to continue lifestyle recommendations and biofeedback techniques to help manage and prevent headaches, along with daily amitriptyline for prevention and an abortive cocktail as needed.

3.3. Case Study: Makayla

Makayla is a 13 year-old female with diagnoses of migraine headache, ankle pain, asthma, chronic urticaria, food allergies, and vasomotor rhinitis. She began treatment with a Headache Clinic nurse practitioner for post-concussion syndrome, after sustaining several concussions. She reported that her migraine headaches began at age seven, with worsening of headache frequency and severity after her concussions. Her post-concussive symptoms included daily continuous headaches and severe migraines three to four days per week, accompanied by light, noise, and smell sensitivity, nausea, numbness, weakness, tingling, vestibular dysfunction, daytime sleepiness, fatigue, and allodynia. She did report that school had become a major stressor for her with difficulty concentrating and not being able to keep up with the work. However, she denied suicidal ideation or poor mood. At the initial visit, she had missed 15 days of school in one semester and had discontinued sports participation after her concussions. She was referred for vestibular therapy and counseled in lifestyle factors, including nutrition, sleep, hydration, and stress management. Prior to her initial headache visit, Makayla was utilizing ibuprofen or acetaminophen on an as needed basis without relief. Her nurse practitioner initiated tizanidine and magnesium gluconate daily for headache prevention. Additionally, meloxicam daily was initiated for 30 days, and rizatriptan was prescribed as a headache abortive, limited to three times weekly.

Additional therapies included Cefaly, an occipital nerve block, and acupuncture. Cefaly was trialed at her clinic visit, with a subsequent decrease in VAS pain scores from 4 out of 10 to 3 out of 10. She trialed Cefaly during a later clinic visit, with similar results. When Makayla underwent an occipital nerve block with lidocaine and bupivacaine, she developed a delayed hypersensitivity reaction to lidocaine with worsening headaches after the nerve block. She was then prescribed prochlorperazine, diphenhydramine, and a solumedrol dosepak for the severe headache. However, these medications did not result in headache relief. Acupuncture was initiated to include scalp, auricular and extremity points, with six acupuncture sessions over eight weeks. At her first acupuncture visit, her headache decreased from 7 out of 10 to 4 out of 10 on the VAS. Additionally, she received counseling in relaxation, acupressure, and diaphragmatic breathing. The following day, she received intramuscular DHE, metoclopramide, ondansetron, and diphenhydramine along with acupuncture. Her pain decreased from 4 out of 10 to 2 out of 10 on the VAS. On subsequent acupuncture visits, she presented with 3 to 4 out of 10 headache pain, decreasing to 1 to 2 out of 10 on the VAS after acupuncture.

Makayla was also referred for clinical hypnosis with a nurse practitioner trained in pediatric clinic hypnosis. Makayla participated in several 40 min hypnosis sessions that focused on progressive muscle relaxation and imagery of a favorite place. The favorite place was a place known only to Makayla where she felt safe and calm. At the end of the visit she was taught self-hypnosis and self-relaxation techniques to trial at home, and she practiced this twice daily for 30 min. Makayla also began counseling sessions with a psychologist. At follow-up visits, she has reported that her headaches are mild and infrequent, occurring less than four times monthly.

4. Conclusions

Integrative therapies offer non-pharmacological treatment options that effectively reduce headache frequency and severity. The goal of integrative therapies is to empower individuals to take ownership of their health through a holistic patient-provider relationship that emphasizes education and at-home adherence. The CMH Headache Clinic has demonstrated positive outcomes by incorporating integrative therapies into headache treatment plans. Headache treatment in the clinic is as multifaceted as the headaches themselves. The multidisciplinary approach takes this complex etiology into account by addressing factors such as lifestyle, anxiety, and stress, through a variety of services.

Concerns about financing integrative therapies are relevant, as integrative therapies may not be covered by government or commercial insurance. CMH takes part in both government and commercial insurance for reimbursement of integrative services, such as acupuncture, biofeedback and relaxation, and psychology services. While financial sustainability is a main priority for healthcare organizations, incorporating evidenced-based treatments that improve clinical outcomes and quality measures should be prioritized.

Furthermore, future studies on integrative therapies and headaches should include larger sample sizes and randomized controlled trials specific to pediatric patients.

Author Contributions: A.E., A.H., E.P. contributed to the conceptualization of the manuscript, in addition to writing and editing the manuscript. C.T., J.D., M.B., T.W., M.C. and J.B. contributed to the writing and editing of the manuscript.

Acknowledgments: The authors would like to thank the faculty and staff in the Division of Child Neurology at Children's Mercy Hospital for their significant contributions to the success of the Headache Section and Clinics.

References

1. Steiner, T.J.; Stoverner, L.J.; Katsarava, Z.; Lainez, J.M.; Lampl, C.; Lanteri-Minet, M.; Rastenyte, D.; Ruiz de la Torre, E.; Tassorelli, C.; Barre, J.; et al. The impact of headache in Europe: Principal results of the Eurolight project. *J. Headache Pain* **2014**, *15*, 31. [CrossRef] [PubMed]
2. Bille, B. Migraine and tension-type headache in children and adolescents. *Cephalalgia* **1996**, *16*, 78. [CrossRef] [PubMed]
3. Soee, A.B.; Skov, L.; Skovgaard, L.T.; Thomsen, L.L. Headache in children: Effectiveness of multidisciplinary treatment in a tertiary pediatric headache clinic. *Cephalalgia* **2013**, *33*, 1218–1228. [CrossRef] [PubMed]
4. Kabbouche, M.A.; Powers, S.W.; Vockell, A.B.; LeCates, S.L.; Ellinor, P.L.; Segers, A.; Manning, P.; Burdine, D.; Hershey, A.D. Outcome of a multidisciplinary approach to pediatric migraine at 1, 2, and 5 years. *Headache* **2005**, *45*, 1298–1303. [CrossRef] [PubMed]
5. Maizes, V.; Rakel, D.; Niemiec, C. Integrative medicine and patient-centered care. *Explore* **2009**, *5*, 277–289. [CrossRef] [PubMed]
6. Ananth, S. Complementary and Alternative Medicine Survey of Hospitals: Summary of Results. Health Forum and Samueli Institute. 2007. Available online: http://www.samueliinstitute.org/File%20Library/Our%20Research/OHE/CAM_Survey_2010_oct6.pdf (accessed on 5 April 2018).
7. Loder, E.; Burch, R.; Rizzoli, P. The 2012 AHS/AAN guidelines for prevention of episodic migraine: A summary and comparison with other recent clinical practice guidelines. *Headache* **2012**, *52*, 930–945. [CrossRef] [PubMed]
8. Linde, K.; Allais, G.; Brinkhaus, B.; Fei, Y.; Mehring, M.; Vertosick, E.A.; Vickers, A.; White, A.R. Acupuncture for the prevention of episodic migraine. *Cochrane Database Syst. Rev.* **2016**, *28*, CD001218. [CrossRef] [PubMed]
9. Linde, K.; Allais, G.; Brinkhaus, B.; Fei, Y.; Mehring, M.; Shin, B.C.; Vickers, A.; White, A.R. Acupuncture for the prevention of tension-type headache. *Cochrane Database Syst. Rev.* **2016**, *4*, CD007587. [CrossRef] [PubMed]
10. Sasannejad, P.; Saeedi, M.; Shoeibi, A.; Gorji, A.; Abbasi, M.; Foroughipour, M. Lavender essential oil in the treatment of migraine headache: A placebo-controlled clinical trial. *Eur. Neurol.* **2012**, *67*, 288–291. [CrossRef] [PubMed]
11. Stubberud, A.; Varkey, E.; McCrory, D.C.; Pedersen, S.A.; Linde, M. Biofeedback as prophylaxis for pediatric migraine: A meta-analysis. *Pediatrics* **2016**, *138*. [CrossRef] [PubMed]
12. Meyer, B.; Keller, A.; Wöhlbier, H.; Overath, C.H.; Müller, B.; Kropp, P. Progressive muscle relaxation reduces migraine frequency and normalizes amplitudes of contingent negative variation (CNV). *J. Headache Pain* **2016**, *17*, 1–9. [CrossRef] [PubMed]
13. Kohen, D.P. Chronic daily headache: Helping adolescents help themselves with self-hypnosis. *Am. J. Clin. Hypn.* **2011**, *54*, 32–46. [CrossRef] [PubMed]
14. Ng, Q.X.; Venkatanaryanan, N.; Kumar, L. A systematic review and meta-analysis of cognitive behavioral therapy for the management of pediatric migraine. *Headache* **2017**, *57*, 349–362. [CrossRef] [PubMed]

15. Libera, D.D.; Colombo, B.; Pavan, G.; Comi, G. Complementary and alternative medicine (CAM) use in an Italian cohort of pediatric headache patients: The tip of the iceberg. *Neurol. Sci.* **2014**, *35*, 145–148. [CrossRef] [PubMed]
16. Gaul, C.; Visscher, C.M.; Bhola, R.; Sorbi, M.J.; Galli, F.; Rasmussen, A.V.; Jensen, R. Team players against headache: Multidisciplinary treatment of primary headaches and medication overuse headache. *J. Headache Pain* **2011**, *12*, 511–519. [CrossRef] [PubMed]
17. Foley, H.; Steel, A. Patient perceptions of patient-centred care, empathy and empowerment in complementary medicine clinical practice: A cross-sectional study. *Adv. Integr. Med.* **2017**, *4*, 22–30. [CrossRef]
18. Taylor, F.R. Nutraceuticals and headache: The biological basis. *Headache* **2011**, *51*, 484–501. [CrossRef] [PubMed]
19. Littaru, G.P.; Tiano, L. Clinical aspects of coenzyme Q10: An update. *Nutrition* **2010**, *26*, 250–254. [CrossRef] [PubMed]
20. Sun-Edelstein, C.; Mauskop, A. Alternative headache treatments: Nutraceuticals, behavioral and physical treatments. *Headache* **2011**, *51*, 469–483. [CrossRef] [PubMed]
21. Holland, S.; Silberstein, S.; Freitag, F.; Dodick, D.; Argoff, C.; Ashman, E. Evidence-based guideline update: NSAIDs and other complementary treatments for episodic migraine prevention in adults: [RETIRED]. *Neurology* **2012**, *78*, 1346–1353. [CrossRef] [PubMed]
22. Langevin, H.M.; Bouffard, N.A.; Badger, G.J.; Churchill, D.L.; Howe, A.K. Subcutaneous tissue fibroblast cytoskeletal remodeling induced by acupuncture: Evidence for a mechanotransduction-based mechanism. *J. Cell. Physiol.* **2006**, *207*, 767–774. [CrossRef] [PubMed]
23. Langevin, H.M.; Sherman, K.J. Pathophysiological model for chronic low back pain integrating connective tissue and nervous system mechanisms. *Med. Hypotheses* **2007**, *68*, 74–80. [CrossRef] [PubMed]
24. Langevin, H.M.; Yandow, J.A. Relationship of acupuncture points and meridians to connective tissue planes. *Anat. Rec.* **2002**, *269*, 257–265. [CrossRef] [PubMed]
25. Berman, B.M.; Langevin, H.H.; Witt, C.M.; Dubner, R. Acupuncture for chronic low back pain. *N. Engl. J. Med.* **2010**, *363*, 454–461. [CrossRef] [PubMed]
26. National Cancer Institute. Available online: https://www.cancer.gov/about-cancer/treatment/cam/hp/aromatherapy-pdq (accessed on 7 February 2018).
27. Silberstein, S.D.; Edlund, W. Practice parameter: Evidence-based guidelines for migraine headache (an evidence-based review): Report of the Quality Standards Subcommittee of the American Academy of Neurology. *Neurology* **2000**, *55*, 754–762. [CrossRef] [PubMed]
28. Goslin, R.E.; Gray, R.; McCrory, D.; Penzien, D.; Rains, J.; Hasselblad, J. Behavioral and Physical Treatments for Migraine Headache. AHRQ Technical Reviews 1999. Available online: https://www.ncbi.nlm.nih.gov/books/NBK45267/ (accessed on 16 May 2018).
29. Kohen, D.P.; Kaiser, P. Clinical hypnosis with children and adolescents—What? Why? How?: Origins, applications, and efficacy. *Children* **2014**, *1*, 74–98. [CrossRef] [PubMed]
30. Sawni, A.; Breuner, C.C. Clinical hypnosis, an effective mind-body modality for adolescents with behavioral and physical complaints. *Children* **2017**, *4*, 19. [CrossRef] [PubMed]
31. Moura, V.L.; Faurot, K.R.; Gaylord, S.A.; Mann, J.D.; Sill, M.; Lynch, C.; Lee, M.Y. Mind-body interventions for treatment of phantom limb pain in persons with amputation. *Am. J. Phys. Med. Rehabil.* **2012**, *91*, 701. [CrossRef] [PubMed]
32. Wells, R.E.; Smitherman, T.A.; Seng, E.K.; Houle, T.T.; Loder, E.W. Behavioral and Mind/Body interventions in headache: Unanswered questions and future research directions. *Headache* **2014**, *54*, 1107–1113. [CrossRef] [PubMed]
33. Kemper, K.J.; Heyer, G.; Pakalnis, A.; Binkley, P.F. Factors contribute to headache-related disability in teens? *Pediatr. Neurol.* **2016**, *56*, 48–54. [CrossRef] [PubMed]
34. Eccleston, C.; Palermo, T.M.; Williams, A.C.; Lewandowski, H.A.; Morley, S.; Fisher, E.; Law, E. Psychological therapies for the management of chronic and recurrent pain in children and adolescents. *Cochrane Database Syst. Rev.* **2014**, *5*. [CrossRef]
35. Walter, S. Lifestyle behaviors and illness-related factors as predictors of recurrent headache in U.S. adolescents. *J. Neurosci. Nurs.* **2014**, *46*, 337–350. [CrossRef] [PubMed]
36. Guidetti, V.; Dosi, C.; Bruni, O. The relationship between sleep and headache in children: Implications for treatment. *Cephalalgia* **2014**, *34*, 767–776. [CrossRef] [PubMed]

37. Taheri, S. Effect of exclusion of frequent consumed dietary triggers in a cohort of children with chronic primary headache. *Nutr. Health* **2017**, *23*, 47–50. [CrossRef] [PubMed]
38. Lee, M.J.; Choi, H.A.; Choi, H.; Chung, C.S. Caffeine discontinuation improves acute migraine treatment: A prospective clinic-based study. *J. Headache Pain* **2016**, *17*, 71. [CrossRef] [PubMed]
39. Spigt, M.G.; Kuijper, E.C.; Schayck, C.P.; Troost, J.; Knipschild, P.G.; Linssen, V.M.; Knottnerus, J.A. Increasing the daily water intake for the prophylactic treatment of headache: A pilot trial. *Eur. J. Neurol.* **2005**, *12*, 715–718. [CrossRef] [PubMed]
40. Spigt, M.; Weerkamp, N.; Troost, J.; van Schayck, C.P.; Knottnerus, J.A. A randomized trial on the effects of regular water intake in patients with recurrent headaches. *Fam. Pract.* **2012**, *29*, 370–375. [CrossRef] [PubMed]

15

The Role of Mindfulness in Reducing the Adverse Effects of Childhood Stress and Trauma

Robin Ortiz [1] and Erica M. Sibinga [2,*]

1 Departments of Internal Medicine and Pediatrics Johns Hopkins Hospital, 1800 Orleans Street, Baltimore, MD 21231, USA, Robin.Ortiz@jhmi.edu
2 Johns Hopkins School of Medicine, 733 North Broadway, Baltimore, MD 21205, USA
* Correspondence: esibinga@jhmi.edu

Abstract: Research suggests that many children are exposed to adverse experiences in childhood. Such adverse childhood exposures may result in stress and trauma, which are associated with increased morbidity and mortality into adulthood. In general populations and trauma-exposed adults, mindfulness interventions have demonstrated reduced depression and anxiety, reduced trauma-related symptoms, enhanced coping and mood, and improved quality of life. Studies in children and youth also demonstrate that mindfulness interventions improve mental, behavioral, and physical outcomes. Taken together, this research suggests that high-quality, structured mindfulness instruction may mitigate the negative effects of stress and trauma related to adverse childhood exposures, improving short- and long-term outcomes, and potentially reducing poor health outcomes in adulthood. Future work is needed to optimize implementation of youth-based mindfulness programs and to study long-term outcomes into adulthood.

Keywords: trauma; mindfulness; adverse childhood events; resilience; MBSR; mind-body; ACEs; at-risk youth; childhood adversity; toxic stress; allostatic load

---

1. Introduction

The evidence continues to mount that exposure to adverse experiences during childhood has the potential to increase morbidity and mortality both during childhood and across the lifespan into adulthood [1]. Adverse childhood experiences (ACEs) are stressful for children, and include neglect; physical, sexual or emotional abuse; exposure to violence, mental illness, incarceration, or substance abuse in the family; parental absence due to divorce or separation; and low socioeconomic status. Further, significant, traumatic, recurrent, and/or prolonged stress may have a cumulative toxic effect on the child [2,3]. In addition to the psychological toll, stress and toxic stress effect the body through increased allostatic load, the physiologic burden of such stress that may manifest as neuroanatomical changes, increased levels of inflammation, and dysfunction of the hypothalamic-pituitary-adrenal axis [4]. More recent findings are emerging suggesting that resilience, i.e., successful management of and coping with stress, can mitigate the negative consequences of such trauma [5,6]. Findings such as these have sparked a call to action for pediatricians to both recognize that, "many adult diseases should be viewed as developmental disorders that begin early in life and that persistent health disparities associated with poverty, discrimination, or maltreatment could be reduced by the alleviation of toxic stress in childhood" and "to serve as both front-line guardians of healthy child development and strategically positioned, community leaders to inform new science-based strategies that build strong foundations for educational achievement, economic productivity, responsible citizenship, and lifelong health" [2]. This is an emphatic call to work together to enhance the prevention of ACEs, provide early and accessible interventions, and broadly expand the delivery of trauma-informed care. Mindfulness is an evidence-based intervention that supports these important responses to ACEs, fundamentally enhancing self-regulation and resilience in everyday life and in the face of stress and trauma.

This review aims to identify the benefits of mindfulness-based interventions as an approach to mitigating the negative sequelae of childhood trauma by summarizing relevant research in adult and pediatric populations. Additionally, the adaptations for introducing and teaching mindfulness for children and youth will be reviewed. Finally, future directions in the research and clinical realms related to trauma-informed mindfulness interventions will be suggested.

2. ACEs and Trauma

Research suggests that children are often exposed to significant environmental stressors and situational adversities [7]. A Centers for Disease Control and Prevention (CDC) report from five states in 2009 showed that 69% of respondents (n = 26,229) report at least one adverse childhood event (ACE) with 9% experiencing up to five adversities [7]. A smaller study of children found 34% of those screened in school report exposure to at least one trauma and evidence of post-traumatic stress even without a current diagnosis [8]. One of the first studies of ACEs (including traumas such as abuse, neglect, witnessing violence against mother, substance use in the home, household mental illness, parental separation or divorce, or household member incarcerated) showed that not only do ACEs cluster together, but there is a dose response relationship with overall health, such that larger numbers of ACEs are associated with poorer health [1]. Other adversities associated with a risk for exposure to trauma include low socioeconomic status and the associated lower education [9] and risky family environments [10,11]. Such negative experiences in the absence of a protective buffer may manifest as toxic stress, yielding an increased allostatic load to the body causing prolonged activation of physiologic stress responses, which over time may yield poor health outcomes and future illness [3,4,12]. For example, ACEs have been associated with biological markers of disease risk including inflammatory cytokines, metabolic abnormalities, and epigenetic modifications [4,13,14] (Figure 1). Remarkably, such epigenetic modifications may carry across generations, as identified in the glucocorticoid receptor related gene *FKBP5* of holocaust survivors also found in their offspring [15]. Toxic stress can result from different situations, including single stressors that are prolonged in exposure (such as recurrent emotional abuse), multiple stressors that become toxic when aggregated (such as low socioeconomic status), living below the poverty line and having limited educational opportunity, and/or traumatic experiences of greater emotional intensity or severity (such as sexual abuse).

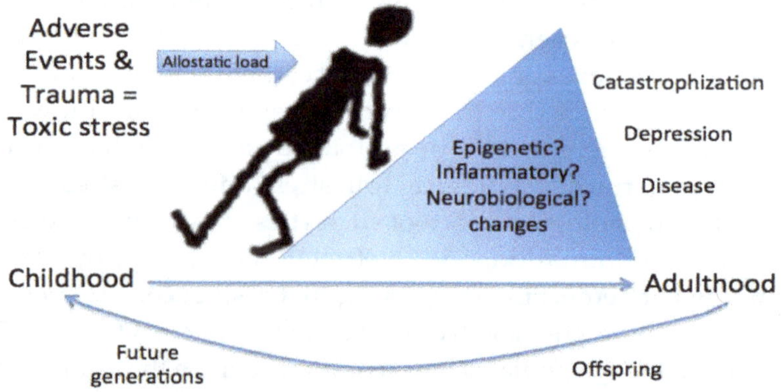

Figure 1. The impact of stress and trauma in childhood. Adverse childhood events, stress, and trauma contribute to toxic stress. Toxic stress that results from prolonged exposure to stress, aggregated trauma experiences, or incidents of significant emotional impact yields an increased allostatic load on the body. Allostatic load, measured by biological markers of disease risk including inflammatory cytokines, neurobiological changes, metabolic abnormalities, and epigenetic modifications, may carry over into future generations.

Specific ACEs, such as those associated with an adverse living environment limited in support and opportunity, have been shown to be associated with negative health outcomes. Such an adverse environment encompasses socioeconomic factors (such as household income, education of parents, and occupational prestige of parents), and risky family environment (such as living with a household member with a substance use disorder, mental illness or history of incarceration, living in a chaotic or disorganized environment, or experiencing violence and lack of parental warmth) [10]. Low socioeconomic status (SES) is associated with reduced access to educational support, or parental involvement in education [16]. Similarly, household chaos is associated with sensitive and harsh parenting, both of which predict childhood misconduct [17]. Low SES also seems to be associated with developmental delay (specifically, a delay in cognitive development of executive functioning including working memory, inhibitory control, and cognitive flexibility), poor conduct, and callous behaviors [17–19]. These lead to consequences of transition to adulthood such that lower SES and early life stress influence both cognitive and associated neurobiological development, which are also associated with poor health outcomes in adulthood and comorbid metabolic and cardiovascular dysfunction [20,21]. Further, adverse living environment, may predispose to the development of characteristics and behaviors that are risk factors for multiple comorbidities, including obesity, smoking, and increased blood pressure trajectory, throughout adolescence into adulthood, and are further specifically associated with metabolic dysfunction and cardiovascular disease in adulthood [10,22–24]. Risky family environments have also been associated with dysfunctional emotional processing, mood disorders, and hypothalamic-pituitary-adrenal (HPA) axis dysfunction [25].

There is diversity in both the types of traumatic experiences that may exist in childhood and the broad systems that may be affected. ACEs are associated with increased poor and risky health behaviors including substance use, smoking, risky sexual activity, and sedentary lifestyle in adulthood. ACEs also show a graded relationship with the presence of mental health disorders, adult ischemic heart disease, cancer, chronic lung disease, skeletal fractures, and liver disease in a study of 9508 Americans in 1998 [1]. In addition, ACEs have also been associated with alcoholism [26], chronic obstructive pulmonary disease [27], autoimmune disease [28], quality of life [29], drug use [23], risk for intimate partner violence [30], sexually transmitted diseases [31], suicide attempts [32], maladjustment and misconduct in and outside of school, as well as risk for incarceration [33,34]. Importantly, many of these conditions begin early in childhood and are reversible or preventable by mitigating risk factors.

Studies have also identified associations between childhood adversity and trauma and specific adult diagnoses including fibromyalgia [35], migraine [36], irritable bowel syndrome [37], insomnia and insufficient sleep [38], cancer [39], cognitive function in mental health disorders [40], as well as learning and behavior problems and obesity in youth [41] and adolescent pregnancy and fetal death [42]. Collectively, this research suggests the significant and pervasive negative impact of childhood ACEs and trauma on short- and long-term health outcomes, and therefore, the necessity and opportunity to prevent and intervene on ACEs, and to provide trauma-informed services broadly to offset the negative consequences in children, the adults they will become, and possibly even future generations.

3. Mindfulness

Mindfulness has origins as a Buddhist concept increased through meditation that has been cultivated into a Western practice of present-focused, non-judgmental awareness [43]. Mindfulness instruction has also been offered through structured training programs such as that developed by Jon Kabat-Zinn in 1979 to enhance non-judgmental attention to the experience of the present moment, entitled Mindfulness Based Stress Reduction (MBSR) [43]. The MBSR program has been shown to increase self-reported mindfulness among participants [44,45]. However, all individuals have the capacity for mindfulness, i.e., non-reactivity, awareness, focus, attention, and nonjudgment [45], though there is variability in the amount and quality of mindfulness among individuals. Therefore, both structured MBSR and unstructured mindfulness practices outside of the MBSR model, may enhance the beneficial characteristics associated with mindfulness.

Structured mindfulness training is available through Kabat-Zinn's MBSR, which typically consists of eight weekly two-and-a-half-hour classes and a full-day retreat, in which participants learn a variety of formal and informal mindfulness practices, learn and discuss the mind-body connection, and have group discussions regarding the challenges to integrating mindfulness into one's life. For particular populations, other programs have been adapted from MBSR, such as Mindfulness-Based Cognitive Therapy (MBCT), shown to be effective in reducing depression recurrences, and one focused on addiction triggers, Mindfulness Based Relapse Prevention (MBRP) [46, 47]. Unstandardized mindfulness may also be offered in other formats such as aspects of educational sessions, art therapy, group therapy, yoga, or other mind-body interventions. Though this review will focus on standardized MBSR and MBSR-related programs to highlight evidence for their practice, there will be brief discussion of the practice and implications of other mindfulness delivery methods.

3.1. Mindfulness in Trauma

Mindfulness instruction has been shown to benefit individuals with a known trauma or ACE. Mindfulness may do this by both an indirect effect of negating the acute response to trauma and stress, but also by inhibiting underlying consequences of chronic exposure to stress and trauma such as psychiatric, metabolic and cardiovascular disease through the influence on lifestyle choices, underlying biochemistry and neurobiology (Figure 2). In 50 women exposed to trauma including witnessing family violence, experiencing childhood physical or sexual abuse, or sudden loss of a loved one, an 8-week MBSR program was associated with decreased symptoms of stress and trauma exposure including perceived stress, depression, trait and state anxiety, emotion dysregulation, and posttraumatic stress symptoms [48]. Additionally, 27 female survivors of sexual abuse in childhood, experienced significantly reduced symptoms of depression, posttraumatic stress disorder (PTSD), and anxiety after an 8-week MBSR intervention [49]. This beneficial effect continued at follow-up 2.5 years later [50], which highlights that mindfulness may have an effect on the formation of related psychiatric comorbidities. This was demonstrated in two populations at risk for high rates of trauma and/or ACEs and related psychiatric disease. In a group of incarcerated women ($n = 33$) improvements in perceived stress, anxiety and depression were seen with a 12-week mindfulness intervention [51]. In a small qualitative study of a population of survivors ($n = 12$) of political violence, when mindfulness was combined with art therapy in a unique 4-day intensive program, themes of resilience emerged [52].

Research also suggests a role for mindfulness to mitigate consequences of toxic stress, by identifying benefit in individuals exposed to high stress environments by both enhancing long-term coping, and influencing the related physiologic effects of stress on the HPA axis. Klatt et al. studied intensive care unit workers finding that a mindfulness intervention was linked to increased resilience [53]. In active duty military personnel preparing for deployment, mindfulness was shown to mitigate the response to stressful experience [54], which suggests that it may both reduce current stress experience and predispose to enhanced coping prior to stress exposure. However, mindfulness, additionally, has lasting effects beyond exposure to prolonged stress as demonstrated by numerous studies in veteran populations and those exposed to war and bereavement. Veterans ($n = 58$) who participated in an 8-week long mindfulness intervention including a day long retreat, saw clinically significant improvements in their Post Traumatic Stress Disorder (PTSD) symptoms up to 17 weeks afterward, and another study suggests a shorter duration ($n = 62$, 4-session program) intervention may also decrease PTSD symptoms though only studied up to 8-weeks post [55,56]. The same group found that mindfulness also decreased cortisol levels in the veterans [57]. To suggest that this may be a global effect, other studies have supported these similar findings. A study that used mindfulness through mantra based meditation also showed decreased PTSD symptoms in veterans [58]. In one of the largest mindfulness studies of the veteran population, a mediation program that elicited mindfulness as an outcome, also reduced PTSD symptoms in 391 veterans in a uniquely implemented Department of Veteran Affairs meditation program through six medical centers [59]. In veterans with mental health comorbidities mindfulness improved sleep quality [60].

These underlying influences of mindfulness may mitigate mental health outcomes, enhance quality of life, and reduce somatic symptoms. A short 4-session intervention incorporating mindfulness in the mind-body approach, modestly increased resilience and also decreased depressive and anxiety symptoms and perceived stress in veterans though only assessed post-intervention [61]. These effects translate to improvements in quality of life [62] with a reduction in somatic symptoms including dizziness, fatigue and tension in addition to depressive symptoms as shown in veterans with PTSD [63]. Undergraduates ages 18–36, who participated in a mindfulness activity interrelated with expressive writing exercises about a past stress or trauma demonstrated decreased physical symptoms, poor sleep, and negative affect; with beneficial findings apparently linked to the mindfulness component, given expressive writing alone was not predictive of improvement [64]. Mindfulness is also inversely associated with functional disability in Iraq and Afghanistan war veterans (n = 115) [65], and with PTSD in a trauma exposed Iranian population (n = 1708) [66]. It may also offer protection in burn-out and compassion fatigue, such as in a study of traumatic bereavement workers [67].

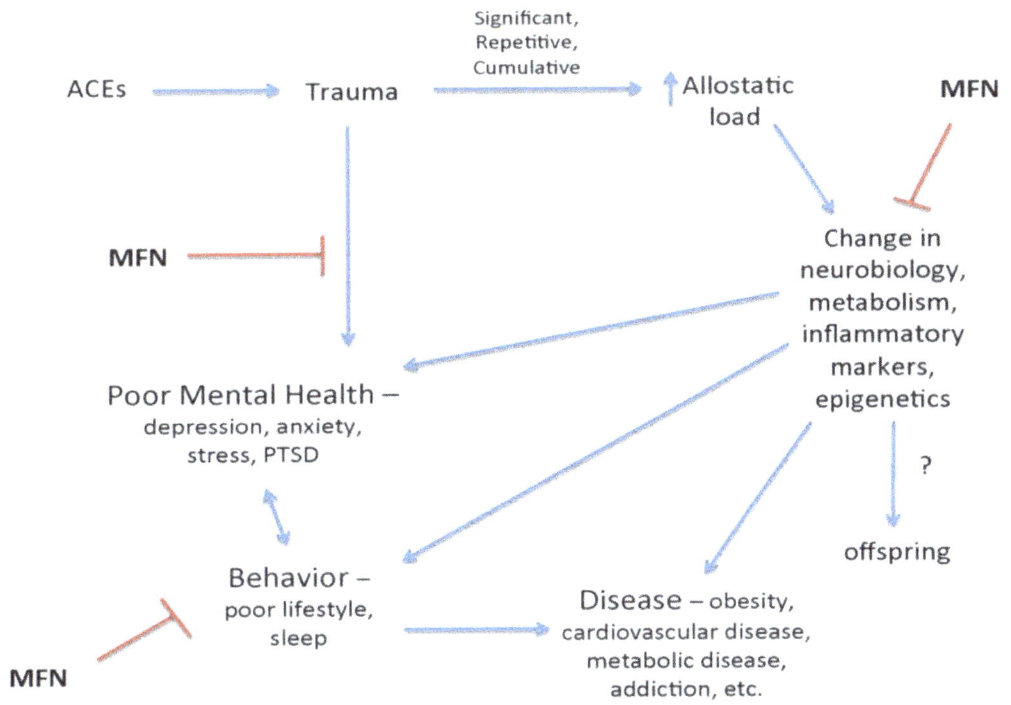

Figure 2. The negative impact of adverse childhood events (ACEs) and trauma in childhood is reduced by mindfulness (MFN). Mindfulness has been shown to mitigate the psychological, behavioral, and physiological changes associated with ACEs and trauma and increased allostatic load. MFN, specifically, reduces symptoms of depression and posttraumatic stress disorder (PTSD) associated with stress and trauma, and is inversely associated with poor health behavior and biological makers of metabolic, neurologic, and inflammatory dysfunction and disease. Stress has been demonstrated to be associated with epigenetic modifications that may persist in offspring, therefore, mindfulness interventions may reduce these negative influences.

Further, research has shown that these beneficial effects of mindfulness may be generalizable to healthy populations, regardless of known exposure to stress and trauma. In large meta-analyses, mindfulness was shown to reduce stress in healthy adult individuals [68] and to reduce anxiety, depression, and pain in diverse clinical populations [69]. Mindfulness is inversely related to anxiety, experiential avoidance, distress and uncertainty, external stimulus reactivity (poorer executive control), and persistence of negative affect [70,71]. Mindfulness programs can improve coping and resiliency in specific conditions including quality of life in patients with multiple sclerosis [72], depression and anxiety in patients with cancer [73], and specifically in trauma-exposed individuals with human immunodeficiency virus (HIV), can reduce PTSD symptoms [74].

Importantly, the beneficial effects of mindfulness on psychological and somatic symptoms and foundations for disease extend beyond negating the psychological impact of stress and may influence physiologic dysfunction (Figure 2). In general, mindfulness has been modestly associated with alterations in markers of inflammation, cell-mediated immunity, and biological aging [75]. Specifically, in women with interpersonal trauma (n = 50), not only were their psychological symptoms improved, as discussed above, but their inflammatory cytokine, interleukin-6 (IL-6) levels decreased [48]. Mindfulness has neurobiological modification potential as demonstrated by enhanced resting state functional connectivity as well as executive control via the dorsolateral prefrontal cortex, both coinciding with decreased levels of peripheral IL-6 levels [76]. Such biomarkers may be modulated by epigenetic changes through, histone-modifying enzymes also found to be associated with mindfulness interventions [77]. These neurobiological changes may represent modifications that can influence behavior and disease risk factors in adults and possibly the predisposition to disease in children, especially those at higher risk when exposed to stress, trauma, and/or toxic stress.

Though children may be exposed to different types of trauma then adults, these studies collectively suggest that mindfulness may serve to buffer the effects of stress and trauma in children and into adulthood.

3.2. *Mindfulness in Youth*

Recent mindfulness studies in youth, specifically in populations with known trauma exposure or populations at high risk for ACEs suggest promise in improving a variety of outcomes, including mental health symptoms, behavior and quality of life, and coping (Table 1). In one randomized control trial (RCT) of a population of urban youth in a low-income environment, middle-school age male children (n = 41) underwent a 12-week school-based mindfulness intervention that resulted in decreased negative coping [78]. The group additionally yielded decreases in anxiety and rumination and possibly school related stress response as suggested by a flatter cortisol curve over the course of the study (three months) and school term compared to the attention, social experience and time matched control, health education group. A larger RCT in two urban public middle schools (n = 300) showed that the 12-week, school-based MBSR program led to reduced depression, self-hostility, negative affect, negative coping, rumination, somatization, and post-trauma stress symptoms [79]. Additionally, one study of mindfulness in youth in foster care, ages 14–21 (n = 42), showed a trend toward post-intervention changes in state anxiety, qualitative gains in-group effectiveness in social gains, and coping with stress was observed [80].

These studies with foster care youth and in urban low-resourced areas likely represent children affected by or at risk for on-going stresses, and/or trauma [78–82], especially illustrated by the reduction in post-stress trauma symptoms in the MBSR arm. Other studies also support the promising hypothesis that mindfulness may offer coping skills, emotional processing and resilience. Many of these studies are done in the school environment. In a RCT of 522 children ages 12–16, the mindfulness arm post-intervention outcomes included lower stress, greater well-being, and fewer depressive symptoms [83]. It is important to note that the control group in this study was a usual school curriculum and did not control for peer experience, attention, or time. In a study of 101 sixth grade children, a 6-week mindfulness curriculum decreased suicidal ideation and self-harm [84] compared to a matched experiential activity control group. Though this study did not show an effect on internalizing or externalizing problems, others have demonstrated it to improve classroom behavior, and attention [85,86] (Table 1). Mindfulness may also offset the psychiatric comorbidities accompanied by traumatic experiences that impact the lives of youth in and outside of the classroom. Biegel and colleagues showed that 104 adolescents ages 14–18 benefited with improved state anxiety, sleep, stress, self-esteem, psychiatric symptoms (such as somatization and hostility) and global assessment functioning [87].

Though mindfulness has been demonstrated to be beneficial across a variety of domains when taught directly to youth, it may also influence youth outcomes when those surround them learn mindfulness, such as teachers and parents [88]. A study by Singh and colleagues demonstrated that an intervention administered to preschool teachers resulted in decreases in difficult behaviors, decreases in negative interactions, and an increase in compliance among students [89]. Similarly, Jennings and colleagues observed that mindfulness training improved teacher well-being and characteristics of impactful teaching including improved efficacy, and reduced stress ($n = 35$) [90].

Resilience in children may also arise through mindful parenting. Less parenting stress, increased parental warmth, and increased parental attention to their children may also contribute to buffering against the poor health outcomes associated with ACEs [10,91]. Given the number of studies that suggest mindfulness may reduce parental dismissal of their children, mindful parenting may also contribute to resilience against trauma [92]. Mindfulness in parents was associated with each individual's positive perspective on quality of the relationship in black families of stepparents and their child [93]. Mindfulness in parents also may be protective against poor psychobehavioral outcomes in children as has been demonstrated by an inverse association between internalizing and externalizing problems in youth across multiple age groups (young childhood, middle childhood, and adolescence, $n = 215$) [94]. Mindful parenting interventions may improve parent-child relationship qualities [94], but there is mixed evidence regarding the effectiveness of mindful parenting in general depending on the outcomes of interest [92]. However, one study specifically showed benefit that may be extrapolated to relate to parenting children exposed to ACEs. Parents in inner-city methadone programs demonstrated reduced ratings on the Child Abuse Potential Inventory indicating lower potential for physical abuse [95], and therefore show promise to reducing the sequelae of ACEs.

Table 1. Beneficial outcomes seen in research of mindfulness programs for children and youth.

Outcome	Reference
Decreased anxiety	Sibinga et al., 2013 [78] Jee et al., 2015 [80]
Decreased rumination	Sibinga et al., 2013 [78]
Decreased school related stress, coping with stress	Sibinga et al., 2013 [78] Jee et al., 2015 [80]
Flatter cortisol curve	Sibinga et al., 2013 [78]
Lower levels of somatization	Sibinga et al., 2016 [79] Biegel et al., 2009 [87]
Decreased depressive symptoms	Sibinga et al., 2016 [79] Kuyken et al., 2013 [83]
Effectiveness in social gains	Jee et al., 2015 [80]
Classroom behavior	Black et al., 2015 [86] van de Weijer-Bergsma et al., 2012 [85]
Decreased hostility	Biegel et al., 2009 [87] Sibinga et al., 2016 [79]
Decreased suicidal ideation	Britton et al., 2014 [84]
Decreased self-harm	Britton et al., 2014 [84]
Reduced child abuse potential by parents	Dawe and Harnett, 2007 [95]
Conflict avoidance	Sibinga et al., 2014 [81]
Improved attention	van de Weijer-Bergsma et al., 2012 [85]
Greater well-being	Kuyken et al., 2013 [83]
Decreased post traumatic symptoms severity	Sibinga et al., 2016 [79]

In summary, high-quality structured mindfulness programs for youth show promise by reducing mood and emotion dysregulation (decrease depressive, self-hostility, PTSD, anxiety and negative affect symptoms), negative-coping with stress, and improved school adaptation (classroom behavior and discipline, social and academic competence), and attention, mitigating negative effects and potential exacerbations of ACEs. Mindfulness has also been shown to benefit those important to youth, including parents and teachers.

3.3. Resilience and Mindfulness

In order to understand how the practice of mindfulness might be offered as an intervention mitigating the relationship between childhood trauma and health outcomes, one must appreciate the contribution of mindfulness to enhancing resiliency [6]. Resilience is buffering, through successful coping, against adverse outcomes after exposure to traumatic experiences. Conceptually, the lack of resilience may predispose to conditions like PTSD and further unfavorable health consequences as seen in those who experience trauma. In an adult urban inner-city population resilience was found to be inversely associated with symptoms of PTSD [5] and depression, but childhood trauma was positively associated with the presence of PTSD and depression symptoms [96]. Further, there may be neurobiological underpinnings to the buffering effect of resilience on ACEs. Though ACEs have been associated with neurocognitive impairment, trait resilience is associated with better neurocognitive skills such as non-verbal memory [20,21,97]. Importantly, a limitation to exploring this concept is the assessment of resilience, which in research investigations is done by collecting data on related concepts such as perseverance and self-confidence as assessed by the Connor-Davidson-Resilience Scale (CD-RISC) questionnaire, or other concepts measures like coping, social support, emotional and behavioral reactivity, and compassion [98,99]. Nonetheless, enhancing these important domains through mindfulness may serve collectively or independently as buffers against trauma.

Mindfulness may increase resilience in those who have experienced trauma, because it offers an alternative to the common psychological dissociation that occurs after trauma, which can prevent healthy processing or coping [100]. The mindfulness characteristics of accepting without judgment, and acting with awareness are inversely associated with PTSD symptoms [101]. This is likely due to the mindfulness teaching of non-judgmental acceptance of painful and unpleasant thoughts, as well as feelings and practice of decreased reactivity to them [102]. In a cross-sectional study of 125 individuals with substance dependence and a history of trauma, the characteristic of mindfulness was inversely associated with thought suppression, which may represent a form of dissociation and which was strongly associated with PTSD symptoms [103]. Accordingly, trait mindfulness was also associated with decreased cravings.

4. Mindfulness Program Considerations

4.1. Mindfulness Practice and Instructor Training

Mindfulness instruction as a practice has taken on many forms, but MBSR is structured as a 26-h (eight 2.5 h sessions with 1 full day) involving mindful exercises, such as body-scans, mindful breathing, and yoga with meditation instruction, group discussions and encouragement of home practice [43,104]. However, some programs have found effect with as few as 12-h of instruction, with no clear association between hours of instruction and effect size of post-MBSR effects, but studies are varied and limited in their duration of effect [105]. Britton et al. implemented a 15-min daily 6-week course in children, and Kalmanowitz et al. demonstrated that even a 4-day long intensive program in adults demonstrated benefit [52,84].

There is no centralized credentialing required for teaching mindfulness. While there are certificate programs to become an MBSR instructor [106], many programs have branched off from Jon Kabat-Zinn's original model and even studies of mindfulness interventions vary in the qualifications of those implementing instruction to subjects. It is a further challenge to find practitioners that have completed both MBSR and trauma-informed training, and still further, rarely so with specific qualifications to work with youth. Importantly, even trauma therapists who offer mindfulness in practice, have varying degrees of self-practice that may impact their level of involvement [107].

There have been attempts at unique modifications to programming for children or those with special focused needs (Tables 2 and 3). Some studies have specifically involved instructors who have had years of experience specifically with children [78–82]. One study partnered a mental health therapist with adolescents in the community to co-facilitate a mindfulness meditation practice, though the study does not comment on the level of experience of the mental health therapist with mindfulness [108]. For mindfulness training implementation in schools, many programs have branched from the classic MBSR program as described by Meiklejohn et al., 2012 [109]. For example, The Mindfulness in Schools Project (UK based), based on MBSR, is one that has been studied with successful outcomes including fewer depressive symptoms in adolescents, and the Mindful Schools (US based) improved teacher-based perceptions of classroom behavior in a 6th grade public elementary school children [110,111]. Many similar programs to The Mindfulness in Schools Project and Mindful Schools, as seen in Table 3, share in their methodology that mindfulness trained individuals lead practices in the school environment and also educate teachers to lead students [109].

Though many studies have administered mindfulness interventions to teachers, showing benefits for teaching work-environment and temperament [88], none have assessed associated student outcomes directly as a result of the teachers training in isolation. However, the training of teachers is a promising approach to improved classroom outcomes. One study cited by Gouda et al., 2016, showed that schoolteachers (n = 82) had self-reported improvements in mood as well as measures of improved emotional regulation (decreased reactivity, increased compassion) as compared to controls, though the subjects were all female [112], and another showing decreased distress [113]. A smaller study (n = 15) with similar outcome measures also suggested reduction in burnout [114]. Based on such studies, programs have launched to improve classroom learning environments such as the "Cultivating Awareness and Resilience in Education" Program [90]. Since, a larger combined RCT recently showed improvements in schoolteacher sleep and work satisfaction and decreased bad mood, but this was of a workplace mindfulness training not specific to educational environments [115]. Though only one small case study in preschool students showed decrease in negative social interactions [89], taken with the teacher trials, these studies suggest that it may be worth considering that future studies assess the effects and consider if training teachers alone may impact resiliency against ACEs. Therefore, perhaps implementation of programming for both students and teachers is ideal, as found by Gouda et al., 2016 in that both students and teachers showed improvement in interpersonal problems, and affect, whereas students also showed improved school-specific self-efficacy by specific developed self-assessment questionnaires [88]. It is important to keep in mind that lack of benefit of mindfulness in schools programs can be due to lack of teacher experience [116].

Even outside of the school, teacher-led environment, children are never cared for in isolation. It may be beneficial to consider methodology of mindfulness implementation that addresses their caretakers. Given that mindful parenting yields reduced parental stress, with increased parental warmth toward their children [10,91], suggests that mindful parenting training should also be included in interventions for youth. However, many caretakers are involved in influencing children. As examples, one intervention partnered therapists with peer instructors, and another allowed time for individualized intervention for youth (average age 11.5 years) and their parents, then partnered them for family intervention [88,108,117]. The intervention to strengthen families (n = 9) involved seven 2-h sessions with the first hour individualized between youth and their parents and the second hour for family training. It also allowed time for mindful parenting training with teaching and practice exercises on being mindful (attentive, reducing emotional reactivity, being less judgmental) [117], demonstrating how a holistic approach including caretakers, parents and children may be implemented.

Table 2. Variations in mindfulness programs and implementation.

Population	Program	Instruction	Setting	Duration	Reference
Public urban middle school (5th–8th grade; avg. 12 years), *n* = 300	Adapted MBSR	Trained MBSR instructors and personal practice 10+ years	School	12 weekly 50-min sessions	Sibinga et al., 2016 [79]
Foster care youth ages 14–21, *n* = 42	Adapted MBSR	Psychologist with expertise in mindfulness, two pediatrician lead group activities	Conference room of a joint family visitation and clinic space	10 weekly 2-h sessions	Jee et al., 2015 [80]
Kindergarten through 6th grade, low-income and ethnic minority students, *n* = 409	Mindful Schools (MS) Program or MS Plus	MS instructor with 3–20 years mindful meditation experience and classroom teacher facilitated	School	5-week (MS) or 7-week (MS Plus), 15-min sessions running three times per week	Black and Fernando, 2014 [118]
Ages 13–21, underserved youth, *n* = 43	Adapted MBSR	Instructors trained in MBSR, 10+ years' experience	Primary care pediatric clinic	8 weekly 2-h sessions	Sibinga et al., 2014 [81]
Middle-school, urban youth, *n* = 41	Adapted MBSR	Trained MBSR instructor, 10+ years' experience	School	12 weekly 50-min sessions	Sibinga et al., 2013 [78]
Adolescents ages 12–16 years, multiple schools, *n* = 522	School teacher facilitated adapted MBSR (Mindfulness in Schools Project – UK)	Teachers trained by instructors with MBSR training	School	9-week	Kuyken et al., 2013 [83]
6th grade students, *n* = 101	Meditation instruction and student writing exercises	One teacher with meditation training and 5+ years' experience, one teacher who completed MBSR course, no experience	School	Daily for 6 weeks	Britton et al., 2014 [84]
Adolescents ages 14–18, *n* = 104	Adapted MBSR	Instructors MBSR trained	Outpatient psychiatric facility	8-week, 2 h/week, home 20–25 min homework daily	Biegel et al., 2009 [87]
Age 11–15 years, with ADHD, parents, and tutors; *n* = 38	Adapted MBSR combining Mindfulness in Schools Project, and methods for children with ADHD	Instructors trained in MBSR	Group program at an academic treatment center	8-week	van de Weijer-Bergsma et al., 2012 [85]
Ages 13–21, HIV infected, *n* = 11	Adapted MBSR	Instructor trained in MBSR, prior experience	Group at specialty HIV clinic	Eight 2-h sessions and a 3-h retreat	Sibinga et al., 2008 [82]

MBSR, Mindfulness Based Stress Reduction; ADHD, attention-deficit/hyperactivity disorder; HIV, human immunodeficiency virus.

Table 3. Examples of structured mindfulness programs for children.

Program Title	Website
Inner Resilience Program	http://www.innerresilience-tidescenter.org/
Wellness and Resilience Program	http://sbsd.schoolfusion.us/modules/cms/pages.phtml?pageid=195404&SID
Mindful Schools	www.mindfulschools.org
Learning to Breathe	www.learning2breathe.org
Mindfulness in Schools Project (".b", or "Stop and Be!" curriculum)	www.mindfulnessinschools.org
Still Quiet Place	www.stillquietplace.com
Stressed Teens	www.stressedteens.com
Wellness Works in Schools	www.wellnessworksinschools.com
Center for Mindful Awareness	www.centerformindfulawareness.org

The type and location of intervention taught varies tremendously in the literature. As discussed and seen in Table 2, many interventions are integrated directly into school curriculum [88], but also have been offered as extracurricular, in the clinic setting (primary care and specialty), during incarceration, and to parents [81,82,85,87,95,108,119]. Some offer mindfulness only as an addition to a structured and detailed training program with other included skillsets including cognitive therapy, behavioral therapy, resilience training for healthy behaviors, and meditation [6,108,119,120]. There is no study to date that has compared settings, but variation may be dependent on population and outcome of interest. For example, if targeting improvements in mood dysfunction, this has been seen across settings by various different outcome measures for PTSD, depression and anxiety. Attention and behavior outcomes are more commonly measures in studies of school-based interventions, though importantly, there is no evidence that interventions outside of school would not produce effects in the school environment. Given the broad exposure to traumas and ACEs, and the generalizable benefits of mindfulness, mindfulness programs offered through school and/or primary care sites may be most suited to reaching the broadest population of children.

The methods of mindfulness implementation may vary given the diversity of existing academic curricula and environments for youth. Generally, schools offer the most appropriate environment to reach a broad spectrum of children across developmental stages, diagnoses, and socioeconomic circumstances, as well as stressor exposure [116]. Incorporation of mindfulness practice directly into the school curriculum addresses the suggestion of the school environment as a means to reach broad categories of children [78,79,81,86,88]. Examples of broad reaching implementations were postulated by Britton et al. who allotted half a semester on a course to mindfulness with the second half preserved for other curriculum and a mid-year switch of groups, or by Johnstone et al., who proposes to complete a study with a 2-semester health class incorporating eight weeks of mindfulness into the class [84,121]. Kuyken et al. replaced studies in either religious studies or personal, social and health education, offering the idea that perhaps mindfulness could be offered as an elective course in the curriculum [83].

Though the school environment offers a promising delivery format for teaching mindfulness, other methods have been suggested. Home practice is one such model and may offer shorter study formats requiring as little as 5 min [122]. Some formats have even bridged home study with one-on-one in home training [95]. Clinic groups if advertised as a 'social' group rather than a 'stress management' group may pose another potential format [80]. To enhance participation regardless of the format studies have implemented facilitating transportation to class, reminder phone calls, and providing snacks, for example [123]. Other organizations are implementing mindfulness into women and children's shelters and community centers [124].

In school, home and clinic environments, a generalized training in mindfulness allows for broad population applicability, but individualized programs also may be helpful in certain specified populations. An example of individualization of mindfulness intervention methodology for a unique trauma exposed population was accomplished by a program that identified reactivity as a problem in incarcerated individuals and tailored the program "S.T.I.C". S.T.I.C. involves the following steps: stop, take a breath, imagine, and choose, allowing the mindfulness and attention to be directed at consequences and redirection of choices [119]. Though S.T.I.C. was individualized by targeting a specific population, personalization can also be accomplished in school or clinic settings by narrowing the target population such as by diagnosis or age. For example, one study clustered female students with any eating disorder history into a mindfulness program finding improved psychosocial outcomes relative to control by six months post-intervention [120]. Grouping by diagnosis has also been beneficial in the diagnoses of attention-deficit/hyperactivity disorder (ADHD), HIV, or psychiatric conditions [82,85,87], with incorporation of mindfulness into existing therapeutic interventions like cognitive or rehabilitation therapy, MBCT or MBRP, specifically. The RAP Club was offered exclusively to 7th and 8th grade students and catered to adolescent specific life challenges in the program design [108], whereas others incorporated simplistic terminology that can be applied to younger and older students such as, "FOFBOC: Feet on the floor and bum on chair", and "Beditation" referring to a body scan done while lying down [116]. Finally, mindfulness technique has been applied in combination with other therapies including sound and music, touch, walking, daily routines, and even "mindful texting" to allow for the inclusion of mindfulness in regular activities with the idea of "checking in" with the self as much as possible throughout the day [125]. For translating concepts of mindfulness to children, metaphors can be helpful and many children's books are available including those authored by Thich Nhat Hahn, a Buddhist monk who has helped bring the practice of mindfulness to western society with John Kabat-Zinn [126].

4.2. Trauma-Informed Care

Per the Substance Abuse and Mental Health Services Administration (SAMHSA) a program that is trauma-informed realizes trauma prevalence and its common adverse effects, recognizes signs and symptoms of trauma, responds with standard operating procedures, and seeks to resist re-traumatization. SAMHSA provides various examples of well-known trauma-informed intervention programs and they all include general principals of safety, connection and trustworthiness, collaboration, empowerment, and current and historical societal and cultural competency [127]. Formal mindfulness instructor training incorporates a number of these elements and lays the foundation for mindfulness as a trauma-informed care (TIC) practice.

In trauma-informed care, an intervention may be primary (preventive), secondary (reduction of severity and acuity of consequences), or tertiary (treatment of long-term sequelae) [128]. Though it is important for clinicians involved in intervention administration to be cognizant of the above principals of TIC, this does not necessarily mean that the specific stressors or traumas need to be identified for mindfulness to have a beneficial effect, though this has not specifically studied. There is a high prevalence of stress and trauma, with up to 34% of children in school reporting exposure to at least one trauma and evidence of post-traumatic stress even without a current diagnosis [8]. Further, it is known that abuse and trauma is underreported [129] and poorly recalled [130]. Even when reported, child memory of trauma can include intrusions or inaccurate recall [131], and symptoms of PTSD are often poorly recognized by parents [132]. In studies assessing previous trauma, methods of quantification vary widely from general indication of trauma domain to specifics of traumatic event(s). Further, PTSD may mask itself through generalized somatic complaints in children including trouble sleeping, low energy, stomach pain, dizziness, and headaches [133]. Taken together, these studies suggest that one cannot rely on always and accurately identifying the presence of traumatic experience in children. Yet, mindfulness may have an impact in children whether they report a trauma exposure, or not. Trait mindfulness is associated with resilience in face of adverse events, and is associated with strong cognitive abilities, and mindfulness interventions can reduce somatic manifestations of psychiatric undertones [6,70,71,87,134,135]. In populations with high likelihood of ACEs, such as low-income urban areas, school-based mindfulness instruction provided to all students (primary prevention) has been shown to improve psychological symptoms and coping and to reduce post-trauma stress symptoms [79]. Therefore, mindfulness interventions that lead to enhanced coping and resilience can be beneficial when offered to all children regardless of specific identification of trauma exposure.

5. Conclusions and Future Directions

In conclusion, research has demonstrated that high-quality, structured mindfulness interventions improve mental, behavioral, and physical outcomes in youth. Further, these results in combination with the well-studied interventions in adults suggest promise in preventing the poor health outcomes associated with trauma exposure in childhood. Future work should aim to optimize the implementation of high-quality mindfulness programs in youth populations. Further research should explore the mechanisms of mindfulness and the long-term outcomes of mindfulness interventions in childhood into adulthood, as well as outcomes in offspring.

References

1. Felitti, V.J.; Anda, R.F.; Nordenberg, D.; Williamson, D.F.; Spitz, A.M.; Edwards, V.; Koss, M.P.; Marks, J.S. Relationship of childhood abuse and household dysfunction to many of the leading causes of death in adults. The adverse childhood experiences (ACE) study. *Am. J. Prev. Med.* **1998**, *14*, 245–258. [CrossRef]
2. Shonkoff, J.P.; Garner, A.S.; Committee on Psychosocial Aspects of Child and Family Healty; Committee on Early Childhood Adoption, and Dependent Care; Section on Developmental and Behavioral Pediatrics. The lifelong effects of early childhood adversity and toxic stress. *Pediatrics* **2012**, *129*, e232–e246. [CrossRef] [PubMed]
3. Johnson, S.B.; Riley, A.W.; Granger, D.A.; Riis, J. The science of early life toxic stress for pediatric practice and advocacy. *Pediatrics* **2013**, *131*, 319–327. [CrossRef] [PubMed]
4. Danese, A.; McEwen, B.S. Adverse childhood experiences, allostasis, allostatic load, and age-related disease. *Physiol. Behav.* **2012**, *106*, 29–39. [CrossRef] [PubMed]
5. Wrenn, G.L.; Wingo, A.P.; Moore, R.; Pelletier, T.; Gutman, A.R.; Bradley, B.; Ressler, K.J. The effect of resilience on posttraumatic stress disorder in trauma-exposed inner-city primary care patients. *J. Natl. Med. Assoc.* **2011**, *103*, 560–566. [CrossRef]
6. Chandler, G.E.; Roberts, S.J.; Chiodo, L. Resilience intervention for young adults with adverse childhood experiences. *J. Am. Psychiatr. Nurses Assoc.* **2015**, *21*, 406–416. [CrossRef] [PubMed]
7. *Adverse Childhood Experiences Reported by Adults—Five States, 2009*; CDC: Atlanta, GA, USA, 2010; pp. 1609–1613.
8. Gonzalez, A.; Monzon, N.; Solis, D.; Jaycox, L.; Langley, A.K. Trauma exposure in elementary school children: Description of screening procedures, level of exposure, and posttraumatic stress symptoms. *Sch. Ment. Health* **2016**, *8*, 77–88. [CrossRef] [PubMed]
9. Umeda, M.; Oshio, T.; Fujii, M. The impact of the experience of childhood poverty on adult health-risk behaviors in japan: A mediation analysis. *Int. J. Equity Health* **2015**, *14*, 145. [CrossRef] [PubMed]
10. Carroll, J.E.; Gruenewald, T.L.; Taylor, S.E.; Janicki-Deverts, D.; Matthews, K.A.; Seeman, T.E. Childhood abuse, parental warmth, and adult multisystem biological risk in the coronary artery risk development in young adults study. *Proc. Natl. Acad. Sci. USA* **2013**, *110*, 17149–17153. [CrossRef] [PubMed]
11. Harter, S.L. Psychosocial adjustment of adult children of alcoholics: A review of the recent empirical literature. *Clin. Psychol. Rev.* **2000**, *20*, 311–337. [CrossRef]
12. Garner, A.S.; Shonkoff, J.P.; Committee on Psychosocial Aspects of Child and Family Health; Committee on Early Childhood, Adoption, and Dependent Care; Section on Developmental and Behavioral Pediatrics. Early childhood adversity, toxic stress, and the role of the pediatrician: Translating developmental science into lifelong health. *Pediatrics* **2012**, *129*, e224–e231. [PubMed]
13. Danese, A.; Moffitt, T.E.; Harrington, H.; Milne, B.J.; Polanczyk, G.; Pariante, C.M.; Poulton, R.; Caspi, A. Adverse childhood experiences and adult risk factors for age-related disease: Depression, inflammation, and clustering of metabolic risk markers. *Arch. Pediatr. Adolesc. Med.* **2009**, *163*, 1135–1143. [CrossRef] [PubMed]

14. Demetriou, C.A.; van Veldhoven, K.; Relton, C.; Stringhini, S.; Kyriacou, K.; Vineis, P. Biological embedding of early-life exposures and disease risk in humans: A role for DNA methylation. *Eur. J. Clin. Investig.* **2015**, *45*, 303–332. [CrossRef] [PubMed]
15. Yehuda, R.; Daskalakis, N.P.; Bierer, L.M.; Bader, H.N.; Klengel, T.; Holsboer, F.; Binder, E.B. Holocaust exposure induced intergenerational effects on *FKBP5* methylation. *Biol. Psychiatry* **2016**, *80*, 372–380. [CrossRef] [PubMed]
16. Benner, A.D.; Boyle, A.E.; Sadler, S. Parental involvement and adolescents' educational success: The roles of prior achievement and socioeconomic status. *J. Youth Adolesc.* **2016**, *45*, 1053–1064. [CrossRef] [PubMed]
17. Mills-Koonce, W.R.; Willoughby, M.T.; Garrett-Peters, P.; Wagner, N.; Vernon-Feagans, L.; Family Life Project Key Investigators. The interplay among socioeconomic status, household chaos, and parenting in the prediction of child conduct problems and callous-unemotional behaviors. *Dev. Psychopathol.* **2016**, *28*, 757–771. [CrossRef] [PubMed]
18. Potijk, M.R.; Kerstjens, J.M.; Bos, A.F.; Reijneveld, S.A.; de Winter, A.F. Developmental delay in moderately preterm-born children with low socioeconomic status: Risks multiply. *J. Pediatr.* **2013**, *163*, 1289–1295. [CrossRef] [PubMed]
19. Ursache, A.; Noble, K.G.; Pediatric Imaging, Neurocognition and Genetics Study. Socioeconomic status, white matter, and executive function in children. *Brain Behav.* **2016**, *6*, e00531. [CrossRef] [PubMed]
20. Ursache, A.; Noble, K.G. Neurocognitive development in socioeconomic context: Multiple mechanisms and implications for measuring socioeconomic status. *Psychophysiology* **2016**, *53*, 71–82. [CrossRef] [PubMed]
21. Saleh, A.; Potter, G.G.; McQuoid, D.R.; Boyd, B.; Turner, R.; MacFall, J.R.; Taylor, W.D. Effects of early life stress on depression, cognitive performance and brain morphology. *Psychol. Med.* **2017**, *47*, 171–181. [CrossRef] [PubMed]
22. Scharoun-Lee, M.; Adair, L.S.; Kaufman, J.S.; Gordon-Larsen, P. Obesity, race/ethnicity and the multiple dimensions of socioeconomic status during the transition to adulthood: A factor analysis approach. *Soc. Sci. Med.* **2009**, *68*, 708–716. [CrossRef] [PubMed]
23. Anda, R.F.; Croft, J.B.; Felitti, V.J.; Nordenberg, D.; Giles, W.H.; Williamson, D.F.; Giovino, G.A. Adverse childhood experiences and smoking during adolescence and adulthood. *JAMA* **1999**, *282*, 1652–1658. [CrossRef] [PubMed]
24. Su, S.; Wang, X.; Pollock, J.S.; Treiber, F.A.; Xu, X.; Snieder, H.; McCall, W.V.; Stefanek, M.; Harshfield, G.A. Adverse childhood experiences and blood pressure trajectories from childhood to young adulthood: The Georgia stress and heart study. *Circulation* **2015**, *131*, 1674–1681. [CrossRef] [PubMed]
25. Taylor, S.E.; Lerner, J.S.; Sage, R.M.; Lehman, B.J.; Seeman, T.E. Early environment, emotions, responses to stress, and health. *J. Personal.* **2004**, *72*, 1365–1393. [CrossRef] [PubMed]
26. Rothman, E.F.; Edwards, E.M.; Heeren, T.; Hingson, R.W. Adverse childhood experiences predict earlier age of drinking onset: Results from a representative us sample of current or former drinkers. *Pediatrics* **2008**, *122*, e298–e304. [CrossRef] [PubMed]
27. Yao, H.; Rahman, I. Current concepts on the role of inflammation in COPD and lung cancer. *Curr. Opin. Pharmacol.* **2009**, *9*, 375–383. [CrossRef] [PubMed]
28. Li, M.; Zhou, Y.; Feng, G.; Su, S.B. The critical role of toll-like receptor signaling pathways in the induction and progression of autoimmune diseases. *Curr. Mol. Med.* **2009**, *9*, 365–374. [CrossRef] [PubMed]
29. Salinas-Miranda, A.A.; Salemi, J.L.; King, L.M.; Baldwin, J.A.; Berry, E.L.; Austin, D.A.; Scarborough, K.; Spooner, K.K.; Zoorob, R.J.; Salihu, H.M. Adverse childhood experiences and health-related quality of life in adulthood: Revelations from a community needs assessment. *Health Qual. Life Outcomes* **2015**, *13*, 123. [CrossRef] [PubMed]
30. Mair, C.; Cunradi, C.B.; Todd, M. Adverse childhood experiences and intimate partner violence: Testing psychosocial mediational pathways among couples. *Ann. Epidemiol.* **2012**, *22*, 832–839. [CrossRef] [PubMed]
31. Hillis, S.D.; Anda, R.F.; Felitti, V.J.; Nordenberg, D.; Marchbanks, P.A. Adverse childhood experiences and sexually transmitted diseases in men and women: A retrospective study. *Pediatrics* **2000**, *106*, E11. [CrossRef] [PubMed]
32. Fuller-Thomson, E.; Baird, S.L.; Dhrodia, R.; Brennenstuhl, S. The association between adverse childhood experiences (ACES) and suicide attempts in a population-based study. *Child Care Health Dev.* **2016**, *42*, 725–734. [CrossRef] [PubMed]

33. Duke, N.N.; Pettingell, S.L.; McMorris, B.J.; Borowsky, I.W. Adolescent violence perpetration: Associations with multiple types of adverse childhood experiences. *Pediatrics* **2010**, *125*, e778–e786. [CrossRef] [PubMed]
34. Skarupski, K.A.; Parisi, J.M.; Thorpe, R.; Tanner, E.; Gross, D. The association of adverse childhood experiences with mid-life depressive symptoms and quality of life among incarcerated males: Exploring multiple mediation. *Aging Ment. Health* **2016**, *20*, 655–666. [CrossRef] [PubMed]
35. Ortiz, R.; Ballard, E.D.; Machado-Vieira, R.; Saligan, L.N.; Walitt, B. Quantifying the influence of child abuse history on the cardinal symptoms of fibromyalgia. *Clin. Exp. Rheumatol.* **2016**, *34*, S59–S66. [PubMed]
36. Tietjen, G.E.; Khubchandani, J.; Herial, N.A.; Shah, K. Adverse childhood experiences are associated with migraine and vascular biomarkers. *Headache* **2012**, *52*, 920–929. [CrossRef] [PubMed]
37. Park, S.H.; Videlock, E.J.; Shih, W.; Presson, A.P.; Mayer, E.A.; Chang, L. Adverse childhood experiences are associated with irritable bowel syndrome and gastrointestinal symptom severity. *Neurogastroenterol. Motil.* **2016**, *28*, 1252–1260. [CrossRef] [PubMed]
38. Bader, K.; Schafer, V.; Schenkel, M.; Nissen, L.; Schwander, J. Adverse childhood experiences associated with sleep in primary insomnia. *J. Sleep Res.* **2007**, *16*, 285–296. [CrossRef] [PubMed]
39. Brown, M.J.; Thacker, L.R.; Cohen, S.A. Association between adverse childhood experiences and diagnosis of cancer. *PLoS ONE* **2013**, *8*, e65524. [CrossRef] [PubMed]
40. Poletti, S.; Colombo, C.; Benedetti, F. Adverse childhood experiences worsen cognitive distortion during adult bipolar depression. *Compr. Psychiatry* **2014**, *55*, 1803–1808. [CrossRef] [PubMed]
41. Burke, N.J.; Hellman, J.L.; Scott, B.G.; Weems, C.F.; Carrion, V.G. The impact of adverse childhood experiences on an urban pediatric population. *Child Abus. Negl.* **2011**, *35*, 408–413. [CrossRef] [PubMed]
42. Hillis, S.D.; Anda, R.F.; Dube, S.R.; Felitti, V.J.; Marchbanks, P.A.; Marks, J.S. The association between adverse childhood experiences and adolescent pregnancy, long-term psychosocial consequences, and fetal death. *Pediatrics* **2004**, *113*, 320–327. [CrossRef] [PubMed]
43. Kabat-Zinn, J. *Full Catastrophe Living: Using the Wisdom of Your Body and Mind to Face Stress, Pain, and Illness*; Dell Publishing: New York, NY, USA, 1990.
44. Carmody, J.; Baer, R.A. Relationships between mindfulness practice and levels of mindfulness, medical and psychological symptoms and well-being in a mindfulness-based stress reduction program. *J. Behav. Med.* **2008**, *31*, 23–33. [CrossRef] [PubMed]
45. Baer, R.A.; Smith, G.T.; Hopkins, J.; Krietemeyer, J.; Toney, L. Using self-report assessment methods to explore facets of mindfulness. *Assessment* **2006**, *13*, 27–45. [CrossRef] [PubMed]
46. Batink, T.; Peeters, F.; Geschwind, N.; van Os, J.; Wichers, M. How does MBCT for depression work? Studying cognitive and affective mediation pathways. *PLoS ONE* **2013**, *8*, e72778. [CrossRef] [PubMed]
47. Bowen, S.; Chawla, N.; Collins, S.E.; Witkiewitz, K.; Hsu, S.; Grow, J.; Clifasefi, S.; Garner, M.; Douglass, A.; Larimer, M.E.; et al. Mindfulness-based relapse prevention for substance use disorders: A pilot efficacy trial. *Subst. Abus.* **2009**, *30*, 295–305. [CrossRef] [PubMed]
48. Gallegos, A.M.; Lytle, M.C.; Moynihan, J.A.; Talbot, N.L. Mindfulness-based stress reduction to enhance psychological functioning and improve inflammatory biomarkers in trauma-exposed women: A pilot study. *Psychol Trauma* **2015**, *7*, 525–532. [CrossRef]
49. Kimbrough, E.; Magyari, T.; Langenberg, P.; Chesney, M.; Berman, B. Mindfulness intervention for child abuse survivors. *J. Clin. Psychol.* **2010**, *66*, 17–33. [PubMed]
50. Earley, M.D.; Chesney, M.A.; Frye, J.; Greene, P.A.; Berman, B.; Kimbrough, E. Mindfulness intervention for child abuse survivors: A 2.5-year follow-up. *J. Clin. Psychol.* **2014**, *70*, 933–941. [CrossRef] [PubMed]
51. Ferszt, G.G.; Miller, R.J.; Hickey, J.E.; Maull, F.; Crisp, K. The impact of a mindfulness based program on perceived stress, anxiety, depression and sleep of incarcerated women. *Int. J. Environ. Res. Public Health* **2015**, *12*, 11594–11607. [CrossRef] [PubMed]
52. Kalmanowitz, D.L.; Ho, R.T. Art therapy and mindfulness with survivors of political violence: A qualitative study. *Psychol. Trauma* **2016**. [CrossRef] [PubMed]
53. Klatt, M.; Steinberg, B.; Duchemin, A.M. Mindfulness in motion (MIM): An onsite mindfulness based intervention (MBI) for chronically high stress work environments to increase resiliency and work engagement. *J. Vis. Exp.* **2015**, e52359. [CrossRef] [PubMed]

54. Johnson, D.C.; Thom, N.J.; Stanley, E.A.; Haase, L.; Simmons, A.N.; Shih, P.A.; Thompson, W.K.; Potterat, E.G.; Minor, T.R.; Paulus, M.P. Modifying resilience mechanisms in at-risk individuals: A controlled study of mindfulness training in marines preparing for deployment. *Am. J. Psychiatry* **2014**, *171*, 844–853. [CrossRef] [PubMed]
55. Polusny, M.A.; Erbes, C.R.; Thuras, P.; Moran, A.; Lamberty, G.J.; Collins, R.C.; Rodman, J.L.; Lim, K.O. Mindfulness-based stress reduction for posttraumatic stress disorder among veterans: A randomized clinical trial. *JAMA* **2015**, *314*, 456–465. [CrossRef] [PubMed]
56. Possemato, K.; Bergen-Cico, D.; Treatman, S.; Allen, C.; Wade, M.; Pigeon, W. A randomized clinical trial of primary care brief mindfulness training for veterans with PTSD. *J. Clin. Psychol.* **2016**, *72*, 179–193. [CrossRef]
57. Bergen-Cico, D.; Possemato, K.; Pigeon, W. Reductions in cortisol associated with primary care brief mindfulness program for veterans with PTSD. *Med. Care* **2014**, *52*, S25–S31. [CrossRef] [PubMed]
58. Bormann, J.E.; Oman, D.; Walter, K.H.; Johnson, B.D. Mindful attention increases and mediates psychological outcomes following mantram repetition practice in veterans with posttraumatic stress disorder. *Med. Care* **2014**, *52*, S13–S18. [CrossRef] [PubMed]
59. Heffner, K.L.; Crean, H.F.; Kemp, J.E. Meditation programs for veterans with posttraumatic stress disorder: Aggregate findings from a multi-site evaluation. *Psychol. Trauma* **2016**, *8*, 365–374. [CrossRef] [PubMed]
60. Kluepfel, L.; Ward, T.; Yehuda, R.; Dimoulas, E.; Smith, A.; Daly, K. The evaluation of mindfulness-based stress reduction for veterans with mental health conditions. *J. Holist Nurs.* **2013**, *31*, 248–255. [CrossRef]
61. Sylvia, L.G.; Bui, E.; Baier, A.L.; Mehta, D.H.; Denninger, J.W.; Fricchione, G.L.; Casey, A.; Kagan, L.; Park, E.R.; Simon, N.M. Resilient warrior: A stress management group to improve psychological health in service members. *Glob. Adv. Health Med.* **2015**, *4*, 38–42. [CrossRef] [PubMed]
62. Azad Marzabadi, E.; Hashemi Zadeh, S.M. The effectiveness of mindfulness training in improving the quality of life of the war victims with post traumatic stress disorder (PTSD). *Iran. J. Psychiatry* **2014**, *9*, 228–236. [PubMed]
63. Omidi, A.; Mohammadi, A.; Zargar, F.; Akbari, H. Efficacy of mindfulness-based stress reduction on mood states of veterans with post-traumatic stress disorder. *Arch. Trauma Res.* **2013**, *1*, 151–154. [CrossRef] [PubMed]
64. Poon, A.; Danoff-Burg, S. Mindfulness as a moderator in expressive writing. *J. Clin. Psychol.* **2011**, *67*, 881–895. [CrossRef] [PubMed]
65. Dahm, K.A.; Meyer, E.C.; Neff, K.D.; Kimbrel, N.A.; Gulliver, S.B.; Morissette, S.B. Mindfulness, self-compassion, posttraumatic stress disorder symptoms, and functional disability in U.S. Iraq and Afghanistan war veterans. *J. Trauma. Stress* **2015**, *28*, 460–464. [CrossRef] [PubMed]
66. Basharpoor, S.; Shafiei, M.; Daneshvar, S. The comparison of experiential avoidance, [corrected] mindfulness and rumination in trauma-exposed individuals with and without posttraumatic stress disorder (PTSD) in an Iranian sample. *Arch. Psychiatr. Nurs.* **2015**, *29*, 279–283. [CrossRef]
67. Thieleman, K.; Cacciatore, J. Witness to suffering: Mindfulness and compassion fatigue among traumatic bereavement volunteers and professionals. *Soc. Work* **2014**, *59*, 34–41. [CrossRef]
68. Chiesa, A.; Serretti, A. Mindfulness-based stress reduction for stress management in healthy people: A review and meta-analysis. *J. Altern. Complement. Med.* **2009**, *15*, 593–600. [CrossRef]
69. Goyal, M.; Singh, S.; Sibinga, E.M.; Gould, N.F.; Rowland-Seymour, A.; Sharma, R.; Berger, Z.; Sleicher, D.; Maron, D.D.; Shihab, H.M.; et al. Meditation programs for psychological stress and well-being: A systematic review and meta-analysis. *JAMA Intern. Med.* **2014**, *174*, 357–368. [CrossRef] [PubMed]
70. Mahoney, C.T.; Segal, D.L.; Coolidge, F.L. Anxiety sensitivity, experiential avoidance, and mindfulness among younger and older adults: Age differences in risk factors for anxiety symptoms. *Int. J. Aging Hum. Dev.* **2015**, *81*, 217–240. [CrossRef] [PubMed]
71. Patterson, P.; McDonald, F.E. "Being mindful": Does it help adolescents and young adults who have completed cancer treatment? *J. Pediatr. Oncol. Nurs.* **2015**, *32*, 189–194. [CrossRef] [PubMed]
72. Senders, A.; Bourdette, D.; Hanes, D.; Yadav, V.; Shinto, L. Perceived stress in multiple sclerosis: The potential role of mindfulness in health and well-being. *J. Evid. Based Complemen. Altern. Med.* **2014**, *19*, 104–111. [CrossRef] [PubMed]
73. Sharplin, G.R.; Jones, S.B.; Hancock, B.; Knott, V.E.; Bowden, J.A.; Whitford, H.S. Mindfulness-based cognitive therapy: An efficacious community-based group intervention for depression and anxiety in a sample of cancer patients. *Med. J. Aust.* **2010**, *193*, S79–S82. [PubMed]

74. Gonzalez, A.; Locicero, B.; Mahaffey, B.; Fleming, C.; Harris, J.; Vujanovic, A.A. Internalized Hiv stigma and mindfulness: Associations with PTSD symptom severity in trauma-exposed adults with HIV/AIDS. *Behav. Modif.* **2016**, *40*, 144–163. [CrossRef] [PubMed]
75. Black, D.S.; Slavich, G.M. Mindfulness meditation and the immune system: A systematic review of randomized controlled trials. *Ann. N. Y. Acad. Sci.* **2016**, *1373*, 13–24. [CrossRef] [PubMed]
76. Creswell, J.D.; Taren, A.A.; Lindsay, E.K.; Greco, C.M.; Gianaros, P.J.; Fairgrieve, A.; Marsland, A.L.; Brown, K.W.; Way, B.M.; Rosen, R.K.; et al. Alterations in resting-state functional connectivity link mindfulness meditation with reduced interleukin-6: A randomized controlled trial. *Biol. Psychiatry* **2016**, *80*, 53–61. [CrossRef] [PubMed]
77. Kaliman, P.; Alvarez-Lopez, M.J.; Cosin-Tomas, M.; Rosenkranz, M.A.; Lutz, A.; Davidson, R.J. Rapid changes in histone deacetylases and inflammatory gene expression in expert meditators. *Psychoneuroendocrinology* **2014**, *40*, 96–107. [CrossRef] [PubMed]
78. Sibinga, E.M.; Perry-Parrish, C.; Chung, S.E.; Johnson, S.B.; Smith, M.; Ellen, J.M. School-based mindfulness instruction for urban male youth: A small randomized controlled trial. *Prev. Med.* **2013**, *57*, 799–801. [CrossRef] [PubMed]
79. Sibinga, E.M.; Webb, L.; Ghazarian, S.R.; Ellen, J.M. School-based mindfulness instruction: An RCT. *Pediatrics* **2016**, *137*. [CrossRef] [PubMed]
80. Jee, S.H.; Couderc, J.P.; Swanson, D.; Gallegos, A.; Hilliard, C.; Blumkin, A.; Cunningham, K.; Heinert, S. A pilot randomized trial teaching mindfulness-based stress reduction to traumatized youth in foster care. *Complement. Ther. Clin. Pract.* **2015**, *21*, 201–209. [CrossRef]
81. Sibinga, E.M.; Perry-Parrish, C.; Thorpe, K.; Mika, M.; Ellen, J.M. A small mixed-method RCT of mindfulness instruction for urban youth. *Explore* **2014**, *10*, 180–186. [CrossRef] [PubMed]
82. Sibinga, E.M.; Stewart, M.; Magyari, T.; Welsh, C.K.; Hutton, N.; Ellen, J.M. Mindfulness-based stress reduction for hiv-infected youth: A pilot study. *Explore* **2008**, *4*, 36–37. [CrossRef] [PubMed]
83. Kuyken, W.; Weare, K.; Ukoumunne, O.C.; Vicary, R.; Motton, N.; Burnett, R.; Cullen, C.; Hennelly, S.; Huppert, F. Effectiveness of the mindfulness in schools programme: Non-randomised controlled feasibility study. *Br. J. Psychiatry* **2013**, *203*, 126–131. [CrossRef] [PubMed]
84. Britton, W.B.; Lepp, N.E.; Niles, H.F.; Rocha, T.; Fisher, N.E.; Gold, J.S. A randomized controlled pilot trial of classroom-based mindfulness meditation compared to an active control condition in sixth-grade children. *J. Sch. Psychol.* **2014**, *52*, 263–278. [CrossRef] [PubMed]
85. Van de Weijer-Bergsma, E.; Formsma, A.R.; de Bruin, E.I.; Bogels, S.M. The effectiveness of mindfulness training on behavioral problems and attentional functioning in adolescents with adhd. *J. Child Fam. Stud.* **2012**, *21*, 775–787. [CrossRef] [PubMed]
86. Black, D.S.; O'Reilly, G.A.; Olmstead, R.; Breen, E.C.; Irwin, M.R. Mindfulness meditation and improvement in sleep quality and daytime impairment among older adults with sleep disturbances: A randomized clinical trial. *JAMA Intern. Med.* **2015**, *175*, 494–501. [CrossRef] [PubMed]
87. Biegel, G.M.; Brown, K.W.; Shapiro, S.L.; Schubert, C.M. Mindfulness-based stress reduction for the treatment of adolescent psychiatric outpatients: A randomized clinical trial. *J. Consult. Clin. Psychol.* **2009**, *77*, 855–866. [CrossRef] [PubMed]
88. Gouda, S.; Luong, M.T.; Schmidt, S.; Bauer, J. Students and teachers benefit from mindfulness-based stress reduction in a school-embedded pilot study. *Front. Psychol.* **2016**, *7*, 590. [CrossRef] [PubMed]
89. Singh, N.N.; Lancioni, G.E.; Winton, A.S.W.; Karazsia, B.T.; Singh, J. Mindfulness training for teachers changes the behavior of their preschool students. *Res. Human Dev.* **2013**, *10*, 211–233. [CrossRef]
90. Jennings, P.A.; Frank, J.L.; Snowberg, K.E.; Coccia, M.A.; Greenberg, M.T. Improving classroom learning environments by cultivating awareness and resilience in education (care): Results of a randomized controlled trial. *Sch. Psychol. Q.* **2013**, *28*, 374–390. [CrossRef]
91. Bethell, C.; Gombojav, N.; Solloway, M.; Wissow, L. Adverse childhood experiences, resilience and mindfulness-based approaches: Common denominator issues for children with emotional, mental, or behavioral problems. *Child Adolesc. Psychiatr. Clin. N. Am.* **2016**, *25*, 139–156. [CrossRef] [PubMed]
92. Townshend, K.; Jordan, Z.; Stephenson, M.; Tsey, K. The effectiveness of mindful parenting programs in promoting parents' and children's wellbeing: A systematic review. *JBI Database Syst. Rev. Implement. Rep.* **2016**, *14*, 139–180. [CrossRef] [PubMed]

93. Parent, J.; Clifton, J.; Forehand, R.; Golub, A.; Reid, M.; Pichler, E.R. Parental mindfulness and dyadic relationship quality in low-income cohabiting black stepfamilies: Associations with parenting experienced by adolescents. *Couple Fam. Psychol.* **2014**, *3*, 67–82. [CrossRef] [PubMed]
94. Parent, J.; McKee, L.G.; J, N.R.; Forehand, R. The association of parent mindfulness with parenting and youth psychopathology across three developmental stages. *J. Abnorm Child Psychol.* **2016**, *44*, 191–202. [CrossRef] [PubMed]
95. Dawe, S.; Harnett, P. Reducing potential for child abuse among methadone-maintained parents: Results from a randomized controlled trial. *J. Subst. Abus. Treat.* **2007**, *32*, 381–390. [CrossRef] [PubMed]
96. Wingo, A.P.; Wrenn, G.; Pelletier, T.; Gutman, A.R.; Bradley, B.; Ressler, K.J. Moderating effects of resilience on depression in individuals with a history of childhood abuse or trauma exposure. *J. Affect. Disord.* **2010**, *126*, 411–414. [CrossRef] [PubMed]
97. Wingo, A.P.; Fani, N.; Bradley, B.; Ressler, K.J. Psychological resilience and neurocognitive performance in a traumatized community sample. *Depress Anxiety* **2010**, *27*, 768–774. [CrossRef] [PubMed]
98. Connor, K.M.; Davidson, J.R. Development of a new resilience scale: The Connor-Davidson Resilience Scale (CD-RISC). *Depress Anxiety* **2003**, *18*, 76–82. [CrossRef] [PubMed]
99. Sinclair, V.G.; Wallston, K.A. The development and psychometric evaluation of the brief resilient coping scale. *Assessment* **2004**, *11*, 94–101. [CrossRef] [PubMed]
100. Thompson, R.W.; Arnkoff, D.B.; Glass, C.R. Conceptualizing mindfulness and acceptance as components of psychological resilience to trauma. *Trauma Violence Abus.* **2011**, *12*, 220–235. [CrossRef] [PubMed]
101. Vujanovic, A.A.; Youngwirth, N.E.; Johnson, K.A.; Zvolensky, M.J. Mindfulness-based acceptance and posttraumatic stress symptoms among trauma-exposed adults without axis i psychopathology. *J. Anxiety Disord.* **2009**, *23*, 297–303. [CrossRef] [PubMed]
102. Perry-Parrish, C.; Copeland-Linder, N.; Webb, L.; Sibinga, E.M. Mindfulness-based approaches for children and youth. *Curr. Probl. Pediatr. Adolesc. Health Care* **2016**, *46*, 172–178. [CrossRef] [PubMed]
103. Garland, E.L.; Roberts-Lewis, A. Differential roles of thought suppression and dispositional mindfulness in posttraumatic stress symptoms and craving. *Addict. Behav.* **2013**, *38*, 1555–1562. [CrossRef] [PubMed]
104. Kabat-Zinn, J. An outpatient program in behavioral medicine for chronic pain patients based on the practice of mindfulness meditation: Theoretical considerations and preliminary results. *Gen. Hosp. Psychiatry* **1982**, *4*, 33–47. [CrossRef]
105. Carmody, J.; Baer, R.A. How long does a mindfulness-based stress reduction program need to be? A review of class contact hours and effect sizes for psychological distress. *J. Clin. Psychol.* **2009**, *65*, 627–638. [CrossRef] [PubMed]
106. Mindfulness-Based Professional Education. Available online: http://www.umassmed.edu/cfm/training/ (accesses on 20 December 2016).
107. Waelde, L.C.; Thompson, J.M.; Robinson, A.; Iwanicki, S. Trauma therapists' clinical applications, training, and personal practice of mindfulness and meditation. *Mindfulness* **2016**, *7*, 622–629. [CrossRef] [PubMed]
108. Mendelson, T.; Tandon, S.D.; O'Brennan, L.; Leaf, P.J.; Ialongo, N.S. Brief report: Moving prevention into schools: The impact of a trauma-informed school-based intervention. *J. Adolesc.* **2015**, *43*, 142–147. [CrossRef] [PubMed]
109. Meiklejohn, J.; Phillips, C.; Freedman, M.L.; Griffin, M.L.; Biegel, G.; Roach, A.; Frank, J.; Burke, C.; Pinger, L.; Soloway, G.; et al. Integrating mindfulness training into k-12 education: Fostering the resilience of teachers and students. *Mindfulness* **2012**, *3*, 291–307. [CrossRef]
110. Mindful in Schools Project. Available online: https://mindfulnessinschools.org (accesses on 20 December 2016).
111. Mindful Schools. Available online: http://www.mindfulschools.org/ (accesses on 20 December 2016).
112. Kemeny, M.E.; Foltz, C.; Cavanagh, J.F.; Cullen, M.; Giese-Davis, J.; Jennings, P.; Rosenberg, E.L.; Gillath, O.; Shaver, P.R.; Wallace, B.A.; et al. Contemplative/emotion training reduces negative emotional behavior and promotes prosocial responses. *Emotion* **2012**, *12*, 338–350. [CrossRef] [PubMed]
113. Franco, C.; Manas, I.; Cangas, A.J.; Moreno, E.; Gallego, J. Reducing teachers' psychological distress through a mindfulness training program. *Span. J. Psychol.* **2010**, *13*, 655–666. [CrossRef] [PubMed]
114. Flook, L.; Goldberg, S.B.; Pinger, L.; Bonus, K.; Davidson, R.J. Mindfulness for teachers: A pilot study to assess effects on stress, burnout and teaching efficacy. *Mind Brain Educ.* **2013**, *7*. [CrossRef] [PubMed]
115. Crain, T.L.; Schonert-Reichl, K.A.; Roeser, R.W. Cultivating teacher mindfulness: Effects of a randomized controlled trial on work, home, and sleep outcomes. *J. Occup. Health Psychol.* **2016**. [CrossRef] [PubMed]

116. Johnson, C.; Burke, C.; Brinkman, S.; Wade, T. Effectiveness of a school-based mindfulness program for transdiagnostic prevention in young adolescents. *Behav. Res. Ther.* **2016**, *81*, 1–11. [CrossRef] [PubMed]
117. Duncan, L.G.; Coatsworth, J.D.; Greenberg, M.T. Pilot study to gauge acceptability of a mindfulness-based, family-focused preventive intervention. *J. Prim. Prev.* **2009**, *30*, 605–618. [CrossRef] [PubMed]
118. Black, D.S.; Fernando, R. Mindfulness Training and Classroom Behavior Among Lower-Income and Ethnic Minority Elementary School Children. *J. Child. Fam. Stud.* **2014**, *23*, 1242–1246. [CrossRef] [PubMed]
119. Himelstein, S.; Saul, S.; Garcia-Romeu, A.; Pinedo, D. Mindfulness training as an intervention for substance user incarcerated adolescents: A pilot grounded theory study. *Subst. Use Misuse* **2014**, *49*, 560–570. [CrossRef] [PubMed]
120. Atkinson, M.J.; Wade, T.D. Mindfulness-based prevention for eating disorders: A school-based cluster randomized controlled study. *Int. J. Eat. Disord.* **2015**, *48*, 1024–1037. [CrossRef] [PubMed]
121. Johnstone, J.M.; Roake, C.; Sheikh, I.; Mole, A.; Nigg, J.T.; Oken, B. School-based mindfulness intervention for stress reduction in adolescents: Design and methodology of an open-label, parallel group, randomized controlled trial. *Contemp. Clin. Trials Commun.* **2016**, *4*, 99–104. [CrossRef] [PubMed]
122. Lee, L.; Semple, R.J.; Rosa, D.; Miller, L. Mindfulness-based cognitive therapy for children: Results of a pilot study. *J. Cogn. Psychother.* **2008**, *22*, 15–28. [CrossRef]
123. Kerrigan, D.; Johnson, K.; Stewart, M.; Magyari, T.; Hutton, N.; Ellen, J.M.; Sibinga, E.M. Perceptions, experiences, and shifts in perspective occurring among urban youth participating in a mindfulness-based stress reduction program. *Complement. Ther. Clin. Pract.* **2011**, *17*, 96–101. [CrossRef] [PubMed]
124. Connolly, A. Center for mindful awareness. Available online: http://centerformindfulawareness.org/ (accessed on 20 December 2016).
125. Thompson, M.; Gauntlett-Gilbert, J. Mindfulness with children and adolescents: Effective clinical application. *Clin. Child Psychol. Psychiatry* **2008**, *13*, 395–407. [CrossRef] [PubMed]
126. Hanh, T.N. *Planting Seeds: Practicing Mindfulness with Children*; Parallax Press: Berkeley, CA, USA, 2007.
127. Trauma-informed approach and trauma-specific interventions. Available online: https://www.samhsa.gov/nctic/trauma-interventions (accessed on 20 December 2016).
128. Oral, R.; Ramirez, M.; Coohey, C.; Nakada, S.; Walz, A.; Kuntz, A.; Benoit, J.; Peek-Asa, C. Adverse childhood experiences and trauma informed care: The future of health care. *Pediatr. Res.* **2016**, *79*, 227–233. [CrossRef] [PubMed]
129. Luce, H.; Schrager, S.; Gilchrist, V. Sexual assault of women. *Am. Fam. Physician* **2010**, *81*, 489–495. [PubMed]
130. Williams, L.M. Recall of childhood trauma: A prospective study of women's memories of child sexual abuse. *J. Consult. Clin. Psychol.* **1994**, *62*, 1167–1176. [CrossRef] [PubMed]
131. Howe, M.L.; Courage, M.L.; Peterson, C. Intrusions in preschoolers' recall of traumatic childhood events. *Psychon. Bull. Rev.* **1995**, *2*, 130–134. [CrossRef] [PubMed]
132. Meiser-Stedman, R.; Smith, P.; Yule, W.; Glucksman, E.; Dalgleish, T. Posttraumatic stress disorder in young children 3 years posttrauma: Prevalence and longitudinal predictors. *J. Clin. Psychiatry* **2016**. [CrossRef] [PubMed]
133. Zhang, Y.; Zhang, J.; Zhu, S.; Du, C.; Zhang, W. Prevalence and predictors of somatic symptoms among child and adolescents with probable posttraumatic stress disorder: A cross-sectional study conducted in 21 primary and secondary schools after an earthquake. *PLoS ONE* **2015**, *10*, e0137101. [CrossRef] [PubMed]
134. Keng, S.L.; Tong, E.M. Riding the tide of emotions with mindfulness: Mindfulness, affect dynamics, and the mediating role of coping. *Emotion* **2016**, *16*, 706–718. [CrossRef] [PubMed]
135. Teper, R.; Inzlicht, M. Meditation, mindfulness and executive control: The importance of emotional acceptance and brain-based performance monitoring. *Soc. Cogn. Affect. Neurosci.* **2013**, *8*, 85–92. [CrossRef] [PubMed]

16

Integrative Pediatrics: Successful Implementation of Integrative Medicine in a German Hospital Setting—Concept and Realization

Marion Eckert [1,*], Catharina Amarell [1], Dennis Anheyer [2], Holger Cramer [2] and Gustav Dobos [2]

1 Kinderkrankenhaus St. Marien, Grillparzerstr. 9, 84036 Landshut, Germany; catharina.amarell@st-marien-la.de
2 Department of Internal and Integrative Medicine, Kliniken Essen-Mitte, Faculty of Medicine, University of Duisburg-Essen, Am Deimelsberg 34a, 45276 Essen, Germany; D.Anheyer@kliniken-essen-mitte.de (D.A.); H.Cramer@kliniken-essen-mitte.de (H.C.); g.dobos@kliniken-essen-mitte.de (G.D.)
* Correspondence: dr-eckert@t-online.de

Abstract: Complementary and Alternative Medicine (CAM) has not been systematically institutionalized in pediatric hospital care in Germany so far. For the responsible implementation and systematic evaluation of CAM in pediatric care, a model project was initialized in three different pediatric hospitals in Germany, one of them being the "Kinderkrankenhaus St. Marien" in Landshut, Germany. During this project, a concept of the implementation process was developed based on clinical care, teaching, and scientific evaluation. A project group was formed in St. Marien, which included leaders of the hospital, physicians, nurses, and physiotherapists. Over a period of three years, pediatric treatment modalities of the CAM-spectrum were systematically integrated into routine pediatric care and a new integrative medicine department was established. CAM is now being applied in an inpatient as well as outpatient setting, in addition to conventional medical treatments. The modalities now applied include Traditional Chinese Medicine (TCM), relaxation, hypnosis, reflexology, wraps and poultices, aromatherapy, homeopathy, yoga, and herbal medicine. Studies were initiated in some areas. The process and concept leading up to this successful implementation will be described in this article. We show that with motivated team players and structured proceedings, implementation of integrative medicine in a children's hospital can be successful.

Keywords: integrative medicine; pediatrics; clinical practice

---

1. Introduction

Integrative Medicine (IM) is an emerging field, even if the increasingly wide use of Complementary and Alternative Medicine (CAM) and its incorporation into conventional medicine has been described in numerous publications [1–3]. IM incorporates the use of methods of the CAM spectrum into conventional medicine in an evidence-based way and integrates the whole person and the environment that person lives in into the treatment of adults as well as children. The Academic Consortium of Integrative Medicine & Health (ACIMH) states that "Integrative Medicine is the practice of medicine that reaffirms the importance of the relationship between practitioner and patient, focuses on the whole person, is informed by evidence, and makes use of all appropriate therapeutic approaches, healthcare professionals and disciplines to achieve optimal health and healing" [4].

Many authors have described the substantial increase in the use of CAM, not only in adults, but also in children [3,5–11], as well as the lack of information the treating physicians receive about the methods used and the possible side-effects that some of these treatments may have [12–14]. A variety of treatment modalities are nowadays applied in integrative medicine in the field of pediatrics [2]. Teaching programs for physicians and residents have been developed to increase their knowledge about and widen their spectrum of CAM treatments [15–17]. Many institutions have implemented integrative medicine in various models, even in hospitals [1,18–20]. Some of them have identified important factors and strategies that are vital for successful implementation [18,19]. Yet, CAM has not been widely systematically institutionalized in pediatric care in Germany so far—in hospitals or private practice.

Our intent was to implement integrative medicine in a pediatric hospital, by building a concept upon our and other's experiences that can be applicable and useful for different hospitals that strive to develop such programs. We also aimed at contributing to scientific insights on the modalities used. Therefore, at the very start of the project, an overview regarding the scientific situation of CAM in pediatrics was compiled and possible indications for CAM in children identified in a multidisciplinary meeting.

2. The Hospital Setting of St. Marien

The Children's Hospital "Kinderkrankenhaus St. Marien" in Landshut, Germany, is an academic teaching hospital of the LMU (Ludwig-Maximilians-University) München. It is equipped with 120 beds. An average of 6500 children are treated annually on the wards and about 16,000 children in the specialized outpatient departments. Seventeen thousand children are seen in the pediatric emergency department annually. A social pediatric center, which takes care of about 5200 patients per year, is affiliated with the hospital.

St. Marien Hospital has always been dedicated to promoting integrative approaches for the medical treatment of children. Besides conventional medicine, additional certifications of attending physicians allowed for naturopathic and homeopathic treatments, even in the years before our project started. For the past 10 years for example, a pediatrician with certification in homeopathy has been employed in the hospital treating inpatients as well as children in the outpatient department. A pediatrician certified in naturopathic medicine had also established policies for the application of naturopathic treatments for pertinent indications like upper airway infections or certain pain conditions.

3. Preparation

Whenever an institution takes a new direction, it is important that its leaders make decisions on the new course of action to be taken from then on. This needs to be communicated and future expectations made clear to the rest of the organization. This also applies to establishing an integrative medical care model within a hospital. Only then does the body of the organization know that a new corporate strategy is being pursued and employees are expected to act upon it in certain ways. In addition, a decision needs to be made on the areas in which CAM is supposed to be integrated in the hospital. The areas can be clinical, teaching, or research [19], depending on the structure of the hospital and interests of the organization. Not every institution will want to or be able to serve all three areas and this is not necessary. Various models, from e.g., focusing on pain management, research orientation, or offering a wide variety of integrative care modalities to patients, can work [19]. Furthermore, there are different approaches that can be taken in order to execute the new strategy. One is a model from "inside" the institution; the other would be a more external approach in which new staff with new skills is employed to start a new venture. We chose the model from inside, in which we built upon the skills and motivation of staff members. This offers the advantage of using existing resources and preventing resistance from staff members on new treatment methods. This has been described as one of the cornerstones of a successful implementation [19].

4. First Steps

First, a project group with members of different disciplines of the hospital with one coordinating leader was formed. This group met once a month to determine next steps to be taken and goals to accomplish.

It was beneficial to have the executive director of the hospital as a part of the group, amongst attending physicians of different disciplines, nursing management, nurses, physiotherapists, and psychologists in order to reach staff members from different disciplines and to build integrative medicine from inside the organization. A new sense of a common comprehensive project led to the necessary enthusiasm in all participants. It was important for the coordinating leader to be an experienced senior pediatrician, also trained in a broad field of complementary medicine, and someone who was accepted by all members of the project group. This leader was responsible for coordinating activities, establishment of contacts, development of next steps, creating questionnaires, communication with other facilities and researchers, networking, and motivation. Leaders from other pediatric integrative medicine programs were contacted and literature was reviewed for advice and ideas on how to successfully establish integrative medicine within a hospital [18,19,21].

The second step involved the determination of resources existing within the hospital. Hospital staff—be it nurses, doctors or physiotherapists—have a variety of additional qualifications in the area of complementary medicine, which they would readily apply in their work. To determine the existing resources, a questionnaire was designed, as other centers had done before in a similar way [22]. The questionnaire included questions about additional qualifications, overall interest in CAM being introduced in the hospital, and interest to use those qualifications in the treatment of children. We found that there was an immense variety of knowledge and skills already present in St. Marien (Table 1), similar to modalities applied in other centers in the US [2]. It was these resources that we utilized to build upon in the process of implementing IM in our institution.

Table 1. Existing staff expertise within St. Marien revealed through questionnaires.

Aromatherapy	Foot Reflexology	Massage
Art therapy	Homeopathy	Music therapy
Biofeedback	Naturopathy	Therapeutic riding
Craniosacral therapy	Nutritional counseling	Yoga

Thirdly we were interested in the assessment of desires of parents. Many studies showed that CAM methods are readily applied in children and that parents also desire the use of CAM in the treatment of their children [3,23]. There are regional differences though, so we wanted to know about the wishes of the parents in the local area as well as their past experiences with CAM and willingness to make additional payments for the integration of CAM in the treatment of their child. Therefore, another questionnaire was created and given to the parents arriving at the hospital. The majority of parents were very approving of CAM treatments for their children. These data will be published in a separate article and therefore will not be further described.

The fourth step was to start educating the nurses, physicians and other staff on different kinds of CAM methods. It is an advantage if there is a culture of regular teaching schedules (like lunch symposia or in-house trainings) already established within the institution. In St. Marien, CAM trainings were included in the in-house trainings taking place regularly. Teachings about aromatherapy, foot reflexology, wraps and poultices, homeopathy, hypnosis, and naturopathic treatment options were given by experts (physicians and nurses) this way. Instructions on the application of acupuncture needles, acupressure, aromatherapy, and homeopathy were also given to smaller groups on the wards. In addition, the staff gained practical experience and training in guided imagery and hypnosis as well as in naturopathic treatments over weekends and in half-day courses. This way, the staff learned about new treatment options and how and when to apply them. Knowledge was disseminated this way and new competencies were acquired (e.g., hypnosis for pain management, acupressure, etc.) and applied by nurses and physicians. Regular refresher teachings, including practical exercises to ensure quality of care, are being given.

In the process, it turned out to be essential to have one responsible, qualified physician, with additional qualifications in naturopathy and Traditional Chinese Medicine (TCM), who was able to anchor CAM deeper on the wards by making sure the new ways of treatment were being applied and by staff were being given repeated teachings. An outpatient clinic for CAM also was established. This is also according to the experience of other medical centers that emphasized on the advantage of having one protagonist leading the initiative in the hospital [19].

In order to publicize our institution's new corporate strategy and promote its presence, different paths were taken, within and outside the hospital. Flyers and posters were designed and displayed in the building, and the hospital website now provides specific details of the CAM services offered and the new department now in operation. A consult service was established and in-house teachings were held regularly. Medical discharge reports now include CAM treatments applied on children, in a bid to inform primary care physicians and make a public statement about the new corporate policy. In addition, articles in magazines and journals were published and interviews videotaped (available online [24,25]). All these efforts help in communicating the significance and new philosophy of the hospital to its staff and the public.

Another important step was creating structures within the hospital. Wards were specialized in different areas like aromatherapy or homeopathy according to interests and competencies of the nurses assigned to the wards. For example, nurses are responsible for keeping a track of stocks of homeopathic remedies or aroma oils, teachings on other wards, etc. CAM was made part of every ward conference meeting held by these nurses. Furthermore, policies for specific treatments were established and were made readily available on the intranet for physicians and nurses to refer to and download. CAM consult services were established across the hospital, as well as a CAM clinic. A curriculum has also been compiled, which every staff member—new and old—is required to go through (it takes approximately 8 h).

5. Financing

The challenge of financing CAM services has been addressed as an issue in most institutions [19,21]. It is absolutely necessary to have enough philanthropic support or available funds at least in the early stages, as financial resources are often scarce and money is needed for salaries, education of staff, and to generate research projects. In our case, this turned out to be the biggest cost factor at the beginning, diminishing over time though, as most staff was trained and the new treatment methods became routine. Trained staff members can now partly assume the teaching of colleagues and therefore diminish the need of external, costly teachers. The clinical care component was self-supporting and not too expensive. In the US as well as in Germany, CAM services are mostly not covered by health insurances. Endowment funding therefore is essential to support sustainability. All of the biggest centers that offer CAM services in the US (e.g., Osher Centers at Harvard and Penny George Institute for Health and Healing) have several million dollars of endowment funding for support. In Germany, foundations can provide substantial monetary inputs. In addition, it turned out beneficial to negotiate special deals with insurance companies that at least many families now profit from. Cost effectiveness of integrative care over time has been demonstrated on numerous occasions [26–28].

6. Results of Our Project

Starting in 2015, complementary medicine was introduced step by step in the routine care of children and an integrative approach was established, which led to the foundation of an integrative medicine department with an attending physician in 2017. One of the first steps we took was identifying the resources present in the hospital, which we could draw upon. A questionnaire for the staff was designed and handed out to all staff members. Questions included the overall interest in the introduction of CAM treatments in the hospital as well as additional certifications of staff members. Seventy-seven percent of those who had answered the questionnaire reported having an interest in CAM methods. While most of them were nursing staff members (58%), 31% were physicians. Areas that garnered most interest were acupuncture, osteopathy, aromatherapy, and naturopathy. As these results will be published in a separate article, they will not be described in detail here.

In the feedback part of the questionnaire, interest in the research topic was evident through several remarks like:

- "I think it is wonderful that our hospital belongs to the more progressive ones. I support CAM treatments 100%."
- "I am VERY happy, that CAM is now being established in our hospital and I hope that nursing staff can participate in trainings and teachings."
- "I think this area is really interesting and important, I would love to receive additional training and participate."

CAM Services Now Offered at St. Marien

Apart from homeopathy, which has a long history at St. Marien, many other treatment modalities were integrated in the everyday care of the children at St. Marien, within three years of our project:

1. Aromatherapy is now being used regularly on hospitalized patients as roll-on sticks and in form of wraps and poultices. One nurse successfully completed her certification as an aromatherapist.
2. Acupuncture points have been taught to nurses and physicians and are now being applied in the form of pyonex press needles inserted in the acupuncture point P6 (pericard 6) to almost all children under anesthesia to prevent post-operative nausea and vomiting. Several studies have shown that P6 can be as effective as antiemetic drugs in preventing post-operative nausea and vomiting [29]. Nurses and doctors have been trained to insert the needles and regular refresher teachings take place.
3. Acupressure points are being taught to children and parents for cough, anxiety, abdominal pain, and nausea.
4. Another treatment modality is foot reflexology according to Hanne Marquardt [30]. Two indications were chosen—abdominal and lung conditions—and their treatment methods were taught to staff and parents. It is now being used regularly. A study was initiated and started in September 2016 to determine the effect of reflexology on children with these conditions.
5. Yoga is being offered in the hospital now and a study was initiated and completed by our research partner in Essen, Germany, about the effect of yoga for headaches in children.
6. Basic hypnotherapy methods (like "the magic glove") were taught to physicians and nurses over the course of two weekends and are now being applied regularly.
7. Wraps and poultices are used in combination with aroma oils in the Newborn Intensive Care Unit (NICU) and the pediatric wards on patients with rheumatic diseases, anxiety, fever, joint pain, sleep problems, abdominal pain, and cough, among others.
8. Two doctors are now consulting on the wards on request for integrative treatment options for a variety of conditions. One of them is a certified homeopath, the other one is certified in naturopathy and TCM.
9. A "handling" course for parents has been held a few times since September 2016 to enable them to touch and move their babies in a more supportive and physiologic way to help their developmental process.
10. Herbal remedies are being applied and medical reference cards (detailing indications and dosage) have been designed for physicians.
11. A multidisciplinary pain management team now applies CAM Methods for treating pain in children.
12. Relaxation techniques of mind-body medicine are applied in the psychosomatic unit and social pediatric center.

7. Discussion

Integrating CAM methods into routine care for children within a hospital to create a real "integrative care" can be challenging. However, through our program, we demonstrated that CAM can successfully be integrated into a pediatric hospital in a relatively short time. The cornerstones that were essential to our process are summarized here and overlap some of which have been described as important components of other successful programs [18,19] as well as learned through personal communications (Kemper 2015).

1. The institution in which methods of the CAM spectrum require establishment has to make a clear decision on the path that should be taken.
2. Institutional support from the executive leader and medical director of the institution is essential. They represent the hospital and determine the overall concept of the institution. In our case, the leaders communicated well with each other about the new business concept, relayed this to their staff and put plans in place for it to be introduced by them. This enabled efficient evolution of the project and offered the prospect of sustainability.
3. It is important to have back-up support within the organization, as leaders can change over time. The project becomes vulnerable if the primary protagonist leaves. At least one well-respected person, preferably a qualified physician, should take the lead in the beginning. This person does not have to be an expert in all offered CAM modalities, but must be willing to cooperate with other CAM experts so that all team members can learn from each other. In St. Marien, two physicians led the project—one in the coordinating role and the other as an integrative physician present and active in the hospital.
4. It is crucial to have philanthropic support or available funds. Financial resources are often scarce and money is required for salaries, education of staff, and to generate research projects.
5. To minimize resistance, it is advisable to build on the prevalent interest of the institution. Depending on the organization, it could be research or clinical applications, or education, or a combination of both. It is easier to first follow that path and strengthen it before starting new ventures. In our case, clinical applications and education of staff were where the most interest was found, followed by research. We followed that interest, used existing resources, and tapped on motivation of the staff members (identified through a questionnaire) and subsequently built the new concept from inside out to keep staff members motivated.
6. It is essential to have motivated, creative colleagues working together, who can solve problems and find solutions one person can't see.
7. Networking with like-minded colleagues and institutions creates motivation and inspiration. Sharing ideas and experiences can help expand the project. In our project, three hospitals were involved and common projects were created and ideas exchanged in regular meetings with all participants. Networking with international colleagues also created inspiration and offered new ideas.
8. It is important to not implement several modalities at once. To have a clear and simple treatment plan in which the patient can develop a relationship with the therapist is better that an overwhelming and expensive plan. In addition, too many new modalities can lead to an overload of the staff and therefore lead to resistance, which is not good for the project. We selected our modalities by identifying evidence-based knowledge and experience present within the hospital. Although there is a lack of evidence in the treatment of children, in accordance with other centers, we did not exclude modalities that had inadequate evidence [19]; instead, we evaluated efficacy by performing meta-analyses and reviews on various topics [31–34].
9. Multidisciplinary meetings can help broaden one's spectrum of knowledge and experiences within the institution.

10. Research programs can be important in some institutions. Academic centers mostly want and need to add research to the project. Again, it is essential to follow the interest of the staff members and collaborate with other disciplines.
11. Education is an important aspect of any facility, be it in the form of lectures for students, training and rotations for staff members, or workshops.
12. Financing is a challenge in all centers. Financial plans have to be made, fundings organized, and payments by patients considered.
13. Cooperation and communication with colleagues in other hospitals as well as in private practices have to be established, in order to ensure complete integration into the field. In Germany, resistance can be quite high if the hospital offers treatments that colleagues in private practices don't. This can hinder the success of the project. A qualified physician or well-respected person has to represent the project in order to raise acceptance and reputation of the institution.

Pediatric Integrative Medicine programs are found in several US medical centers and a few in Europe [18,19,35]. In 2009, nine US medical centers that played an important pioneer role in integrative medicine were interviewed on the critical factors leading to success or failure of the establishment of IM in hospitals in the fields of research, education, and clinical application [19]. Many of the factors discussed are consistent with our findings, and therefore can be considered essential in the process of implementing an integrative medicine program in any institution.

8. Conclusions

Integrative medicine can be established in a pediatric hospital, if there is support from leaders, has a motivated, multidisciplinary team with a qualified leader, and enough philanthropic or institutional initial funding. Regular team meetings to identify and pursue goals, communication of these within the institution, and repeated teaching modules that meet the interest of the staff are essential strategies to ensure motivation and sustainability. Also, the addition of CAM treatments into the curriculum of residents and nurses will allow for an even-deeper anchoring of integrative medicine into the institution. As a next step, new treatment standards and policies encompassing CAM treatments for various conditions can be defined, so they become a natural part of routine care of the hospital. Parental desire for CAM treatments is strong and a variety of indications are suitable for their application.

Author Contributions: M.E. was primarily responsible for the coordination of the project as well as the conception and design of this article. C.A. is the leading physician for integrative medicine at St. Marien and was responsible for the implementation of the new treatment concepts and critically revised the manuscript. D.A. and H.C. were responsible for the scientific supervision of the project, participated in conception and design of the project, and critically revised the manuscript. G.D. initiated and designed the whole project and critically revised the manuscript. All authors approved the final manuscript.

Acknowledgments: We thank Hilary McClafferty and Kathi Kemper for all the support provided during and for the finalization of this project. We also thank Bernhard Brand for the support and encouragement in the realization of new pathways at St. Marien. We also thank Anita Eder, without whom our success would not have been possible.

References

1. Horrigan, B.; Lewis, S.; Abrams, D.I.; Pechura, C. *How Integrative Medicine Is Being Practiced in Clinical Centers across the United States*; The Bravewell Collaborative: Minneapolis, MN, USA, 2012. Available online: http://www.bravewell.org/current_projects/mapping_field/ (accessed on 20 May 2018).
2. Vohra, S.; Surette, S.; Mittra, D.; Rosen, L.D.; Gardiner, P.; Kemper, K.J. Pediatric integrative medicine: Pediatrics' newest subspecialty? *BMC Pediatr.* **2012**, *12*, 123. [CrossRef] [PubMed]

3. Zuzak, T.J.; Boňková, J.; Careddu, D.; Garami, M.; Hadjipanayis, A.; Jazbec, J.; Merrick, J.; Miller, J.; Ozturk, C.; Persson, I.A.; et al. Use of complementary and alternative medicine by children in Europe: Published data and expert perspectives. *Complement. Ther. Med.* **2013**, *21* (Suppl. 1), S34–S47. [CrossRef] [PubMed]
4. Academic Consortium of Integrative Medicine and Health (ACIMH). Definition of Integrative Medicine and Health. Available online: https://www.imconsortium.org/about/about-us.cfm (accessed on 5 June 2018).
5. Du, Y.; Wolf, I.K.; Zhuang, W.; Bodemann, S.; Knöss, W.; Knopf, H. Use of herbal medicinal products among children and adolescents in Germany. *BMC Complement. Altern. Med.* **2014**, *14*, 218. [CrossRef] [PubMed]
6. Du, Y.; Knopf, H. Paediatric homoeopathy in Germany: Results of the German Health Interview and Examination Survey for Children and Adolescents (KiGGS). *Pharmacoepidemiol. Drug Saf.* **2009**, *18*, 370–379. [CrossRef] [PubMed]
7. Du, Y.; Knopf, H. Self-medication among children and adolescents in Germany: Results of the National Health Survey for Children and Adolescents (KiGGS). *Br. J. Clin. Pharmacol.* **2009**, *68*, 599–608. [CrossRef] [PubMed]
8. Italia, S.; Wolfenstetter, S.B.; Teuner, C.M. Patterns of complementary and alternative medicine (CAM) use in children: A systematic review. *Eur. J. Pediatr.* **2014**, *173*, 1413–1428. [CrossRef] [PubMed]
9. Kemper, K.J.; Vohra, S.; Walls, R. American Academy of Pediatrics. The use of complementary and alternative medicine in pediatrics. *Pediatrics* **2008**, *122*, 1374–1386. [CrossRef] [PubMed]
10. Lin, Y.C.; Lee, A.C.; Kemper, K.J.; Berde, C.B. Use of complementary and alternative medicine in pediatric pain management service: A survey. *Pain Med.* **2005**, *6*, 452–458. [CrossRef] [PubMed]
11. Groenewald, C.B.; Beals-Erickson, S.E.; Ralston-Wilson, J.; Rabbitts, J.A.; Palermo, T.M. Complementary and Alternative Medicine Use by Children With Pain in the United States. *Acad. Pediatr.* **2017**, *17*, 785–793. [CrossRef] [PubMed]
12. Sidora-Arcoleo, K.; Yoos, H.L.; Kitzman, H.; McMullen, A.; Anson, E. Don't ask, don't tell: Parental nondisclosure of complementary and alternative medicine and over-the-counter medication use in children's asthma management. *J. Pediatr. Health Care* **2008**, *22*, 221–229. [CrossRef] [PubMed]
13. Lindly, O.; Thorburn, S.; Zuckerman, K. Use and Nondisclosure of Complementary Health Approaches Among US Children with Developmental Disabilities. *J. Dev. Behav. Pediatr.* **2018**, *39*, 217–227. [CrossRef] [PubMed]
14. Sibinga, E.M.; Ottolini, M.C.; Duggan, A.K.; Wilson, M.H. Parent-pediatrician communication about complementary and alternative medicine use for children. *Clin. Pediatr.* **2004**, *43*, 367–373. [CrossRef] [PubMed]
15. McClafferty, H.; Dodds, S.; Brooks, A.J.; Brenner, M.G.; Brown, M.L.; Frazer, P.; Mark, J.D.; Weydert, J.A.; Wilcox, G.M.; Lebensohn, P.; et al. Pediatric Integrative Medicine in Residency (PIMR): Description of a New Online Educational Curriculum. *Children* **2015**, *2*, 98–107. [CrossRef] [PubMed]
16. Lebensohn, P.; Kligler, B.; Brooks, A.J.; Teets, R.; Birch, M.; Cook, P.; Maizes, V. Integrative Medicine in Residency: Feasibility and Effectiveness of an Online Program. *Fam. Med.* **2017**, *49*, 514–521. [PubMed]
17. Academy of Integrative Health & Medicine (AIHM). Available online: https://www.aihm.org (accessed on 20 July 2018).
18. Von Rosenstiel, I.A.; Schats, W.; Bongers, K.; Jong, M.C. Integrative paediatrics: A Dutch experience. *Focus Altern. Complement. Ther.* **2011**, *16*, 22–27. [CrossRef]
19. Vohra, S.; Feldman, K.; Johnston, B.; Waters, K.; Boon, H. Integrating complementary and alternative medicine into academic medical centers: Experience and perceptions of nine leading centers in North America. *BMC Health Serv. Res.* **2005**, *5*, 78. [CrossRef] [PubMed]
20. Highfield, E.S.; McLellan, M.C.; Kemper, K.J.; Risko, W.; Woolf, A.D. Integration of complementary and alternative medicine in a major pediatric teaching hospital: An initial overview. *J. Altern. Complement. Med.* **2005**, *11*, 373–380. [CrossRef] [PubMed]
21. Eisenberg, D.M.; Kaptchuk, T.; Post, D.E.; Hrbek, A.L.; O'connor, B.B.; Osypiuk, K.; Wayne, P.M.; Buring, J.E.; Levy, D.B. Establishing an Integrative Medicine Program within an Academic Health Center: Essential Considerations. *Acad. Med.* **2016**, *91*, 1223–1230. [CrossRef] [PubMed]
22. Kemper, K.J.; Dirkse, D.; Eadie, D.; Pennington, M. What do clinicians want? Interest in integrative health services at a North Carolina academic medical center. *BMC Complement. Altern. Med.* **2007**, *7*, 5. [CrossRef] [PubMed]

23. Sencer, S.F.; Kelly, K.M. Complementary and alternative therapies in pediatric oncology. *Pediatr. Clin. N. Am.* **2007**, *54*, 1043–1060. [CrossRef] [PubMed]
24. Carstens Stiftung. Available online: https://www.carstens-stiftung.de/paediatrie.html (accessed on 20 July 2018).
25. Carstens Stiftung. Available online: https://www.youtube.com/results?search_query=integrative+pädiatrie (accessed on 20 July 2018).
26. Herman, P.M.; Poindexter, B.L.; Witt, C.M.; Eisenberg, D.M. Are complementary therapies and integrative care cost-effective? A systematic review of economic evaluations. *BMJ Open* **2012**, *2*, e001046. [CrossRef] [PubMed]
27. Baars, E.W.; Kooreman, P. A 6-year comparative economic evaluation of healthcare costs and mortality rates of Dutch patients from conventional and CAM GPs. *BMJ Open* **2014**, *4*, e005332. [CrossRef] [PubMed]
28. Deng, G.; Cassileth, B.R. Integrative oncology: Complementary therapies for pain, anxiety, and mood disturbance. *CA Cancer J. Clin.* **2005**, *55*, 109–116. [CrossRef] [PubMed]
29. Lee, A.; Chan, S.K.; Fan, L.T. Stimulation of the wrist acupuncture point PC6 for preventing postoperative nausea and vomiting. *Cochrane Database Syst. Rev.* **2015**, *11*, CD003281. [CrossRef] [PubMed]
30. Lett, A. The scope and limitations of treatment. An interview with Ann Lett, Principle, British School—Reflex Zone Therapy of the Feet. *Complement. Ther. Nurs. Midwifery* **2001**, *7*, 146–149. [CrossRef] [PubMed]
31. Anheyer, D.; Dobos, G.; Cramer, H. Evidenzlage pflanzlicher Präparate in der Anwendung bei Kindern und Jugendlichen. [Herbal medicines in children and adolescents—A narrative overview]. *Zeitschrift für Phytotherapie* **2016**, *6*, 236–241.
32. Anheyer, D.; Lauche, R.; Schumann, D.; Dobos, G.; Cramer, H. Herbal medicines in children with attention deficit hyperactivity disorder: A systematic review. *Complement. Ther. Med.* **2017**, *30*, 14–23. [CrossRef] [PubMed]
33. Anheyer, D.; Frawley, J.; Koch, A.K.; Lauche, R.; Langhorst, J.; Dobos, G.; Cramer, H. Herbal medicines for gastrointestinal disorders in children and adolescents: A systematic review. *Pediatrics* **2017**, *139*, e20170062. [CrossRef] [PubMed]
34. Anheyer, D.; Cramer, H.; Lauche, R.; Saha, F.J.; Dobos, G. Herbal medicine in children with respiratory tract infection: Systematic review and meta-analysis. *Acad. Pediatr.* **2018**, *18*, 8–19. [CrossRef] [PubMed]
35. Winther, C.; Von Rosenstiel, I.; Robinson, N.; Lee, R.; Shah, P.; Bukutu, C.; Koolen, R.; Vlieger, A.; Bongers, K.; Eckert, M.; et al. It'a small world—Pediatric CAM initiatives in the EU. *Focus Altern. Complement. Ther.* **2008**, *13*, 90–94. [CrossRef]

Permissions

All chapters in this book were first published by MDPI; hereby published with permission under the Creative Commons Attribution License or equivalent. Every chapter published in this book has been scrutinized by our experts. Their significance has been extensively debated. The topics covered herein carry significant findings which will fuel the growth of the discipline. They may even be implemented as practical applications or may be referred to as a beginning point for another development.

The contributors of this book come from diverse backgrounds, making this book a truly international effort. This book will bring forth new frontiers with its revolutionizing research information and detailed analysis of the nascent developments around the world.

We would like to thank all the contributing authors for lending their expertise to make the book truly unique. They have played a crucial role in the development of this book. Without their invaluable contributions this book wouldn't have been possible. They have made vital efforts to compile up to date information on the varied aspects of this subject to make this book a valuable addition to the collection of many professionals and students.

This book was conceptualized with the vision of imparting up-to-date information and advanced data in this field. To ensure the same, a matchless editorial board was set up. Every individual on the board went through rigorous rounds of assessment to prove their worth. After which they invested a large part of their time researching and compiling the most relevant data for our readers.

The editorial board has been involved in producing this book since its inception. They have spent rigorous hours researching and exploring the diverse topics which have resulted in the successful publishing of this book. They have passed on their knowledge of decades through this book. To expedite this challenging task, the publisher supported the team at every step. A small team of assistant editors was also appointed to further simplify the editing procedure and attain best results for the readers.

Apart from the editorial board, the designing team has also invested a significant amount of their time in understanding the subject and creating the most relevant covers. They scrutinized every image to scout for the most suitable representation of the subject and create an appropriate cover for the book.

The publishing team has been an ardent support to the editorial, designing and production team. Their endless efforts to recruit the best for this project, has resulted in the accomplishment of this book. They are a veteran in the field of academics and their pool of knowledge is as vast as their experience in printing. Their expertise and guidance has proved useful at every step. Their uncompromising quality standards have made this book an exceptional effort. Their encouragement from time to time has been an inspiration for everyone.

The publisher and the editorial board hope that this book will prove to be a valuable piece of knowledge for researchers, students, practitioners and scholars across the globe.

List of Contributors

Xiaojuan Shang and Luquan Chen
Department of Traditional Chinese Medicine, Beijing Tongren Hospital, Capital Medical University, Beijing 100730, China

Gerhard Litscher
Department of Traditional Chinese Medicine, Beijing Tongren Hospital, Capital Medical University, Beijing 100730, China
TCM Research Center Graz, Research Unit of Biomedical Engineering in Anesthesia and Intensive Care Medicine, and Research Unit for Complementary and Integrative Laser Medicine, Medical University of Graz, 8036 Graz, Austria
Department of Anesthesiology, Beijing Tongren Hospital, Capital Medical University, Beijing 100730, China
Department of Acupuncture and Moxibustion, Dongfang Hospital Affiliated to Beijing University of Chinese Medicine, Beijing 100078, China

Yanxia Sun and Chuxiong Pan
Department of Anesthesiology, Beijing Tongren Hospital, Capital Medical University, Beijing 100730, China

Cun-Zhi Liu
Department of Acupuncture and Moxibustion, Dongfang Hospital Affiliated to Beijing University of Chinese Medicine, Beijing 100078, China

Daniela Litscher
TCM Research Center Graz, Research Unit of Biomedical Engineering in Anesthesia and Intensive Care Medicine, and Research Unit for Complementary and Integrative Laser Medicine, Medical University of Graz, 8036 Graz, Austria

Lu Wang
Department of Traditional Chinese Medicine, Beijing Tongren Hospital, Capital Medical University, Beijing 100730, China
TCM Research Center Graz, Research Unit of Biomedical Engineering in Anesthesia and Intensive Care Medicine, and Research Unit for Complementary and Integrative Laser Medicine, Medical University of Graz, 8036 Graz, Austria
Department of Anesthesiology, Beijing Tongren Hospital, Capital Medical University, Beijing 100730, China

Suzi Tortora
Memorial Sloan Kettering Cancer Center, New York, NY 10021, USA
The Andréa Rizzo Foundation, Charlestown, RI 02813, USA

Kate Shafto
Department of Internal Medicine and Pediatrics, University of Minnesota, Minneapolis, MN 55455, USA
Division of Pediatric Anesthesia and Pain Medicine, Department of Anesthesiology, Perioperative and Pain Medicine, School of Medicine, Stanford University, Palo Alto, CA 94304, USA
Department of Pain Medicine, Palliative Care and Integrative Medicine, Children's Hospitals and Clinics of Minnesota, Minneapolis, MN 55404, USA

Melanie L. Brown
Department of Pediatrics, The University of Chicago, Chicago, IL 60637, USA
Department of Pain, Palliative Care and Integrative Medicine, Children's Hospitals and Clinics of Minnesota, Minneapolis, MN 55404, USA
Department of Pediatrics, University of Minnesota, Minneapolis, MN 55455, USA

Enrique Rojas and Suzanne Gouda
Department of Pediatrics, The University of Chicago, Chicago, IL 60637, USA

Anava A. Wren
Department of Pediatrics, Division of Pediatric Gastroenterology, Hepatology and Nutrition, Stanford University, Palo Alto, CA 94305, USA

Alexandra C. Ross
Department of Pediatrics, Child and Adolescent Headache Program, University of California San Francisco, San Francisco, CA 94158, USA

Genevieve D'Souza, Christina Almgren and Amanda Feinstein
Department of Anesthesiology Perioperative and Pain Medicine, Stanford University, Palo Alto, CA 94305, USA

Amanda Marshall
Centre for Clinical Brain Sciences, University of Edinburgh, Edinburgh EH16 4SB, UK

Anna Esparham
Division of Child Neurology-Headache Section, Children's Mercy Hospital, University of Missouri School of Medicine-Kansas City, Kansas City, MO 64108, USA
Children's Mercy Hospital, University of Missouri-Kansas City School of Medicine, Division of Child Neurology, 2401 Gillham Rd., Kansas City, MO 64108, USA

Sanghamitra M. Misra
Mobile Clinic Program, Texas Children's Hospital, Baylor College of Medicine, Houston, TX 77054, USA

Erica Sibinga
Department of Pediatrics, Johns Hopkins School of Medicine, Baltimore, MD 21205, USA

Timothy Culbert
Integrative Medicine, Prairie Care, University of Minnesota Medical School, Chaska, MN 55318, USA

Kathi Kemper
Department of Pediatrics, College of Medicine, Ohio State University, Columbus, OH 43210, USA

Hilary McClafferty
Department of Medicine, Arizona Center for Integrative Medicine, University of Arizona, Tucson, AZ 85724, USA

Sunita Vohra
Integrative Health Institute, CARE Program, PedCAM Network, Department of Pediatrics, Medicine, and Psychiatry, Faculty of Medicine and Dentistry, University of Alberta, Edmonton, AB T6G 2C8, Canada

Lawrence Rosen
Whole Child Center, Oradell, NJ 07649, USA

Ina Stephens
Department of Pediatrics, University of Virginia Medical Center, Charlottesville, VA 22903, USA

Melanie Anheyer
Elisabeth Krankenhaus, 45138 Essen, Germany

Robert A. Pendergrast Jr.
Department of Pediatrics, Medical College of Georgia, Augusta University, 1120 15th Street, Augusta, GA 30912, USA

Anna-Kaisa Niemi
Department of Pediatrics, Division of Neonatal & Developmental Medicine, Stanford University, Palo Alto, CA 94304, USA

Gautam Ramesh
School of Medicine, University of California, San Diego, La Jolla, CA 92093, USA

Dana Gerstbacher
Division of Rheumatology, Department of Pediatrics, School of Medicine, Stanford University, Palo Alto, CA 94304, USA

Jenna Arruda
Department of Pediatrics, School of Medicine, Stanford University, Palo Alto, CA 94304, USA

John Mark
Division of Pulmonary Medicine, Department of Pediatrics, School of Medicine, Stanford University, Palo Alto, CA 94304, USA

Ann Ming Yeh
Division of Gastroenterology, Hepatology and Nutrition, Department of Pediatrics, School of Medicine, Stanford University, Palo Alto, CA 94304, USA
Department of Pediatrics, Division of Pediatric Gastroenterology, Hepatology and Nutrition, Stanford University, Palo Alto, CA 94304, USA

Avneet K. Mangat
Faculty of Science, University of Alberta, Edmonton, AB T6G 2R3, Canada
Centre for the Studies of Asphyxia and Resuscitation, Neonatal Research Unit, Royal Alexandra Hospital, Edmonton, AB T6G 2R3, Canada

Ju-Lee Oei and Im Quah-Smith
School of Women's and Children's Health, University of New South Wales, Kensington, NSW 2031, Australia

Kerry Chen
Faculty of Medicine, University of New South Wales, Kensington, NSW 2033, Australia

Georg M. Schmölzer
Centre for the Studies of Asphyxia and Resuscitation, Neonatal Research Unit, Royal Alexandra Hospital, Edmonton, AB T6G 2R3, Canada
Department of Pediatrics, University of Alberta, Edmonton, AB T6G 2R3, Canada

Anava Wren
Department of Pediatrics, Division of Pediatric Gastroenterology, Hepatology and Nutrition, Stanford University, Palo Alto, CA 94304, USA

Robin Ortiz
Departments of Internal Medicine and Pediatrics Johns Hopkins Hospital, 1800 Orleans Street, Baltimore, MD 21231, USA

Brenda Golianu
Department of Anesthesia, Perioperative and Pain Medicine, Stanford University, Palo Alto, CA 94304, USA
Division of Pediatric Anesthesia and Pain Medicine, Department of Anesthesiology, Perioperative and Pain Medicine, School of Medicine, Stanford University, Palo Alto, CA 94304, USA

Anne Herbert, Emily Pierzchalski, Catherine Tran, Jennifer Dilts, Madeline Boorigie, Tammie Wingert, Mark Connelly and Jennifer Bickel
Children's Mercy Hospital, University of Missouri-Kansas City School of Medicine, Division of Child Neurology, 2401 Gillham Rd., Kansas City, MO 64108, USA

Erica M. Sibinga
Johns Hopkins School of Medicine, 733 North Broadway, Baltimore, MD 21205, USA

Marion Eckert and Catharina Amarell
Kinderkrankenhaus St. Marien, Grillparzerstr. 9, 84036 Landshut, Germany

Dennis Anheyer, Holger Cramer and Gustav Dobos
Department of Internal and Integrative Medicine, Kliniken Essen-Mitte, Faculty of Medicine, University of Duisburg-Essen, Am Deimelsberg 34a, 45276 Essen, Germany

Index

www.ingramcontent.com/pod-product-compliance
Lightning Source LLC
LaVergne TN
LVHW082148200926
848484LV00008B/2123
* 9 7 9 8 8 8 7 4 0 1 4 7 8 *